The Challenges of COVID-19 with Obesity-Related Cancers

The Challenges of COVID-19 with Obesity-Related Cancers

Editors

Maria Dalamaga
Narjes Nasiri-Ansari
Nikolaos Spyrou

MDPI • Basel • Beijing • Wuhan • Barcelona • Belgrade • Manchester • Tokyo • Cluj • Tianjin

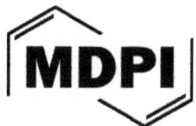

Editors

Maria Dalamaga
Department of Biological
Chemistry, Medical School
University of Athens
Athens
Greece

Narjes Nasiri-Ansari
Department of Biological
Chemistry, Medical School
University of Athens
Athens
Greece

Nikolaos Spyrou
Tisch Cancer Institute
Mount Sinai School of
Medicine
New York
United States

Editorial Office
MDPI
St. Alban-Anlage 66
4052 Basel, Switzerland

This is a reprint of articles from the Special Issue published online in the open access journal *Cancers* (ISSN 2072-6694) (available at: www.mdpi.com/journal/cancers/special_issues/covid_obesity_cancer).

For citation purposes, cite each article independently as indicated on the article page online and as indicated below:

LastName, A.A.; LastName, B.B.; LastName, C.C. Article Title. *Journal Name* **Year**, *Volume Number*, Page Range.

ISBN 978-3-0365-7351-9 (Hbk)
ISBN 978-3-0365-7350-2 (PDF)

© 2023 by the authors. Articles in this book are Open Access and distributed under the Creative Commons Attribution (CC BY) license, which allows users to download, copy and build upon published articles, as long as the author and publisher are properly credited, which ensures maximum dissemination and a wider impact of our publications.

The book as a whole is distributed by MDPI under the terms and conditions of the Creative Commons license CC BY-NC-ND.

Contents

About the Editors vii

Preface to "The Challenges of COVID-19 with Obesity-Related Cancers" ix

Maria Dalamaga, Narjes Nasiri-Ansari and Nikolaos Spyrou
Perspectives and Challenges of COVID-19 with Obesity-Related Cancers
Reprinted from: *Cancers* **2023**, *15*, 1771, doi:10.3390/cancers15061771 1

Parham Habibzadeh, Hassan Dastsooz, Mehdi Eshraghi, Marek J. Łos, Daniel J. Klionsky and Saeid Ghavami
Autophagy: The Potential Link between SARS-CoV-2 and Cancer
Reprinted from: *Cancers* **2021**, *13*, 5721, doi:10.3390/cancers13225721 9

Karlen Stade Bader-Larsen, Elisabeth Anne Larson, Maria Dalamaga and Faidon Magkos
A Narrative Review of the Safety of Anti-COVID-19 Nutraceuticals for Patients with Cancer
Reprinted from: *Cancers* **2021**, *13*, 6094, doi:10.3390/cancers13236094 21

Muna Almasri, Khalifa Bshesh, Wafa Khan, Malik Mushannen, Mohammad A. Salameh and Ameena Shafiq et al.
Cancer Patients and the COVID-19 Vaccines: Considerations and Challenges
Reprinted from: *Cancers* **2022**, *14*, 5630, doi:10.3390/cancers14225630 43

Jennyfa K. Ali and John C. Riches
The Impact of the COVID-19 Pandemic on Oncology Care and Clinical Trials
Reprinted from: *Cancers* **2021**, *13*, 5924, doi:10.3390/cancers13235924 75

Jonathan Cottenet, Solène Tapia, Patrick Arveux, Alain Bernard, Tienhan Sandrine Dabakuyo-Yonli and Catherine Quantin
Effect of Obesity among Hospitalized Cancer Patients with or without COVID-19 on a National Level
Reprinted from: *Cancers* **2022**, *14*, 5660, doi:10.3390/cancers14225660 87

María Sereno, Ana María Jimenez-Gordo, Javier Baena-Espinar, Carlos Aguado, Xabier Mielgo and Ana Pertejo et al.
A Multicenter Analysis of the Outcome of Cancer Patients with Neutropenia and COVID-19 Optionally Treated with Granulocyte-Colony Stimulating Factor (G-CSF): A Comparative Analysis
Reprinted from: *Cancers* **2021**, *13*, 4205, doi:10.3390/cancers13164205 103

Caterina Cariti, Martina Merli, Gianluca Avallone, Marco Rubatto, Elena Marra and Paolo Fava et al.
Melanoma Management during the COVID-19 Pandemic Emergency: A Literature Review and Single-Center Experience
Reprinted from: *Cancers* **2021**, *13*, 6071, doi:10.3390/cancers13236071 117

Maria V. Deligiorgi, Gerasimos Siasos, Lampros Vakkas and Dimitrios T. Trafalis
Charting the Unknown Association of COVID-19 with Thyroid Cancer, Focusing on Differentiated Thyroid Cancer: A Call for Caution
Reprinted from: *Cancers* **2021**, *13*, 5785, doi:10.3390/cancers13225785 129

Dimitrios Tsilingiris, Narjes Nasiri-Ansari, Nikolaos Spyrou, Faidon Magkos and Maria Dalamaga
Management of Hematologic Malignancies in the Era of COVID-19 Pandemic: Pathogenetic Mechanisms, Impact of Obesity, Perspectives, and Challenges
Reprinted from: *Cancers* **2022**, *14*, 2494, doi:10.3390/cancers14102494 . . . . **157**

Anastasia Prodromidou, Aristotelis-Marios Koulakmanidis, Dimitrios Haidopoulos, Gregg Nelson, Alexandros Rodolakis and Nikolaos Thomakos
Where Enhanced Recovery after Surgery (ERAS) Protocols Meet the Three Major Current Pandemics: COVID-19, Obesity and Malignancy
Reprinted from: *Cancers* **2022**, *14*, 1660, doi:10.3390/cancers14071660 . . . . **181**

Zoe Petropoulou, Nikolaos Arkadopoulos and Nikolaos V. Michalopoulos
Breast Cancer and COVID-19: Challenges in Surgical Management
Reprinted from: *Cancers* **2022**, *14*, 5360, doi:10.3390/cancers14215360 . . . . **193**

Nikolaos Pararas, Anastasia Pikouli, Dimitrios Papaconstantinou, Georgios Bagias, Constantinos Nastos and Andreas Pikoulis et al.
Colorectal Surgery in the COVID-19 Era: A Systematic Review and Meta-Analysis
Reprinted from: *Cancers* **2022**, *14*, 1229, doi:10.3390/cancers14051229 . . . . **201**

About the Editors

Maria Dalamaga

Prof. Dr. Maria Dalamaga is a Physician, Clinical Pathologist–Epidemiologist, Professor of Biological Chemistry—Clinical Biochemistry at the Medical School of the University of Athens (NKUA) in Greece. She graduated from the Medical School of the University of Ioannina, the National School of Public Health, and completed her PhD at the Medical School of the NKUA and the Hellenic Pasteur Institute. With scholarships from the Harvard and Onassis Foundations, she graduated from the Harvard School of Public Health with a Master's Degree in Epidemiology. She completed her service as a rural physician at the Milea-Health Center of Metsovo, where she was declared an Honorary Citizen. She specialized in Clinical Pathology at the NIMTS and Evangelismos General Hospitals. She has been a Fellow of the College of American Pathologists and has received a Fellowship in Clinical Chemistry from the European Board of Medical Biopathology. She has worked as a clinical pathologist at the IASO General Hospital and as a National Health Service Consultant and, later, academic physician at the Attikon University General Hospital. She has been honored with 47 Greek and international awards and 7 scholarships, among which includes the First Section Science Award from the Academy of Athens, the Choremeio and Empeirikio Foundation awards, and the Fulbright Research Award as a Visiting Scholar at the Harvard Medical School/Massachusetts General Hospital. She is the Editor-in-Chief of *Metabolism Open* (Elsevier), the Section Editor of *Current Obesity Reports* and *Current Nutrition Reports* (Springer), a Guest Editor in high-impact journals (*Seminars in Cancer Biology* and *Cancers*), and the President of the Hellenic Society of Medical Biochemistry. She has more than 210 publications in reputable international journals (>7510 citations, h-index: 47) and 27 monographs and chapters in collective volumes or books. Her research work is focused on cardiometabolic biomarkers, adipose tissue, and obesity. She is married and is the mother of two children.

Narjes Nasiri-Ansari

Dr. Narjes Nasiri Ansari is a Post-Doctoral Fellow in the Department of Biological Chemistry, Medical School, National and Kapodistrian University of Athens-Greece. Dr. Nasiri-Ansari obtained her PhD degree from the Faculty of Medicine, University of Athens, and her research interests include an understanding of the underlying molecular mechanisms of cardio-metabolic disorders, as well as the role of circadian clock system dysregulation during tumorigenesis processes. Her research on the role of circadian clock dysregulation on the pathogenesis of endometriosis was acknowledged by the young investigator award from the European Society of Endocrinology. So far, she has published over 30 research and review articles, and she has served as a co-guest editor in three different journals.

Nikolaos Spyrou

Nikolaos Spyrou is a Post-Doctoral Fellow of the Mount Sinai Acute Graft Versus Host Disease International Consortium of the Tisch Cancer Institute. He conducts translational research focusing on prognostic biomarker algorithms in hematology/oncology and hematopoietic transplantation. He graduated from the Academy of Military Medicine of the Aristotle University of Thessaloniki. He has a Master's Degree in Bioinformatics from the University of Athens. He will soon be a resident of the Internal Medicine Residency program, Physician Scientist Track of the Mount Sinai Hospital.

Preface to "The Challenges of COVID-19 with Obesity-Related Cancers"

The COVID-19 pandemic has taken place at a time when the worldwide prevalence rate of overweight and obesity is greater than 39% and 13%, respectively, for adults, and cancer is a leading cause of death globally. The emergence of COVID-19 has created an unprecedented threat worldwide, overwhelming health care systems in the majority of countries. COVID-19 had devastating effects on oncologic patients, with an important number of missed diagnoses and delayed treatments attributed mainly to patient's reluctance to seek medical care and to health care systems under pressure. Throughout the pandemic, particularly during the first phases, there were significant delays in cancer screening and surveillance that resulted in delayed diagnoses particularly in obesity-associated cancers, an increased rate of patients diagnosed in an emergency setting, a plethora of diagnoses of advanced stage malignancies with higher tumor burden, and delays in the treatment of patients with newly diagnosed cancers.

This reprint emphasizes the perspectives and challenges surrounding COVID-19 and obesity-related cancers, including but not limited to the risk factors of severe COVID-19 in cancer patients; the complications of COVID-19 in cancer patients; the challenges in cancer treatment and surgery; guidelines for cancer care during COVID-19; delayed diagnosis and suboptimal cancer management; the impact of COVID-19 on cancer screening, early diagnosis and cancer presentation; immune response after SARS-CoV-2 infection and vaccination in cancer patients; psychological distress among cancer survivors; telehealth in cancer care; the role of diet and nutraceuticals in the prevention of severe COVID-19 and cancer; and the effects of COVID-19 pandemic on cancer research.

Overall, this volume on "The Challenges of COVID-19 with Obesity-Related Cancers" represents a useful tool in providing a valuable addition to COVID-19 research on pathogenesis, prevention and management in cancer patients. It is useful to all students, researchers and clinicians involved or interested in the mechanisms by which obesity and cancer contribute to the severity of COVID-19 and may serve as a foundation for stimulating further research on this subject. We have been fortunate to assemble articles authored by an international group of authors with expertise in prevention, public health, infectious diseases, nutrition, oncology/hematology and surgery, and we are grateful for their contribution. We welcome feedback on this volume and appreciate the support and encouragement received during the publication of this volume. Finally, without the understanding and support of our families, the compilation of this encompassing book would have not been possible.

Maria Dalamaga, Narjes Nasiri-Ansari, and Nikolaos Spyrou
Editors

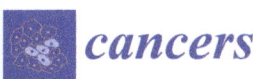

Editorial

Perspectives and Challenges of COVID-19 with Obesity-Related Cancers

Maria Dalamaga [1,*], Narjes Nasiri-Ansari [1] and Nikolaos Spyrou [2]

1. Department of Biological Chemistry, School of Medicine, National and Kapodistrian University of Athens, 75 Mikras Asias, 11527 Athens, Greece
2. Tisch Cancer Institute Icahn School of Medicine at Mount Sinai, 1190 One Gustave L. Levy Place, New York, NY 10029, USA
* Correspondence: madalamaga@med.uoa.gr

The emergence of COVID-19 has created an unprecedented threat worldwide, involving overwhelmed health-care systems in the majority of countries [1,2]. Cancer screening and delivering care in oncologic patients has been a challenging task based on the balance between the risk of mortality from untreated malignancy versus the risk of severity of COVID-19 and death in immunocompromised individuals [3].

The COVID-19 pandemic has taken place at a time when the worldwide prevalence rate of overweight and obesity is greater than 39% and 13%, respectively, for adults, and cancer is a leading cause of death globally based on recent WHO data [4,5]. Obesity has become a major global public health concern related to a variety of disorders, including metabolic syndrome, type 2 diabetes mellitus, cardiovascular disease, nonalcoholic fatty liver disease, polycystic ovary syndrome, autoimmune disorders and cancer [6–13].

Interestingly, a growing body of evidence has shown that obesity and increased visceral fat are strongly and independently linked with adverse outcomes and death due to COVID-19 [14–18]. Moreover, there is convincing evidence that excess body weight is associated with an increased risk for cancer of at least 13 anatomic sites, including endometrial, esophageal, renal and pancreatic adenocarcinomas; hepatocellular carcinoma; gastric cardia cancer; meningioma; multiple myeloma; colorectal, postmenopausal breast, ovarian, gallbladder and thyroid cancers [19–21].

Two umbrella reviews and meta-analyses on the association between pre-existing health conditions and severe outcomes from COVID-19 have shown that other than diabetes, obesity, heart failure, chronic obstructive pulmonary disease and dementia, active cancer was also linked with a higher risk of death, particularly in Europe and North America [22,23]. Oncologic patients may be more susceptible to SARS-CoV-2 infection. Evidence is mixed regarding COVID-19 severity in cancer patients [24–26], while COVID-19 outcomes in these patients are improved with an earlier diagnosis, the availability of effective COVID-19 vaccines, the advent of the omicron outbreak and the timely use of anti-viral therapy [24,27]. Despite all the abovementioned factors, most studies have highlighted an elevated risk of severe COVID-19 in patients with active cancer, particularly in non-vaccinated individuals [22,23,25,28,29]. The risk may vary by type and stage of cancer and treatment. Particularly, older age, hematologic malignancies, lung cancer, advanced or progressive cancer, active chemotherapy, comorbid conditions, including obesity, and smoking are associated with severe COVID-19 [30–37].

COVID-19 had devastating effects on cancer patients, with an immense number of missed diagnoses and delayed treatments attributed mainly to patient's reluctance to seek medical care and to health systems under pressure [38]. Throughout the pandemic and particularly during the first and second phases, there were significant delays in cancer screening and surveillance that resulted in delayed diagnoses, particularly in obesity-associated cancers, an increased rate of patients diagnosed in an emergency setting, a

Citation: Dalamaga, M.; Nasiri-Ansari, N.; Spyrou, N. Perspectives and Challenges of COVID-19 with Obesity-Related Cancers. *Cancers* **2023**, *15*, 1771. https://doi.org/10.3390/cancers15061771

Received: 6 March 2023
Revised: 7 March 2023
Accepted: 10 March 2023
Published: 15 March 2023

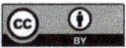

Copyright: © 2023 by the authors. Licensee MDPI, Basel, Switzerland. This article is an open access article distributed under the terms and conditions of the Creative Commons Attribution (CC BY) license (https://creativecommons.org/licenses/by/4.0/).

plethora of diagnoses of advanced stage malignancies with higher tumor burden as well as delays in the treatment of patients with newly diagnosed cancers [39–44]. In the initial phase of the pandemic, collective data from 200 sources in 17 European countries have shown that an estimated 100 million screening tests were not performed while up to 50% of all cancer patients were affected by treatment delays [45].

Generally, therapeutic management of oncologic patients with COVID-19 is similar to that used for the general population. In the outpatient setting, available treatment options comprise antiviral agents, such as nirmatrelvir-ritonavir, remdesivir and molnupiravir, as well as monoclonal antibodies active against prevalent variants [46,47]. Persistent SARS-CoV-2 infection may uncommonly occur in immunocompromised patients, particularly those with severe B-cell depletion due to cancer treatment (e.g., rituximab, hematopoietic cell transplantation, etc.) [46,48,49].

Overall, when cancer treatment is indicated according to consensus guidelines, it should be administered without delay [50]. In most hematologic cancers, the efficacy of treatment favors the adoption of curative approaches, despite the infectious risk of COVID-19; however, decisions should be made on a case-by-case basis [51]. In patients who have tested positive for SARS-CoV-2, immune checkpoint inhibitors (ICIs) should be postponed until recovery [50]. Transplantation/cellular therapy should be delayed for 2–3 weeks and until patients are asymptomatic; however, decisions should be made on a case-by-case basis (e.g., prolonged viral shedding should be taken into consideration) [52]. In cases where treatment is not urgent as in indolent lymphomas, treatment can be deferred until nasopharyngeal sampling is negative and symptoms have resolved; less immunosuppressive therapies can also be prioritized [53]. Moreover, in the absence of urgent treatment indication, an individual treatment deferral after anti-SARS-CoV-2 vaccination (at least one injection) may be considered [53]. Therapeutic decisions to proceed with systemic therapies should be preceded by a multidisciplinary discussion, risk/benefit analysis and discussion with the patient.

Up-to-date COVID-19 vaccination is recommended to all patients with active or prior malignancy in order to prevent severe SARS-CoV-2 infection. Data have indicated that vaccine efficacy is relatively diminished in patients with active cancer in comparison to individuals without cancer, especially in patients with hematologic malignancies, and particularly those on anti-CD20 antibody treatment [54–56]. Patients with hematologic malignancies present lower seroconversion rates post-vaccination, potentially leading to inferior COVID-19 outcomes despite vaccination, and an elevated risk for breakthrough infections [57–59]. Figure 1 depicts the main challenges of COVID-19 associated with cancer.

This Special Issue places emphasis on the challenges surrounding COVID-19 and obesity-related cancers, including, but not limited to: risk factors of severe COVID-19 in cancer patients; complications of COVID-19 in cancer patients; challenges in cancer treatment and surgery; guidelines for cancer care during COVID-19; delayed diagnosis and suboptimal cancer management; impact of COVID-19 on cancer screening, early diagnosis and cancer presentation; immune response after SARS-CoV-2 infection and vaccination in cancer patients; psychological distress among cancer survivors; telehealth in cancer care; role of diet and nutraceuticals in the prevention of severe COVID-19 and cancer as well as effects of COVID-19 pandemic on cancer research.

Although SARS-CoV-2 mainly affects the lower respiratory tract, it can initiate system-wide pathophysiological alterations and dysfunctional immune responses. Habibzadeh et al. reviewed the potential effects of autophagy on cancer development and outcomes [60]. Various SARS-CoV-2 proteins interact with different components of the cellular autophagy pathway and could lead to long-term defects in the cellular autophagy machinery. The authors hypothesize that these defects could mediate alterations in cell proliferation, immunity against cancer cells, cell metabolism and cancer drug efficacy that could eventually impact on carcinogenesis and responsiveness to cancer therapy.

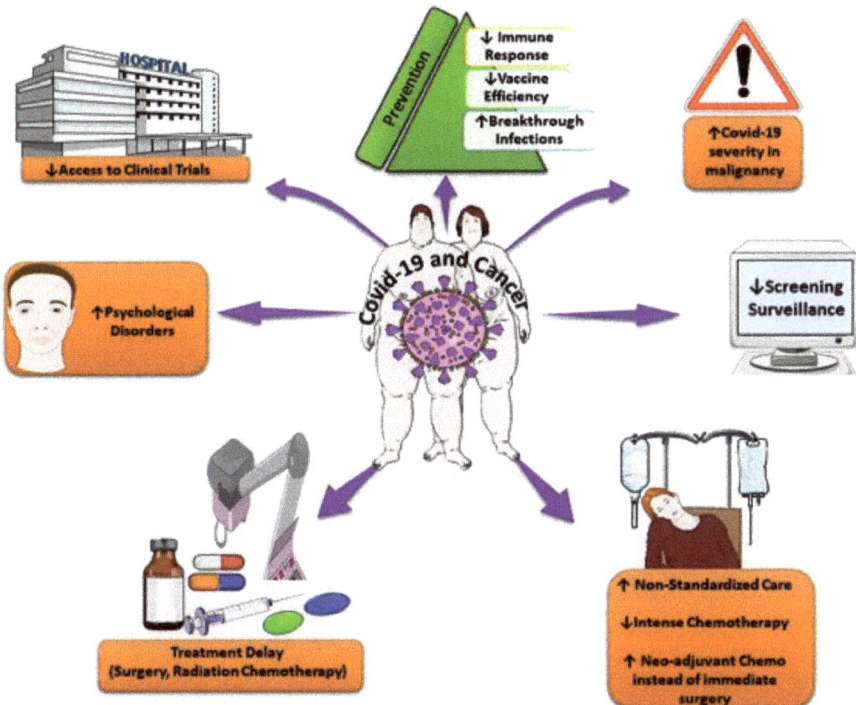

Figure 1. Main challenges of COVID-19 associated with cancer. This image was derived from the free medical site http://smart.servier.com/ (accessed on 2 March 2023) by Servier, licensed under a Creative Commons Attribution 3.0 Unported License.

The lack of medications for COVID-19 in the early phases of the pandemic led the public to seek alternative therapies, including nutraceuticals. Bader-Larsen et al. evaluated the safety of "anti-COVID-19" nutraceuticals in patients with cancer [61]. They reported that the use of vitamin C, vitamin D and selenium supplements is likely safe at typically recommended doses. However, they cast caution on the use of omega-3 fatty acids and zinc, as potential risks may outweigh the benefits derived from their use.

Almasri and colleagues reviewed the evidence on the immune response rates and safety profiles of COVID-19 vaccines in patients with hematologic and solid malignancies [62]. In comparison to the general population, lower seropositivity following vaccination was associated with malignancy as well as with hematologic malignancy compared to solid cancers. Patients receiving active chemotherapy, radiotherapy and immunosuppressive therapy generally displayed lower seropositivity rates compared to healthy controls, a phenomenon not observed in patients who received checkpoint inhibitors, endocrine therapies and cyclin-dependent kinase inhibitors. Nevertheless, cancer patients demonstrated the ability to mount safe and effective immune responses to COVID-19 vaccines. Adverse events were comparable to those of the general population; however, inflammatory lymphadenopathy following vaccination was commonly reported and may be mistaken for a lymphadenopathy of malignant etiology. Finally, the authors suggested that vaccination should be promoted, and reluctance to receive it should be addressed in this population.

The SARS-CoV-2 pandemic brought multi-dimensional disruptions in oncology. Ali and Riches reviewed the changes that affected the care of cancer patients as well as clinical trials [63]. The pandemic disrupted routine cancer screenings and decreased the potential for early cancer detection, resulting in many thousands of missed cancer diagnoses. Initially, clinical trials were significantly impacted, resulting in the cessation of trial initiation and recruitment, particularly in oncology clinical trials. Clinical trial practices and protocols underwent significant changes, including a reduction in in-person appointments, use of telemedicine and remote monitoring systems, to minimize the risk of exposure to the virus. Cottenet et al. studied the effect of obesity on the risk of intensive care unit (ICU) admission, severe complications and in-hospital mortality, in 992,899 cancer patients hospitalized with or without COVID-19 from the French national administrative database [64]. The authors found that obese cancer patients had an increased risk of admission to the ICU and severe complications, regardless of the type of obesity. Severe obesity was associated with an increased risk of in-hospital mortality, particularly in patients with hematological cancers. This study showed that among hospitalized cancer patients with or without COVID-19, increased vigilance is needed for obese patients, both in epidemic and non-epidemic periods. Lastly, Sereno et al. conducted a retrospective study in 943 cancer patients, of whom 83 (11.3%) were neutropenic and infected with COVID-19, looking at the effect of G-CSF treatment on outcomes during the first phase of the pandemic [65]. They observed a significant effect of the number of days of G-CSF treatment on severe disease and mortality, suggesting that prolonged treatment could be disadvantageous for these patients.

The management of many diseases was altered after the COVID-19 outbreak. Obesity has a great impact on COVID-19 patients' outcome while it affects the etiopathogenesis of various types of cancers, including melanoma, thyroid (TC) and hematological cancers. Cariti et al. critically evaluated whether screening, diagnosis and treatment of melanoma have been changed by the COVID-19 pandemic as well as the implications of these changes [66]. The authors found that during the pandemic, there was a delay in the diagnosis of new melanoma cases. After detection, the management of early-stage and advanced melanoma cases was fully guaranteed, whereas the follow-up visits of disease-free patients were delayed or replaced by teleconsultation when possible. The authors reported their valuable experience in the management of patients with melanoma during the COVID-19 pandemic, in a dermatological clinic in Northern Italy.

The interplay between obesity, TC and COVID-19 was extensively evaluated by Deligiorgi et al. [67]. Obesity is associated with an increased risk of differentiated TC (DTC). The authors summarized exciting, published data on the association between COVID-19 and TC into four sections: (i) the interrelationship between obesity, immunity, inflammation and oxidative stress, underlying this association; (ii) the challenging management of (D)TC in the COVID-19 era; (iii) the impact of COVID-19 on (D)TC and vice versa; and (iv) the oncogenic potential of SARS-CoV-2. The researchers highlighted the importance of evidence-based, risk-stratified and consensus-based decision making for providing the safest premium-quality care for (D)TC patients, with or without COVID-19.

Both obesity and hematological cancers are well-known risk factors for severe SARS-CoV-2 infection. Tsilingiris and colleagues comprehensively summarized the evidence linking obesity to the development of hematological cancers as well as their interconnection with severe COVID-19. They analyzed various challenges associated with the management of patients suffering from hematological cancers, including prevention, diagnosis and therapeutic approaches [46]. They thoroughly highlighted the unsolved issues and challenges that need to be overcome in the ongoing COVID-19 pandemic. The co-existence of obesity and hematological malignancies in the frame of SARS-CoV-2 infection may theoretically confer an adverse prognosis. Recent global-scale data have shown that the diagnosis of multiple myeloma has been missed or delayed in the early COVID-19 era compared with the previous year, while a decreased survival among newly diagnosed cases has been noted. The field of hemato-oncology has already overcome the initial blow to a great degree and adjusted to the new reality brought forward by COVID-19. Nonetheless, there is a need for continued appraisal and update of numerous aspects of therapeutic management. Many issues need to be determined, including the optimal timing of hematology–oncology therapy initiation, the post-treatment follow-up and the timely therapeutical planning, including allogeneic hematopoietic stem cell transplantation in the case of infections that emerge during the active medical therapy.

Apart from the abovementioned therapeutic approaches in oncologic patients during the COVID-19 pandemic, special attention must be given to patients who need oncological surgery because of the modification of treatment guidelines, the reduced access of patients to healthcare resources and the postponement of surgery. Prodromidou and colleagues studied how Enhanced Recovery after Surgery (ERAS) protocols may provide optimal management of patients with obesity and malignancy during the COVID-19 pandemic, with a special focus on patients who required surgery for gynecologic malignancy [68]. They highlighted the importance of the establishment of protective measures before surgery in order to reduce the exposure of cancer patients to SARS-CoV-2 while simultaneously improving vaccination access. Finally, the authors emphasized that ERAS protocols may play a crucial role in the management of patients with gynecologic cancer based on their efficiency in many surgical fields, such as general surgery and orthopedics, during the COVID-19 pandemic.

Breast cancer patients and caregivers were also tremendously affected by the healthcare crisis in multiple domains and ways. Petropoulou et al. summarized the challenges in breast cancer management and the subsequent implications in clinical practice [69]. Similar to other obesity-related cancers, screening, diagnosis and surgical intervention were the most affected domains, causing a serious psychological burden to patients. The aftermath of diagnostic and surgical delays is yet to be assessed, while alterations in the treatment plans and the introduction of new therapeutic schemes, such as the extensive use of neoadjuvant hormonal therapy and the significant reduction in the first-line surgical approach, may open a novel era in the management of breast cancer.

Furthermore, the COVID-19 pandemic resulted in changes in surgical practice involving colorectal malignancies. In a systemic review and meta-analysis of ten studies including 26,808 patients, Pararas et al. evaluated the impact of the COVID-19 pandemic on the management of colorectal cancer, the third-most-common cancer worldwide, which is also associated with obesity [70]. The authors found that the number of patients presenting with metastases during the pandemic was significantly increased, with no differences regarding the extent of the primary tumor and the nodal status. In addition, patients with colorectal cancer during the pandemic were more likely to undergo palliative interventions or receive neoadjuvant treatment.

Finally, we expect that these manuscripts contributed by experts in this field will provide useful resources to physicians and scientists interested in the interplay of COVID-19 and obesity-related cancer, as well as the development of relevant preventive and therapeutic strategies.

Author Contributions: M.D., N.N.-A. and N.S. were involved in the preparation and promotion of the Special Issue as well as the writing and review of the Editorial. All authors have read and agreed to the published version of the manuscript.

Funding: This research did not receive any specific grant from funding agencies in the public, commercial or not-for-profit sectors.

Conflicts of Interest: The authors declare no conflict of interest.

References

1. Han, X.; Shi, S.K.; Zhao, J.; Nogueira, L.M.; Bandi, P.; Fedewa, S.A.; Jemal, A.; Yabroff, K.R. The first year of the COVID-19 pandemic and health among cancer survivors in the United States. *Cancer* **2022**, *128*, 3727–3733. [CrossRef] [PubMed]
2. Syriga, M.; Karampela, I.; Dalamaga, M.; Karampelas, M. The effect of COVID-19 pandemic on the attendance and clinical outcomes of patients with ophthalmic disease: A mini-review. *Metab. Open* **2021**, *12*, 100131. [CrossRef] [PubMed]
3. Lewis, M.A. Between Scylla and Charybdis—Oncologic Decision Making in the Time of COVID-19. *N. Engl. J. Med.* **2020**, *382*, 2285–2287. [CrossRef] [PubMed]
4. WHO. Cancer. Available online: https://www.who.int/news-room/fact-sheets/detail/cancer (accessed on 20 February 2023).
5. WHO. Obesity and Overweight. Available online: https://www.who.int/news-room/fact-sheets/detail/obesity-and-overweight (accessed on 20 February 2023).

6. Dalamaga, M.; Papadavid, E.; Basios, G.; Vaggopoulos, V.; Rigopoulos, D.; Kassanos, D.; Trakakis, E. Ovarian SAHA syndrome is associated with a more insulin-resistant profile and represents an independent risk factor for glucose abnormalities in women with polycystic ovary syndrome: A prospective controlled study. *J. Am. Acad. Dermatol.* **2013**, *69*, 922–930. [CrossRef] [PubMed]
7. Hroussalas, G.; Kassi, E.; Dalamaga, M.; Delimaris, I.; Zachari, A.; Dionyssiou-Asteriou, A. Leptin, soluble leptin receptor, adiponectin and resistin in relation to OGTT in overweight/obese postmenopausal women. *Maturitas* **2008**, *59*, 339–349. [CrossRef] [PubMed]
8. Marouga, A.; Dalamaga, M.; Kastania, A.N.; Antonakos, G.; Thrasyvoulides, A.; Kontelia, G.; Dimas, C.; Vlahakos, D.V. Correlates of serum resistin in elderly, non-diabetic patients with chronic kidney disease. *Clin. Lab.* **2013**, *59*, 1121–1128. [CrossRef]
9. Papadavid, E.; Katsimbri, P.; Kapniari, I.; Koumaki, D.; Karamparpa, A.; Dalamaga, M.; Tzannis, K.; Betaoumpas, D.; Rigopoulos, D. Prevalence of psoriatic arthritis and its correlates among patients with psoriasis in Greece: Results from a large retrospective study. *J. Eur. Acad. Dermatol. Venereol.* **2016**, *30*, 1749–1752. [CrossRef]
10. Paroutoglou, K.; Papadavid, E.; Christodoulatos, G.S.; Dalamaga, M. Deciphering the Association Between Psoriasis and Obesity: Current Evidence and Treatment Considerations. *Curr. Obes. Rep.* **2020**, *9*, 165–178. [CrossRef]
11. Powell-Wiley, T.M.; Poirier, P.; Burke, L.E.; Despres, J.P.; Gordon-Larsen, P.; Lavie, C.J.; Lear, S.A.; Ndumele, C.E.; Neeland, I.J.; Sanders, P.; et al. Obesity and Cardiovascular Disease: A Scientific Statement From the American Heart Association. *Circulation* **2021**, *143*, e984–e1010. [CrossRef]
12. Tsigalou, C.; Vallianou, N.; Dalamaga, M. Autoantibody Production in Obesity: Is There Evidence for a Link Between Obesity and Autoimmunity? *Curr. Obes. Rep.* **2020**, *9*, 245–254. [CrossRef]
13. Vallianou, N.; Dalamaga, M.; Stratigou, T.; Karampela, I.; Tsigalou, C. Do Antibiotics Cause Obesity Through Long-term Alterations in the Gut Microbiome? A Review of Current Evidence. *Curr. Obes. Rep.* **2021**, *10*, 244–262. [CrossRef] [PubMed]
14. Dalamaga, M.; Christodoulatos, G.S.; Karampela, I.; Vallianou, N.; Apovian, C.M. Understanding the Co-Epidemic of Obesity and COVID-19: Current Evidence, Comparison with Previous Epidemics, Mechanisms, and Preventive and Therapeutic Perspectives. *Curr. Obes. Rep.* **2021**, *10*, 214–243. [CrossRef] [PubMed]
15. Karampela, I.; Vallianou, N.; Magkos, F.; Apovian, C.M.; Dalamaga, M. Obesity, Hypovitaminosis D, and COVID-19: The Bermuda Triangle in Public Health. *Curr. Obes. Rep.* **2022**, *11*, 116–125. [CrossRef] [PubMed]
16. Kritis, P.; Karampela, I.; Kokoris, S.; Dalamaga, M. The combination of bromelain and curcumin as an immune-boosting nutraceutical in the prevention of severe COVID-19. *Metab. Open* **2020**, *8*, 100066. [CrossRef] [PubMed]
17. Tsilingiris, D.; Dalamaga, M.; Liu, J. SARS-CoV-2 adipose tissue infection and hyperglycemia: A further step towards the understanding of severe COVID-19. *Metab. Open* **2022**, *13*, 100163. [CrossRef]
18. Tsilingiris, D.; Vallianou, N.G.; Karampela, I.; Dalamaga, M. Vaccine induced thrombotic thrombocytopenia: The shady chapter of a success story. *Metab. Open* **2021**, *11*, 100101. [CrossRef]
19. Argyrakopoulou, G.; Dalamaga, M.; Spyrou, N.; Kokkinos, A. Gender Differences in Obesity-Related Cancers. *Curr. Obes. Rep.* **2021**, *10*, 100–115. [CrossRef]
20. Christodoulatos, G.S.; Antonakos, G.; Karampela, I.; Psallida, S.; Stratigou, T.; Vallianou, N.; Lekka, A.; Marinou, I.; Vogiatzakis, E.; Kokoris, S.; et al. Circulating Omentin-1 as a Biomarker at the Intersection of Postmenopausal Breast Cancer Occurrence and Cardiometabolic Risk: An Observational Cross-Sectional Study. *Biomolecules* **2021**, *11*, 1609. [CrossRef]
21. Dalamaga, M.; Karmaniolas, K.; Chamberland, J.; Nikolaidou, A.; Lekka, A.; Dionyssiou-Asteriou, A.; Mantzoros, C.S. Higher fetuin-A, lower adiponectin and free leptin levels mediate effects of excess body weight on insulin resistance and risk for myelodysplastic syndrome. *Metabolism* **2013**, *62*, 1830–1839. [CrossRef]
22. Arayici, M.E.; Basbinar, Y.; Ellidokuz, H. The impact of cancer on the severity of disease in patients affected with COVID-19: An umbrella review and meta-meta-analysis of systematic reviews and meta-analyses involving 1,064,476 participants. *Clin. Exp. Med.* **2022**. [CrossRef]
23. Treskova-Schwarzbach, M.; Haas, L.; Reda, S.; Pilic, A.; Borodova, A.; Karimi, K.; Koch, J.; Nygren, T.; Scholz, S.; Schonfeld, V.; et al. Pre-existing health conditions and severe COVID-19 outcomes: An umbrella review approach and meta-analysis of global evidence. *BMC Med.* **2021**, *19*, 212. [CrossRef] [PubMed]
24. OnCovid Study, G.; Pinato, D.J.; Patel, M.; Scotti, L.; Colomba, E.; Dolly, S.; Loizidou, A.; Chester, J.; Mukherjee, U.; Zambelli, A.; et al. Time-Dependent COVID-19 Mortality in Patients With Cancer: An Updated Analysis of the OnCovid Registry. *JAMA Oncol.* **2022**, *8*, 114–122. [CrossRef] [PubMed]
25. Sengar, M.; Chinnaswamy, G.; Ranganathan, P.; Ashok, A.; Bhosale, S.; Biswas, S.; Chaturvedi, P.; Dhamne, C.; Divatia, J.; D'Sa, K.; et al. Outcomes of COVID-19 and risk factors in patients with cancer. *Nat. Cancer* **2022**, *3*, 547–551. [CrossRef]
26. Van Dam, P.A.; Huizing, M.; Mestach, G.; Dierckxsens, S.; Tjalma, W.; Trinh, X.B.; Papadimitriou, K.; Altintas, S.; Vermorken, J.; Vulsteke, C.; et al. SARS-CoV-2 and cancer: Are they really partners in crime? *Cancer Treat. Rev.* **2020**, *89*, 102068. [CrossRef] [PubMed]
27. Tagliamento, M.; Gennari, A.; Lambertini, M.; Salazar, R.; Harbeck, N.; Del Mastro, L.; Aguilar-Company, J.; Bower, M.; Sharkey, R.; Dalla Pria, A.; et al. Pandemic Phase-Adjusted Analysis of COVID-19 Outcomes Reveals Reduced Intrinsic Vulnerability and Substantial Vaccine Protection From Severe Acute Respiratory Syndrome Coronavirus 2 in Patients With Breast Cancer. *J. Clin. Oncol.* **2023**, JCO2201667. [CrossRef]

28. Pinato, D.J.; Aguilar-Company, J.; Ferrante, D.; Hanbury, G.; Bower, M.; Salazar, R.; Mirallas, O.; Sureda, A.; Plaja, A.; Cucurull, M.; et al. Outcomes of the SARS-CoV-2 omicron (B.1.1.529) variant outbreak among vaccinated and unvaccinated patients with cancer in Europe: Results from the retrospective, multicentre, OnCovid registry study. *Lancet Oncol.* **2022**, *23*, 865–875. [CrossRef]
29. Song, Q.; Bates, B.; Shao, Y.R.; Hsu, F.C.; Liu, F.; Madhira, V.; Mitra, A.K.; Bergquist, T.; Kavuluru, R.; Li, X.; et al. Risk and Outcome of Breakthrough COVID-19 Infections in Vaccinated Patients With Cancer: Real-World Evidence From the National COVID Cohort Collaborative. *J. Clin. Oncol.* **2022**, *40*, 1414–1427. [CrossRef]
30. Carrara, E.; Razzaboni, E.; Azzini, A.M.; De Rui, M.E.; Pinho Guedes, M.N.; Gorska, A.; Giannella, M.; Bussini, L.; Bartoletti, M.; Arbizzani, F.; et al. Predictors of clinical evolution of SARS-CoV-2 infection in hematological patients: A systematic review and meta-analysis. *Hematol. Oncol.* **2023**, *41*, 16–25. [CrossRef]
31. Chavez-MacGregor, M.; Lei, X.; Zhao, H.; Scheet, P.; Giordano, S.H. Evaluation of COVID-19 Mortality and Adverse Outcomes in US Patients With or Without Cancer. *JAMA Oncol.* **2022**, *8*, 69–78. [CrossRef]
32. Kouhpayeh, H. Clinical features predicting COVID-19 mortality risk. *Eur. J. Transl. Myol.* **2022**, *32*, 10268. [CrossRef]
33. Lunski, M.J.; Burton, J.; Tawagi, K.; Maslov, D.; Simenson, V.; Barr, D.; Yuan, H.; Johnson, D.; Matrana, M.; Cole, J.; et al. Multivariate mortality analyses in COVID-19: Comparing patients with cancer and patients without cancer in Louisiana. *Cancer* **2021**, *127*, 266–274. [CrossRef]
34. Mileham, K.F.; Bruinooge, S.S.; Aggarwal, C.; Patrick, A.L.; Davis, C.; Mesenhowski, D.J.; Spira, A.; Clayton, E.J.; Waterhouse, D.; Moore, S.; et al. Changes Over Time in COVID-19 Severity and Mortality in Patients Undergoing Cancer Treatment in the United States: Initial Report From the ASCO Registry. *JCO Oncol. Pract.* **2022**, *18*, e426–e441. [CrossRef] [PubMed]
35. Vallianou, N.G.; Evangelopoulos, A.; Kounatidis, D.; Stratigou, T.; Christodoulatos, G.S.; Karampela, I.; Dalamaga, M. Diabetes Mellitus and SARS-CoV-2 Infection: Pathophysiologic Mechanisms and Implications in Management. *Curr. Diabetes Rev.* **2021**, *17*, e123120189797. [CrossRef]
36. Varnai, C.; Palles, C.; Arnold, R.; Curley, H.M.; Purshouse, K.; Cheng, V.W.T.; Booth, S.; Campton, N.A.; Collins, G.P.; Hughes, D.J.; et al. Mortality Among Adults With Cancer Undergoing Chemotherapy or Immunotherapy and Infected With COVID-19. *JAMA Netw. Open* **2022**, *5*, e220130. [CrossRef] [PubMed]
37. Wang, Q.; Berger, N.A.; Xu, R. Analyses of Risk, Racial Disparity, and Outcomes Among US Patients With Cancer and COVID-19 Infection. *JAMA Oncol.* **2021**, *7*, 220–227. [CrossRef] [PubMed]
38. The Lancet Oncology. COVID-19 and cancer: 1 year on. *Lancet Oncol.* **2021**, *22*, 411. [CrossRef]
39. Englum, B.R.; Prasad, N.K.; Lake, R.E.; Mayorga-Carlin, M.; Turner, D.J.; Siddiqui, T.; Sorkin, J.D.; Lal, B.K. Impact of the COVID-19 pandemic on diagnosis of new cancers: A national multicenter study of the Veterans Affairs Healthcare System. *Cancer* **2022**, *128*, 1048–1056. [CrossRef]
40. Joung, R.H.; Nelson, H.; Mullett, T.W.; Kurtzman, S.H.; Shafir, S.; Harris, J.B.; Yao, K.A.; Brajcich, B.C.; Bilimoria, K.Y.; Cance, W.G. A national quality improvement study identifying and addressing cancer screening deficits due to the COVID-19 pandemic. *Cancer* **2022**, *128*, 2119–2125. [CrossRef]
41. Kuzuu, K.; Misawa, N.; Ashikari, K.; Kessoku, T.; Kato, S.; Hosono, K.; Yoneda, M.; Nonaka, T.; Matsushima, S.; Komatsu, T.; et al. Gastrointestinal Cancer Stage at Diagnosis Before and During the COVID-19 Pandemic in Japan. *JAMA Netw. Open* **2021**, *4*, e2126334. [CrossRef]
42. Terashima, T.; Konishi, H.; Sato, Y.; Igarashi, M.; Yanagibashi, T.; Konno, R.; Saya, H.; Doki, Y.; Kakizoe, T. Impact of coronavirus disease 2019 on the number of newly diagnosed cancer patients and examinations and surgeries performed for cancer in Japan: A nationwide study. *BMC Cancer* **2022**, *22*, 1303. [CrossRef] [PubMed]
43. Thierry, A.R.; Pastor, B.; Pisareva, E.; Ghiringhelli, F.; Bouche, O.; De La Fouchardiere, C.; Vanbockstael, J.; Smith, D.; Francois, E.; Dos Santos, M.; et al. Association of COVID-19 Lockdown With the Tumor Burden in Patients With Newly Diagnosed Metastatic Colorectal Cancer. *JAMA Netw. Open* **2021**, *4*, e2124483. [CrossRef] [PubMed]
44. Toss, A.; Isca, C.; Venturelli, M.; Nasso, C.; Ficarra, G.; Bellelli, V.; Armocida, C.; Barbieri, E.; Cortesi, L.; Moscetti, L.; et al. Two-month stop in mammographic screening significantly impacts on breast cancer stage at diagnosis and upfront treatment in the COVID era. *ESMO Open* **2021**, *6*, 100055. [CrossRef] [PubMed]
45. Walsh, D. Available online: https://www.euronews.com/next/2021/12/01/cancer-in-europe-the-devastating-impact-of-covid-on-diagnosis-and-treatment-country-by-cou (accessed on 8 February 2023).
46. Tsilingiris, D.; Nasiri-Ansari, N.; Spyrou, N.; Magkos, F.; Dalamaga, M. Management of Hematologic Malignancies in the Era of COVID-19 Pandemic: Pathogenetic Mechanisms, Impact of Obesity, Perspectives, and Challenges. *Cancers* **2022**, *14*, 2494. [CrossRef] [PubMed]
47. Vallianou, N.G.; Tsilingiris, D.; Christodoulatos, G.S.; Karampela, I.; Dalamaga, M. Anti-viral treatment for SARS-CoV-2 infection: A race against time amidst the ongoing pandemic. *Metab. Open* **2021**, *10*, 100096. [CrossRef]
48. DeWolf, S.; Laracy, J.C.; Perales, M.A.; Kamboj, M.; van den Brink, M.R.M.; Vardhana, S. SARS-CoV-2 in immunocompromised individuals. *Immunity* **2022**, *55*, 1779–1798. [CrossRef]
49. Hettle, D.; Hutchings, S.; Muir, P.; Moran, E.; COVID-19 Genomics UK (COG-UK) Consortium. Persistent SARS-CoV-2 infection in immunocompromised patients facilitates rapid viral evolution: Retrospective cohort study and literature review. *Clin. Infect. Pract.* **2022**, *16*, 100210. [CrossRef]

50. Curigliano, G.; Banerjee, S.; Cervantes, A.; Garassino, M.C.; Garrido, P.; Girard, N.; Haanen, J.; Jordan, K.; Lordick, F.; Machiels, J.P.; et al. Managing cancer patients during the COVID-19 pandemic: An ESMO multidisciplinary expert consensus. *Ann. Oncol.* **2020**, *31*, 1320–1335. [CrossRef]
51. El Chaer, F.; Auletta, J.J.; Chemaly, R.F. How I treat and prevent COVID-19 in patients with hematologic malignancies and recipients of cellular therapies. *Blood* **2022**, *140*, 673–684. [CrossRef]
52. Waghmare, A.; Abidi, M.Z.; Boeckh, M.; Chemaly, R.F.; Dadwal, S.; El Boghdadly, Z.; Kamboj, M.; Papanicolaou, G.A.; Pergam, S.A.; Shahid, Z. Guidelines for COVID-19 Management in Hematopoietic Cell Transplantation and Cellular Therapy Recipients. *Biol. Blood Marrow Transplant.* **2020**, *26*, 1983–1994. [CrossRef]
53. Buske, C.; Dreyling, M.; Alvarez-Larran, A.; Apperley, J.; Arcaini, L.; Besson, C.; Bullinger, L.; Corradini, P.; Giovanni Della Porta, M.; Dimopoulos, M.; et al. Managing hematological cancer patients during the COVID-19 pandemic: An ESMO-EHA Interdisciplinary Expert Consensus. *ESMO Open* **2022**, *7*, 100403. [CrossRef]
54. Fendler, A.; Shepherd, S.T.C.; Au, L.; Wilkinson, K.A.; Wu, M.; Schmitt, A.M.; Tippu, Z.; Farag, S.; Rogiers, A.; Harvey, R.; et al. Immune responses following third COVID-19 vaccination are reduced in patients with hematological malignancies compared to patients with solid cancer. *Cancer Cell* **2022**, *40*, 438. [CrossRef] [PubMed]
55. Mair, M.J.; Berger, J.M.; Berghoff, A.S.; Starzer, A.M.; Ortmayr, G.; Puhr, H.C.; Steindl, A.; Perkmann, T.; Haslacher, H.; Strassl, R.; et al. Humoral Immune Response in Hematooncological Patients and Health Care Workers Who Received SARS-CoV-2 Vaccinations. *JAMA Oncol.* **2022**, *8*, 106–113. [CrossRef] [PubMed]
56. Naranbhai, V.; Pernat, C.A.; Gavralidis, A.; St Denis, K.J.; Lam, E.C.; Spring, L.M.; Isakoff, S.J.; Farmer, J.R.; Zubiri, L.; Hobbs, G.S.; et al. Immunogenicity and Reactogenicity of SARS-CoV-2 Vaccines in Patients With Cancer: The CANVAX Cohort Study. *J. Clin. Oncol.* **2022**, *40*, 12–23. [CrossRef]
57. Amanatidou, E.; Gkiouliava, A.; Pella, E.; Serafidi, M.; Tsilingiris, D.; Vallianou, N.G.; Karampela, I.; Dalamaga, M. Breakthrough infections after COVID-19 vaccination: Insights, perspectives and challenges. *Metab. Open* **2022**, *14*, 100180. [CrossRef]
58. Chien, K.S.; Peterson, C.; Young, E.; Chihara, D.; Manasanch, E.E.; Ramdial, J.; Thompson, P.A. Outcomes of Breakthrough COVID-19 Infections in Patients with Hematologic Malignancies. *Blood Adv.* **2023**, *8*, 827. [CrossRef] [PubMed]
59. Wang, L.; Kaelber, D.C.; Xu, R.; Berger, N.A. COVID-19 breakthrough infections, hospitalizations and mortality in fully vaccinated patients with hematologic malignancies: A clarion call for maintaining mitigation and ramping-up research. *Blood Rev.* **2022**, *54*, 100931. [CrossRef] [PubMed]
60. Habibzadeh, P.; Dastsooz, H.; Eshraghi, M.; Los, M.J.; Klionsky, D.J.; Ghavami, S. Autophagy: The Potential Link between SARS-CoV-2 and Cancer. *Cancers* **2021**, *13*, 5721. [CrossRef] [PubMed]
61. Bader-Larsen, K.S.; Larson, E.A.; Dalamaga, M.; Magkos, F. A Narrative Review of the Safety of Anti-COVID-19 Nutraceuticals for Patients with Cancer. *Cancers* **2021**, *13*, 6094. [CrossRef]
62. Almasri, M.; Bshesh, K.; Khan, W.; Mushannen, M.; Salameh, M.A.; Shafiq, A.; Vattoth, A.L.; Elkassas, N.; Zakaria, D. Cancer Patients and the COVID-19 Vaccines: Considerations and Challenges. *Cancers* **2022**, *14*, 5630. [CrossRef]
63. Ali, J.K.; Riches, J.C. The Impact of the COVID-19 Pandemic on Oncology Care and Clinical Trials. *Cancers* **2021**, *13*, 5924. [CrossRef]
64. Cottenet, J.; Tapia, S.; Arveux, P.; Bernard, A.; Dabakuyo-Yonli, T.S.; Quantin, C. Effect of Obesity among Hospitalized Cancer Patients with or without COVID-19 on a National Level. *Cancers* **2022**, *14*, 5660. [CrossRef] [PubMed]
65. Sereno, M.; Jimenez-Gordo, A.M.; Baena-Espinar, J.; Aguado, C.; Mielgo, X.; Pertejo, A.; Alvarez-Alvarez, R.; Sanchez, A.; Lopez, J.L.; Molina, R.; et al. A Multicenter Analysis of the Outcome of Cancer Patients with Neutropenia and COVID-19 Optionally Treated with Granulocyte-Colony Stimulating Factor (G-CSF): A Comparative Analysis. *Cancers* **2021**, *13*, 4205. [CrossRef] [PubMed]
66. Cariti, C.; Merli, M.; Avallone, G.; Rubatto, M.; Marra, E.; Fava, P.; Caliendo, V.; Picciotto, F.; Gualdi, G.; Stanganelli, I.; et al. Melanoma Management during the COVID-19 Pandemic Emergency: A Literature Review and Single-Center Experience. *Cancers* **2021**, *13*, 6071. [CrossRef]
67. Deligiorgi, M.V.; Siasos, G.; Vakkas, L.; Trafalis, D.T. Charting the Unknown Association of COVID-19 with Thyroid Cancer, Focusing on Differentiated Thyroid Cancer: A Call for Caution. *Cancers* **2021**, *13*, 5785. [CrossRef] [PubMed]
68. Prodromidou, A.; Koulakmanidis, A.M.; Haidopoulos, D.; Nelson, G.; Rodolakis, A.; Thomakos, N. Where Enhanced Recovery after Surgery (ERAS) Protocols Meet the Three Major Current Pandemics: COVID-19, Obesity and Malignancy. *Cancers* **2022**, *14*, 1660. [CrossRef]
69. Petropoulou, Z.; Arkadopoulos, N.; Michalopoulos, N.V. Breast Cancer and COVID-19: Challenges in Surgical Management. *Cancers* **2022**, *14*, 5360. [CrossRef] [PubMed]
70. Pararas, N.; Pikouli, A.; Papaconstantinou, D.; Bagias, G.; Nastos, C.; Pikoulis, A.; Dellaportas, D.; Lykoudis, P.; Pikoulis, E. Colorectal Surgery in the COVID-19 Era: A Systematic Review and Meta-Analysis. *Cancers* **2022**, *14*, 1229. [CrossRef]

Disclaimer/Publisher's Note: The statements, opinions and data contained in all publications are solely those of the individual author(s) and contributor(s) and not of MDPI and/or the editor(s). MDPI and/or the editor(s) disclaim responsibility for any injury to people or property resulting from any ideas, methods, instructions or products referred to in the content.

Hypothesis

Autophagy: The Potential Link between SARS-CoV-2 and Cancer

Parham Habibzadeh [1], Hassan Dastsooz [2,3,4], Mehdi Eshraghi [5], Marek J. Łos [6,*], Daniel J. Klionsky [7] and Saeid Ghavami [5,8,9,*]

1. Research Center for Health Sciences, Institute of Health, Shiraz University of Medical Sciences, Shiraz 71348-14336, Iran; Parham.Habibzadeh@yahoo.com
2. Department of Life Sciences and Systems Biology, University of Turin, Via Accademia, Albertina, 13, 10123 Torino, Italy; Hassan.Dastsooz@unito.it
3. IIGM-Italian Institute for Genomic Medicine, c/o IRCCS, Candiolo, 10126 Torino, Italy
4. Candiolo Cancer Institute, FPO-IRCCS, 10060 Torino, Italy
5. Department of Human Anatomy and Cell Science, Rady Faculty of Health Sciences, Max Rady College of Medicine, University of Manitoba, Winnipeg, MB R3E 0J9, Canada; eshraghi.mehdi@gmail.com
6. Biotechnology Center, Silesian University of Technology, 44-100 Gliwice, Poland
7. Life Sciences Institute, University of Michigan, Ann Arbor, MI 48109, USA; klionsky@umich.edu
8. Research Institute of Oncology and Hematology, Cancer Care Manitoba, University of Manitoba, Winnipeg, MB R3E 0V9, Canada
9. Faculty of Medicine, Katowice School of Technology, ul. Rolna 43, 40-555 Katowice, Poland
* Correspondence: Marek.Los@polsl.pl (M.J.Ł.); saeid.ghavami@umanitoba.ca (S.G.)

Simple Summary: Coronavirus disease 2019 (COVID-19) has led to a global crisis. With the increasing number of individuals infected worldwide, the long-term consequences of this disease have become an active area of research. The constellation of symptoms COVID-19 survivors suffer from is commonly referred to as post-acute COVID-19 syndrome in the scientific literature. In this paper, we discuss the potential long-term complications of this infection resulting from the persistence of the viral particles in body tissues interacting with host cells' autophagy machinery in the context of the development of cancer, cancer progression and metastasis, as well as response to treatment. We also propose a structured framework for future studies to investigate the potential impact of COVID-19 infection on cancer.

Abstract: COVID-19 infection survivors suffer from a constellation of symptoms referred to as post-acute COVID-19 syndrome. However, in the wake of recent evidence highlighting the long-term persistence of SARS-CoV-2 antigens in tissues and emerging information regarding the interaction between SARS-CoV-2 proteins and various components of the host cell macroautophagy/autophagy machinery, the unforeseen long-term consequences of this infection, such as increased risk of malignancies, should be explored. Although SARS-CoV-2 is not considered an oncogenic virus, the possibility of increased risk of cancer among COVID-19 survivors cannot be ruled out. Herein, we provide an overview of the possible mechanisms leading to cancer development, particularly obesity-related cancers (e.g., colorectal cancer), resulting from defects in autophagy and the blockade of the autophagic flux, and also immune escape in COVID-19 survivors. We also highlight the potential long-term implications of COVID-19 infection in the prognosis of patients with cancer and their response to different cancer treatments. Finally, we consider future directions for further investigations on this matter.

Keywords: colorectal neoplasms; COVID-19; gastrointestinal neoplasms; immune checkpoint inhibitors; neoplasms; oncogenic viruses; oncolytic virotherapy; post-acute COVID-19 syndrome; reactive oxygen species; tumor escape

1. Introduction

Coronavirus disease 2019 (COVID-19), caused by severe acute respiratory syndrome coronavirus 2 (SARS-CoV-2), has led to unprecedented mortality and morbidity at a global scale. SARS-CoV-2 is a positive-stranded RNA virus belonging to the *Coronaviridae* family, members of which interact with different components of the cellular autophagy machinery [1,2]. A constellation of symptoms, such as fatigue, exhaustion, and shortness of breath, persisting long after the resolution of the acute phase of infection, has been reported among some survivors of this infection [3]. The persistence of symptoms beyond 12 weeks after the initial onset is called post-COVID-19 syndrome [3,4]. However, long-term complications of this infection could extend well beyond these symptoms.

2. Autophagy and Cancer

Autophagy plays a prominent role in maintaining cellular homeostasis through the removal of damaged organelles, abnormal proteins, and invading organisms. Defects in autophagy are associated with various pathological conditions, including cancer [5]. It can lead to accumulation of damaged mitochondria and alter cellular metabolism, leading to a high oxidative state [6]. Furthermore, impairments in autophagy flux can lead to ER stress and subsequent accumulation of chaperone proteins and an eventual rise in the unfolded protein burden [7,8]. This chronic injury to various cellular organelles and proteins and the accumulation of the genetic damage in cells with defective autophagy can lead to the development of pathophysiologies, as evidenced by the detection of loss-of-function mutations in different autophagy genes in various malignancies such as colorectal cancer [9]. However, despite this significant role of autophagy in the initiation of tumors, it is a double-edged sword in cancer, and its role is highly context dependent [10]. Cancer cells are dependent on the cellular autophagy machinery due to their rapid growth and biosynthetic demands [6,8]. Autophagy also plays a significant role in promoting metastasis in certain tumors, particularly in RAS-driven cancers [11]. Conversely, autophagy can also be leveraged to enhance the response to various cancer treatments [12] (Figure 1).

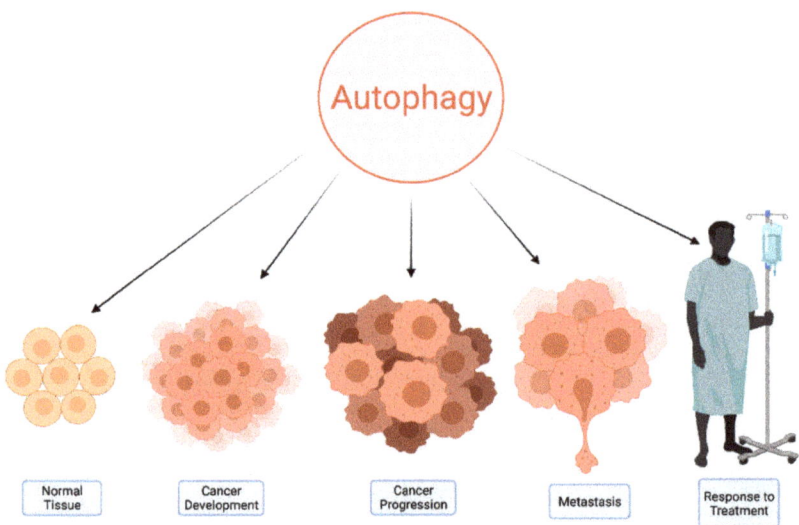

Figure 1. Autophagy has a principle role in both the health and disease states, such as malignancies. This process plays a complex role in various aspects of cancer.

3. Potential Clues and Mechanisms Supporting the Role of SARS-CoV-2 in Oncogenesis

Several oncogenic viruses exert their carcinogenesis through altering autophagy [13]. Although the oncogenic potential of SARS-CoV-2 has not yet been investigated, two other positive-sense single-strand RNA viruses, namely, hepatitis C virus/HCV and human T-cell lymphotropic virus type 1/HTLV-1, exploit the cellular autophagy machinery in order to cause liver cancer and adult T-cell leukemia/lymphoma/ATLL, respectively [13].

Both ACE2 (the major SARS-CoV-2 receptor) and TMPRSS2 (a transmembrane serine protease necessary for viral cell entry) display a very high level of expression in the human gastrointestinal tract [14]. This virus can infect and actively replicate in human enterocytes [14]. A recent study on the gastrointestinal biopsies of 14 individuals performed four months after their COVID-19 diagnosis reported persistence of the viral nucleic acids and antigens in 50% of the cases [15]. Persistent shedding of SARS-CoV-2 viral particles for months after the resolution of the symptoms has also been reported in the nasopharyngeal specimens obtained from individuals with previous infection [16,17]. This continued presence of the viral antigens in different tissues could have serious long-term consequences for survivors of COVID-19 infection.

Interestingly, various SARS-CoV-2 proteins interact with different components of the cellular autophagy pathway (Figure 2). For example, viral ORF3a protein interacts with VPS39, a part of the homotypic fusion and protein sorting/HOPS complex, leading to the inhibition of the fusion of autophagosomes with lysosomes [18]. In addition, SARS-CoV-2 Nsp15 blocks the induction of autophagy, whereas the viral ORF7a protein decreases the acidity of lysosomes, which can interfere with autophagosome–lysosome fusion as well as cargo degradation [19]. Moreover, accumulation of SQSTM1 and an increase in the processed LC3B (LC3B-II) levels have been observed upon SARS-CoV-2 envelope (E) protein overexpression [19,20]. Altogether, these findings indicate that various SARS-CoV-2 antigens block autophagic flux in the infected cells. Conversely, a recent study showed that the protein encoded by viral ORF8 leads to major histocompatibility complex I (MHC-I) degradation in the affected cells by targeting these molecules for lysosomal degradation through the BECN1-dependent autophagy pathway [21].

The persistence of the SARS-CoV-2 antigens in the enterocytes could lead to long-term defects in the cellular autophagy machinery, as evidenced by recent studies. The blockage in the autophagic flux in these cells would lead to the accumulation of SQSTM1/p62 (an autophagic receptor protein), reactive oxygen species, organelle damage, and genetic alterations in response to different stresses, eventually leading to tumorigenesis [22,23]. An approximate 1.5-fold increase in SQSTM1 levels in the presence of SARS-CoV-2 ORF3a, ORF7a, or E proteins has been observed [19]. SQSTM1 plays a significant role in tumor transformation due to its important function as a signaling molecule interacting with many oncogenic pathways, including those involving NFE2L2/NRF2 and NFKB/NF-κB [24]. Several studies also reported evidence of mitochondrial dysfunction, excessive production of reactive oxygen species, ER stress, and unfolded protein responses in the cells infected with SARS-CoV-2 [25–27]. As mentioned, these pathological events could be, in part, a result of disturbed autophagy flux in the cells. Furthermore, disrupted cell cycle regulation due to autophagy defects would lead to the uncontrolled proliferation of cells carrying defective genetic materials, paving the way for the development of cancer [28]. In addition, activation of compensatory mechanisms in colorectal cancer cells in specific contexts secondary to the inhibition of autophagy lead to tumor growth [29]. This could in turn lead to a higher risk of cancer development and more rapid proliferation of tumor cells among COVID-19 survivors.

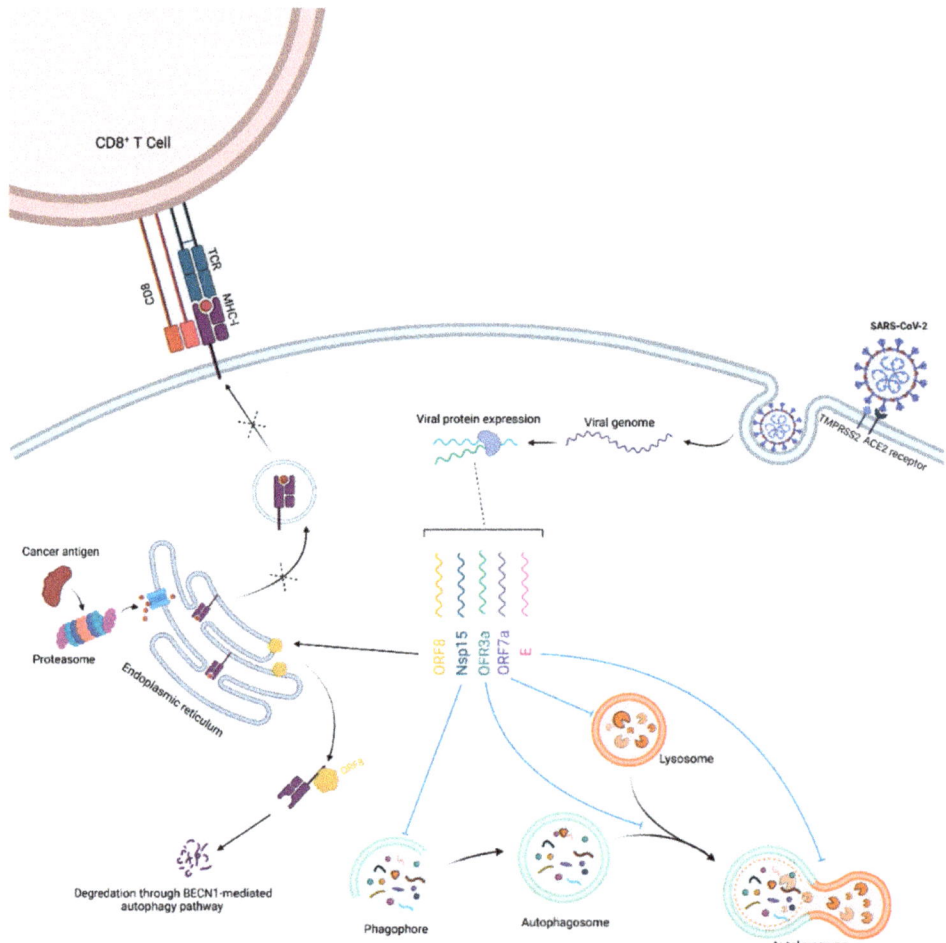

Figure 2. SARS-CoV-2 infects enterocytes through ACE2 receptors and TMPRSS2 expressed on their surface. The release of the viral genome and production of viral proteins (simplified in this schema) will lead to the interaction of various SARS-CoV-2 antigens with the host cell autophagy machinery. Overall, this will induce the blockage of the autophagic flux. The accumulation of reactive oxygen species, damaged cellular proteins and organelles, and acquired genetic defects due to various stressors can lead to the development of malignancies. Furthermore, infection can also interfere with the cellular MHC-I antigen-presentation pathway, blunting the ability of host cytotoxic CD8⁺ T cells to recognize potential oncogenic antigens.

Downregulation of MHC-I is one of the major mechanisms of the immune evasion by tumor cells through escaping detection by CD8$^+$ T-cells and their cytotoxicity [30]. This adaptive immune escape mechanism is observed in many malignancies, including colorectal cancer, and is associated with a poor prognosis [31]. MHC-I degradation through the BECN1-dependent autophagy pathway induced by viral ORF8 could, therefore, provide a fertile soil for carcinogenesis by blunting the ability of the immune system to detect the cancer cells because their neo-antigens are no longer presented on the MHC-I molecules.

It should be noted that SARS-CoV-2 antigens have also been detected in various other human organs, such as the lungs, heart, kidneys, hepatobiliary system, and the lymphatic system [32]. Although most of these findings have been reported in post-mortem studies and the persistence of the viral antigens in these organs among COVID-19 survivors has not so far been assessed due to technical and ethical considerations, it is likely that viral particles could linger in these tissues, continuing to interact with the host cell autophagy machinery and therefore inducing carcinogenesis in various organ systems. Chronic SARS-CoV-2 infection is reported in immunocompromised patients (e.g., due to anti-cancer therapy) and animal models [33–35]. These immunocompromised patients with chronic infection might have a higher risk of cancer, as evidenced in other malignancies with suspected infectious etiology [36].

Interestingly, a recent study has reported that SARS-CoV-2 RNA can integrate into the genome of cultured human cells through reverse transcription. The authors also claimed that they were able to detect viral-host chimeric transcripts in the patient-derived tissues, suggesting that these transcripts are a result of integration of DNA copies of viral sequences in the human genome [37]. However, a later study by another group did not find any evidence for such an event in human cells [38]. Clearly, further large-scale studies are required to investigate if the SARS-CoV-2 genome is able to integrate into the human genome.

A nation-wide population-based study conducted in Denmark investigating mortality rates among patients admitted to the hospitals for non-COVID-19 diseases during the pandemic from March 2019 to January 2021, and found a consistently higher mortality rate among patients with cancer compared with baseline pre-pandemic mortality rates among these patients [39]. Although this observation is likely due to a multitude of factors, it is possible that defects in autophagy and increased tumor immune evasion among patients with certain malignancies who had previously contracted this infection could have led to more a rapid progression of their cancer due to the processes described above. In addition, a 6.9-fold increase in tumor burden has been reported in patients who had been diagnosed with metastatic colorectal cancer after the first lockdown compared with those diagnosed prior to the lockdown [40]. Despite the significant role of the delays in the screening and diagnosis as a result of the COVID-19-related lockdown, the above-mentioned processes could have also contributed to this observation. Notably, patients with cancer remain a vulnerable population for COVID-19 [41].

4. Autophagy and Metabolism

Autophagy plays a fundamental role as a catabolic process recycling intracellular components into breakdown products that could be used in various cellular metabolic pathways [42]. This, in turn, enables cells to survive under metabolic stress conditions (e.g., nutrient deprivation, hypoxia, etc.) [43,44].

Alteration in cellular metabolism is one of the hallmarks of cancer [45]. Unlike normal cells, which mainly rely on mitochondrial oxidative phosphorylation for energy production, most cancer cells depend on aerobic glycolysis (the Warburg effect) [45,46]. Despite being an inefficient pathway for adenosine 5′-triphosphate (ATP) generation, it is thought that it confers an advantage to tumor cells in incorporating nutrients in tumor biomass and cellular proliferation [46]. Considering the diverse role of autophagy in feeding different metabolic pathways through degradation of various cellular substrates, it is not surprising that elevated basal autophagy is seen in many tumor types [8,47].

Furthermore, mitochondrial metabolism plays an important role in various tumor types by redox balance, ATP generation, and synthesis of intermediates required for macromolecule biosynthesis (e.g., nucleotides) [48]. The selective autophagic elimination of the mitochondria (i.e., mitophagy) is a very important cellular process regulating their number and also participating in mitochondria quality control [49]. In addition, mitophagy plays a vital role in the metabolic rewiring of cancer cells aimed at meeting their bioenergetic needs [50].

Considering the paramount role of autophagy in maintaining tissue homeostasis, dysregulation in this process has been linked to cancer development and progression in a context-specific manner [51]. The potential inhibition of the autophagy flux by SARS-CoV-2 antigens can deprive tumor cells of the building blocks essential for unconstrained tumor proliferation and could, therefore, limit tumor growth. However, the accumulation of dysfunctional organelles, particularly dysfunctional mitochondria, as a result of impaired autophagy can pave the way for the development of cancer [52] (Figure 3).

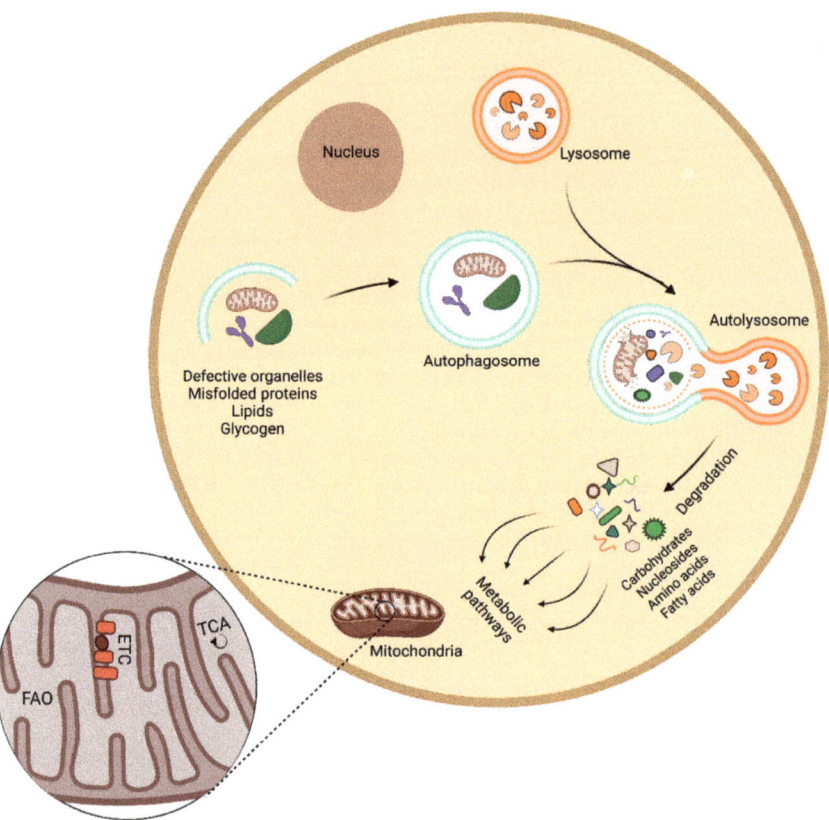

Figure 3. Autophagy and cell metabolism in cancer. Autophagy plays an important role in removing defective cellular organelles and macromolecules and recycling them for further use in different metabolic pathways. Mitochondria are the primary cellular organelles responsible for various cellular metabolic pathways including fatty acid oxidation (FAO), the tricarboxylic acid (TCA) cycle, and the electron transport chain (ETC). Impaired production of metabolic intermediates important for cellular proliferation can lead to a metabolic crisis and subsequently limit tumor growth. Conversely, excessive production of reactive oxygen species and the resultant oxidative damage can lead to tumorigenesis.

Obesity is correlated with elevated systemic oxidative stress [53]. The excessive nutrients supply, overwhelming the cellular Krebs cycle and mitochondrial respiratory chain, leads to mitochondrial dysfunction and increases the formation of reactive oxygen species (ROS) [54]. Elevation of intracellular ROS is known to lead to the upregulation of the cellular autophagic response, which subsequently removes defective mitochondria and therefore limits the generation of ROS [55–57]. The potential inhibition of autophagic flux as a result of the persistence of SARS-CoV-2 antigens in different tissues could blunt this protective mechanism and could particularly be more important in the pathogenesis of obesity-related cancers. ROS levels are higher in colorectal cancer cells compared with normal non-cancerous tissues [58]. Furthermore, ROS play a critical role in mediating tumorigenesis and colorectal cancer initiation driven by RAC1 [59]. The effects of ROS extend beyond the initiation of obesity-related cancers; they are anti-apoptotic factors promoting the survival of pancreatic cancer cells [60].

5. Implications for Cancer Treatment

The long-term presence of SARS-CoV-2 antigens in cancer tissues could also have wide-ranging implications for cancer therapy. MHC-I loss or downregulation is a common mechanism for the development of resistance to PDCD1/PD-1 inhibitors among patients with melanoma [61,62]. The same phenomenon could potentially render cancer cells arising in the presence of SARS-CoV-2 antigens resistant to anti-PDCD1 monotherapy as a result of MHC-I degradation through BECN1-dependent autophagy. This outcome could necessitate the use of PDCD1 and CTLA4 blockade combination therapy in such cases, as this treatment strategy does not require MHC-I expression for exerting its therapeutic effects [63].

Lysosomal sequestration of weak base hydrophobic chemotherapeutic agents decreasing their accessibility to their target sites and the resultant decrease in their cytotoxic effects is a significant challenge that culminates in treatment failure and subsequent increase in mortality due to cancer [64]. Lysosomal exocytosis facilitating the clearance of chemotherapeutics accumulated in this organelle is another important component of lysosome-mediated chemotherapy resistance [65]. A recent study has shown that SARS-CoV-2 ORF3a not only inhibits the autophagy flux but also promotes lysosomal exocytosis [66]. This could confer drug resistance to the cancer cells arising in the setting of persistence SARS-CoV-2 ORF3a presence.

Despite the preliminary clues pointing towards the role of the virus in promoting tumor progression described here, rare instances of tumor burden reduction in three patients with colorectal cancer and disease remission in a patient with Hodgkin lymphoma following COVID-19 infection have been reported in the literature [67,68]. Although the over-exuberant immune response instigated by SARS-CoV-2 attacking the tumor cells could have led to this phenomenon [69], the complex role of autophagy in cancer (acting as a double-edged sword) should not be underestimated in interpreting these exceptional cases. These serendipitous observations may partly be due to the blockage of autophagy flux, leading to the deprivation of cancer cells of the essential biosynthetic materials generated by the cellular autophagy machinery required for tumor growth [6,8]. This in turn highlights the therapeutic potential of SARS-CoV-2 in oncolytic virotherapy via blockage of autophagic flux in specific tumor types at certain stages of their natural course. Theoretically, this potential therapeutic strategy could particularly be effective against tumor cells with high autophagy activity.

6. Future Directions

Notwithstanding significant efforts to unravel the role of autophagy in COVID-19 infection, many questions, particularly those surrounding the role of autophagy in the long-term complications of COVID-19, remain unanswered [70,71]. A multidisciplinary approach, involving both clinical and basic science researchers, aimed towards studying the unforeseen long-term consequences of COVID-19 infection in cancer development, tumor progression, metastasis, and response to various cancer therapeutics could eventually piece together different parts of this puzzle, providing a better understanding of the complex interaction between SARS-CoV-2 and cancer.

The potential long-term oncogenic effects of SARS-CoV-2 antigens that inhibit the autophagic flux (e.g., NSP15, ORF3a, etc.) could be investigated through in vitro studies assessing changes in tumor formation following the long-term presence of these antigens in various human cell lines, such as human *KRAS* knockout cells. In addition, studies on patient-derived cancer cell lines could provide valuable insight into the effect of viral antigens and the subsequent blockage of the autophagic flux and MHC-I downregulation on tumor cell response to various cancer treatments and its effect on metastatic potential. Furthermore, although due to the short lifespan of most animal models they may not be suitable for investigating the long-term effects of viral antigens on cancer development, patient-derived mouse xenograft models of different human malignancies that have arisen in the presence of SARS-CoV-2 antigens can provide an ideal framework for exploring tumor growth, metastasis, and the response to different cancer treatments. Comprehensive molecular phenotyping of various human tumors arising in the setting of long-term presence of SARS-CoV-2 antigens and comparing them with malignancies developed in other settings could shed light on the potential biological processes specifically affected (Figure 4).

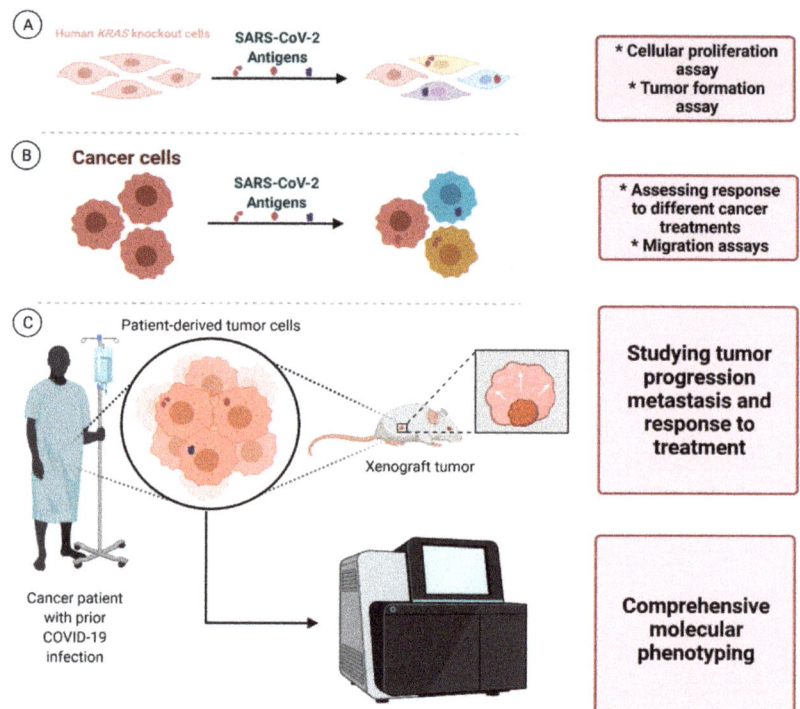

Figure 4. Proposed framework for laboratory-based investigations. (**A**) Investigations that could unravel the potential effects of various SARS-CoV-2 antigens on cellular proliferation and tumor formation in human KRAS knockout cells. (**B**) Using patient-derived cancer cells, the effect of these antigens and the subsequent autophagy blockade and MHC-I downregulation on response to different cancer treatments and metastasis (migration assays) could be studied. (**C**) Furthermore, studying tumor specimens arising in the presence of SARS-CoV-2 antigens using xenograft mouse models and also advanced molecular phenotyping techniques could unravel tumor biological behavior (growth rate, metastasis, etc.), its molecular characteristics, and the underlying factors affecting its response to various cancer therapeutics.

Clinical and epidemiological investigations can also play a principal role in expanding our understanding of this matter. Cohort studies with sufficient follow-up can assess the long-term incidence of various malignancies in different populations and would determine whether prior COVID-19 infection is a risk factor for the development of different cancers adjusting for well-known cancer risk factors. In addition, studying specific subpopulations, such as those with severe infection (i.e., ICU admission), and also patients with primary and secondary immunodeficiency could offer profound insight into the most susceptible populations. Considering the potential far-reaching implications of the infection for patients with active cancer, specific studies focused on this vulnerable population assessing the long-term impact of the infection on the clinical course of their malignancy should be carried out. Prospective studies investigating if prior COVID-19 infection affects the rate of cancer progression, mortality rate, and response to treatment among patients with different malignancies, adjusting for the traditional contributing factors, could provide insight into the possible interaction between SARS-CoV-2 antigens and neoplastic cells (Figure 5).

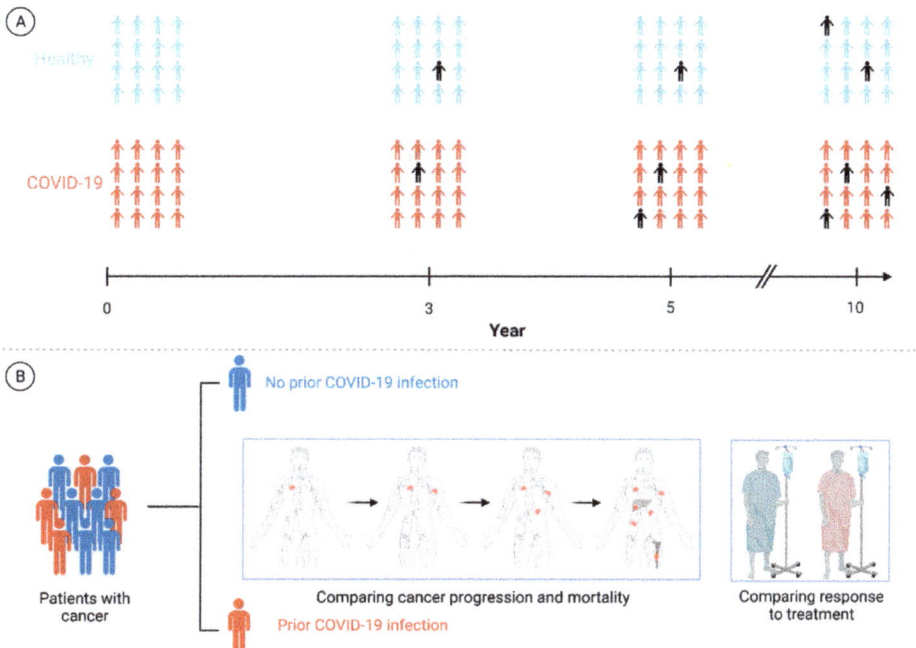

Figure 5. Proposed framework for clinical and population-based investigations. (**A**) Studies that can investigate whether prior COVID-19 infection is a risk factor for development of malignancies in subsequent years. (**B**) Other investigations could also shed light on the potential long-term effects of SARS-CoV-2 antigens present in cancer tissues on cancer progression and mortality rate and the response to different cancer therapeutics. The back icon in (**A**) represents a patient with a new diagnosis of cancer. Please note that the numbers of individuals with cancer in both groups have been arbitrarily chosen and are not based on real-life data. Future investigations will hopefully examine the hypothesis described here.

7. Conclusions

Despite the short amount of time since SARS-CoV-2 was first reported in 2019, scientists around the globe have managed to unravel various aspects of this infectious disease. However, we are still far from a solid understanding of this emerging infection and many important questions, particularly those regarding the long-term complications of this disease, remain unanswered.

In this work, building on the previous investigations demonstrating long-term persistence of the SARS-CoV-2 nucleic acids and antigens in human tissues and also other research studies showing the interaction of the viral particles with the host autophagy machinery, we hypothesize that SARS-CoV-2 could potentially be an oncogenic virus by blocking the autophagic flux, and also leading to immune escape by downregulation of MHC-I. We also propose that the resultant dysregulation in cellular autophagy could affect the response to treatment in cancer cells. Further laboratory-based, clinical, and population-based studies are required to explore this matter.

Author Contributions: Conceptualization, P.H., S.G.; resources, S.G. and M.J.Ł.; writing—original draft preparation, P.H. and H.D.; writing—review and editing, P.H., M.E., D.J.K., M.J.Ł. and S.G.; visualization, P.H., S.G.; supervision, S.G. and M.J.Ł. All authors have read and agreed to the published version of the manuscript.

Funding: This work was supported by grant # 32/007/RGJ21/0034 from Silesian University of Technology and NIH grant GM131919.

Acknowledgments: The authors would like to thank Mohammad Sajadi (Institute of Human Virology, University of Maryland) for his invaluable comments. The figures used in this article were created using BioRender (BioRender.com, accessed on 27 October 2021).

Conflicts of Interest: The authors declare no conflict of interest.

References

1. Miller, K.; McGrath, M.E.; Hu, Z.; Ariannejad, S.; Weston, S.; Frieman, M.; Jackson, W.T. Coronavirus interactions with the cellular autophagy machinery. *Autophagy* **2020**, *16*, 2131–2139. [CrossRef] [PubMed]
2. Habibzadeh, P.; Stoneman, E.K. The Novel Coronavirus: A Bird's Eye View. *Int. J. Occup. Environ. Med.* **2020**, *11*, 65–71. [CrossRef]
3. Nalbandian, A.; Sehgal, K.; Gupta, A.; Madhavan, M.V.; McGroder, C.; Stevens, J.S.; Cook, J.R.; Nordvig, A.S.; Shalev, D.; Sehrawat, T.S.; et al. Post-acute COVID-19 syndrome. *Nat. Med.* **2021**, *27*, 601–615. [CrossRef] [PubMed]
4. Shah, W.; Hillman, T.; Playford, E.D.; Hishmeh, L. Managing the long term effects of covid-19: Summary of NICE, SIGN, and RCGP rapid guideline. *BMJ* **2021**, *372*, n136. [CrossRef] [PubMed]
5. Levine, B.; Kroemer, G. Biological Functions of Autophagy Genes: A Disease Perspective. *Cell* **2019**, *176*, 11–42. [CrossRef] [PubMed]
6. Rabinowitz, J.D.; White, E. Autophagy and metabolism. *Science* **2010**, *330*, 1344–1348. [CrossRef] [PubMed]
7. Hoyer-Hansen, M.; Jaattela, M. Connecting endoplasmic reticulum stress to autophagy by unfolded protein response and calcium. *Cell Death Differ.* **2007**, *14*, 1576–1582. [CrossRef] [PubMed]
8. White, E. The role for autophagy in cancer. *J. Clin. Investig.* **2015**, *125*, 42–46. [CrossRef]
9. Kang, M.R.; Kim, M.S.; Oh, J.E.; Kim, Y.R.; Song, S.Y.; Kim, S.S.; Ahn, C.H.; Yoo, N.J.; Lee, S.H. Frameshift mutations of autophagy-related genes ATG2B, ATG5, ATG9B and ATG12 in gastric and colorectal cancers with microsatellite instability. *J. Pathol.* **2009**, *217*, 702–706. [CrossRef]
10. White, E. Deconvoluting the context-dependent role for autophagy in cancer. *Nat. Rev. Cancer* **2012**, *12*, 401–410. [CrossRef] [PubMed]
11. Lock, R.; Kenific, C.M.; Leidal, A.M.; Salas, E.; Debnath, J. Autophagy-dependent production of secreted factors facilitates oncogenic RAS-driven invasion. *Cancer Discov.* **2014**, *4*, 466–479. [CrossRef] [PubMed]
12. Mulcahy Levy, J.M.; Thorburn, A. Autophagy in cancer: Moving from understanding mechanism to improving therapy responses in patients. *Cell Death Differ.* **2020**, *27*, 843–857. [CrossRef] [PubMed]
13. Vescovo, T.; Pagni, B.; Piacentini, M.; Fimia, G.M.; Antonioli, M. Regulation of Autophagy in Cells Infected With Oncogenic Human Viruses and Its Impact on Cancer Development. *Front. Cell Dev. Biol.* **2020**, *8*, 47. [CrossRef] [PubMed]
14. Zang, R.; Gomez Castro, M.F.; McCune, B.T.; Zeng, Q.; Rothlauf, P.W.; Sonnek, N.M.; Liu, Z.; Brulois, K.F.; Wang, X.; Greenberg, H.B.; et al. TMPRSS2 and TMPRSS4 promote SARS-CoV-2 infection of human small intestinal enterocytes. *Sci. Immunol.* **2020**, *5*, eabc3582. [CrossRef] [PubMed]
15. Gaebler, C.; Wang, Z.; Lorenzi, J.C.C.; Muecksch, F.; Finkin, S.; Tokuyama, M.; Cho, A.; Jankovic, M.; Schaefer-Babajew, D.; Oliveira, T.Y.; et al. Evolution of antibody immunity to SARS-CoV-2. *Nature* **2021**, *591*, 639–644. [CrossRef] [PubMed]
16. Habibzadeh, P.; Mofatteh, M.; Silawi, M.; Ghavami, S.; Faghihi, M.A. Molecular diagnostic assays for COVID-19: An overview. *Crit. Rev. Clin. Lab. Sci.* **2021**, *58*, 385–398. [CrossRef]
17. Habibzadeh, P.; Sajadi, M.M.; Emami, A.; Karimi, M.H.; Yadollahie, M.; Kucheki, M.; Akbarpoor, S.; Habibzadeh, F. Rate of re-positive RT-PCR test among patients recovered from COVID-19. *Biochem. Med.* **2020**, *30*, 030401. [CrossRef]
18. Zhang, Y.; Sun, H.; Pei, R.; Mao, B.; Zhao, Z.; Li, H.; Lin, Y.; Lu, K. The SARS-CoV-2 protein ORF3a inhibits fusion of autophagosomes with lysosomes. *Cell Discov.* **2021**, *7*, 31. [CrossRef] [PubMed]
19. Hayn, M.; Hirschenberger, M.; Koepke, L.; Nchioua, R.; Straub, J.H.; Klute, S.; Hunszinger, V.; Zech, F.; Prelli Bozzo, C.; Aftab, W.; et al. Systematic functional analysis of SARS-CoV-2 proteins uncovers viral innate immune antagonists and remaining vulnerabilities. *Cell Rep.* **2021**, *35*, 109126. [CrossRef] [PubMed]
20. Koepke, L.; Hirschenberger, M.; Hayn, M.; Kirchhoff, F.; Sparrer, K.M. Manipulation of autophagy by SARS-CoV-2 proteins. *Autophagy* **2021**, *17*, 2659–2661. [CrossRef] [PubMed]
21. Zhang, Y.; Chen, Y.; Li, Y.; Huang, F.; Luo, B.; Yuan, Y.; Xia, B.; Ma, X.; Yang, T.; Yu, F.; et al. The ORF8 protein of SARS-CoV-2 mediates immune evasion through down-regulating MHC-Iota. *Proc. Natl. Acad. Sci. USA* **2021**, *118*, e2024202118. [CrossRef]
22. Mathew, R.; Karp, C.M.; Beaudoin, B.; Vuong, N.; Chen, G.; Chen, H.Y.; Bray, K.; Reddy, A.; Bhanot, G.; Gelinas, C.; et al. Autophagy suppresses tumorigenesis through elimination of p62. *Cell* **2009**, *137*, 1062–1075. [CrossRef] [PubMed]
23. Mokarram, P.; Albokashy, M.; Zarghooni, M.; Moosavi, M.A.; Sepehri, Z.; Chen, Q.M.; Hudecki, A.; Sargazi, A.; Alizadeh, J.; Moghadam, A.R.; et al. New frontiers in the treatment of colorectal cancer: Autophagy and the unfolded protein response as promising targets. *Autophagy* **2017**, *13*, 781–819. [CrossRef] [PubMed]
24. Moscat, J.; Diaz-Meco, M.T. p62: A versatile multitasker takes on cancer. *Trends. Biochem. Sci.* **2012**, *37*, 230–236. [CrossRef] [PubMed]

25. Muhammad, Y.; Kani, Y.A.; Iliya, S.; Muhammad, J.B.; Binji, A.; El-Fulaty Ahmad, A.; Kabir, M.B.; Umar Bindawa, K.; Ahmed, A. Deficiency of antioxidants and increased oxidative stress in COVID-19 patients: A cross-sectional comparative study in Jigawa, Northwestern Nigeria. *SAGE Open Med.* **2021**, *9*, 2050312121991246. [CrossRef]
26. Ajaz, S.; McPhail, M.J.; Singh, K.K.; Mujib, S.; Trovato, F.M.; Napoli, S.; Agarwal, K. Mitochondrial metabolic manipulation by SARS-CoV-2 in peripheral blood mononuclear cells of patients with COVID-19. *Am. J. Physiol.-Cell Physiol.* **2021**, *320*, C57–C65. [CrossRef]
27. Rosa-Fernandes, L.; Lazari, L.C.; da Silva, J.M.; de Morais Gomes, V.; Machado, R.R.G.; dos Santos, A.F.; Araujo, D.B.; Coutinho, J.V.P.; Arini, G.S.; Angeli, C.B.; et al. SARS-CoV-2 activates ER stress and Unfolded protein response. *bioRxiv* **2021**. [CrossRef]
28. Mathiassen, S.G.; De Zio, D.; Cecconi, F. Autophagy and the Cell Cycle: A Complex Landscape. *Front. Oncol.* **2017**, *7*, 51. [CrossRef]
29. Lauzier, A.; Normandeau-Guimond, J.; Vaillancourt-Lavigueur, V.; Boivin, V.; Charbonneau, M.; Rivard, N.; Scott, M.S.; Dubois, C.M.; Jean, S. Colorectal cancer cells respond differentially to autophagy inhibition in vivo. *Sci. Rep.* **2019**, *9*, 11316. [CrossRef] [PubMed]
30. Dhatchinamoorthy, K.; Colbert, J.D.; Rock, K.L. Cancer Immune Evasion Through Loss of MHC Class I Antigen Presentation. *Front. Immunol.* **2021**, *12*, 636568. [CrossRef]
31. Simpson, J.A.; Al-Attar, A.; Watson, N.F.; Scholefield, J.H.; Ilyas, M.; Durrant, L.G. Intratumoral T cell infiltration, MHC class I and STAT1 as biomarkers of good prognosis in colorectal cancer. *Gut* **2010**, *59*, 926–933. [CrossRef]
32. Polak, S.B.; Van Gool, I.C.; Cohen, D.; von der Thusen, J.H.; van Paassen, J. A systematic review of pathological findings in COVID-19: A pathophysiological timeline and possible mechanisms of disease progression. *Mod. Pathol.* **2020**, *33*, 2128–2138. [CrossRef]
33. Aydillo, T.; Gonzalez-Reiche, A.S.; Aslam, S.; van de Guchte, A.; Khan, Z.; Obla, A.; Dutta, J.; van Bakel, H.; Aberg, J.; García-Sastre, A.; et al. Shedding of Viable SARS-CoV-2 after Immunosuppressive Therapy for Cancer. *N. Engl. J. Med.* **2020**, *383*, 2586–2588. [CrossRef]
34. Choi, B.; Choudhary, M.C.; Regan, J.; Sparks, J.A.; Padera, R.F.; Qiu, X.; Solomon, I.H.; Kuo, H.-H.; Boucau, J.; Bowman, K.; et al. Persistence and Evolution of SARS-CoV-2 in an Immunocompromised Host. *N. Engl. J. Med.* **2020**, *383*, 2291–2293. [CrossRef]
35. Israelow, B.; Mao, T.; Klein, J.; Song, E.; Menasche, B.; Omer, S.B.; Iwasaki, A. Adaptive immune determinants of viral clearance and protection in mouse models of SARS-CoV-2. *bioRxiv* **2021**. [CrossRef]
36. Grulich, A.E.; van Leeuwen, M.T.; Falster, M.O.; Vajdic, C.M. Incidence of cancers in people with HIV/AIDS compared with immunosuppressed transplant recipients: A meta-analysis. *Lancet* **2007**, *370*, 59–67. [CrossRef]
37. Zhang, L.; Richards, A.; Barrasa, M.I.; Hughes, S.H.; Young, R.A.; Jaenisch, R. Reverse-transcribed SARS-CoV-2 RNA can integrate into the genome of cultured human cells and can be expressed in patient-derived tissues. *Proc. Natl. Acad. Sci. USA* **2021**, *118*, e2105968118. [CrossRef] [PubMed]
38. Smits, N.; Rasmussen, J.; Bodea, G.O.; Amarilla, A.A.; Gerdes, P.; Sanchez-Luque, F.J.; Ajjikuttira, P.; Modhiran, N.; Liang, B.; Faivre, J.; et al. No evidence of human genome integration of SARS-CoV-2 found by long-read DNA sequencing. *Cell Rep.* **2021**, *36*, 109530. [CrossRef]
39. Bodilsen, J.; Nielsen, P.B.; Sogaard, M.; Dalager-Pedersen, M.; Speiser, L.O.Z.; Yndigegn, T.; Nielsen, H.; Larsen, T.B.; Skjoth, F. Hospital admission and mortality rates for non-covid diseases in Denmark during covid-19 pandemic: Nationwide population based cohort study. *BMJ* **2021**, *373*, n1135. [CrossRef] [PubMed]
40. Thierry, A.R.; Pastor, B.; Pisareva, E.; Ghiringhelli, F.; Bouche, O.; De La Fouchardiere, C.; Vanbockstael, J.; Smith, D.; Francois, E.; Dos Santos, M.; et al. Association of COVID-19 Lockdown With the Tumor Burden in Patients With Newly Diagnosed Metastatic Colorectal Cancer. *JAMA Netw. Open* **2021**, *4*, e2124483. [CrossRef]
41. Desai, A.; Sachdeva, S.; Parekh, T.; Desai, R. COVID-19 and Cancer: Lessons From a Pooled Meta-Analysis. *JCO Glob. Oncol.* **2020**, *6*, 557–559. [CrossRef] [PubMed]
42. Levine, B.; Klionsky, D.J. Development by self-digestion: Molecular mechanisms and biological functions of autophagy. *Dev. Cell* **2004**, *6*, 463–477. [CrossRef]
43. Amaravadi, R.; Kimmelman, A.C.; White, E. Recent insights into the function of autophagy in cancer. *Genes. Dev.* **2016**, *30*, 1913–1930. [CrossRef]
44. Ghavami, S.; Yeganeh, B.; Stelmack, G.L.; Kashani, H.H.; Sharma, P.; Cunnington, R.; Rattan, S.; Bathe, K.; Klonisch, T.; Dixon, I.M.; et al. Apoptosis, autophagy and ER stress in mevalonate cascade inhibition-induced cell death of human atrial fibroblasts. *Cell Death Dis.* **2012**, *3*, e330. [CrossRef]
45. Kumar, V.; Abbas, A.K.; Aster, J.C. *Robbins and Cotran Pathologic Basis of Disease*; Elsevier/Saunders: Amsterdam, The Netherlands, 2015.
46. Vander Heiden, M.G.; Cantley, L.C.; Thompson, C.B. Understanding the Warburg effect: The metabolic requirements of cell proliferation. *Science* **2009**, *324*, 1029–1033. [CrossRef]
47. Guo, J.Y.; White, E. Autophagy, Metabolism, and Cancer. *Cold Spring Harb. Symp. Quant. Biol.* **2016**, *81*, 73–78. [CrossRef] [PubMed]
48. Weinberg, S.E.; Chandel, N.S. Targeting mitochondria metabolism for cancer therapy. *Nat. Chem. Biol.* **2015**, *11*, 9–15. [CrossRef]
49. Youle, R.J.; Narendra, D.P. Mechanisms of mitophagy. *Nat. Rev. Mol. Cell Biol.* **2011**, *12*, 9–14. [CrossRef]
50. Vara-Perez, M.; Felipe-Abrio, B.; Agostinis, P. Mitophagy in Cancer: A Tale of Adaptation. *Cells* **2019**, *8*, 493. [CrossRef]

51. Kimmelman, A.C.; White, E. Autophagy and Tumor Metabolism. *Cell Metab.* **2017**, *25*, 1037–1043. [CrossRef]
52. Palikaras, K.; Lionaki, E.; Tavernarakis, N. Mechanisms of mitophagy in cellular homeostasis, physiology and pathology. *Nat. Cell Biol.* **2018**, *20*, 1013–1022. [CrossRef] [PubMed]
53. Keaney, J.F., Jr.; Larson, M.G.; Vasan, R.S.; Wilson, P.W.; Lipinska, I.; Corey, D.; Massaro, J.M.; Sutherland, P.; Vita, J.A.; Benjamin, E.J.; et al. Obesity and systemic oxidative stress: Clinical correlates of oxidative stress in the Framingham Study. *Arter. Thromb. Vasc. Biol.* **2003**, *23*, 434–439. [CrossRef]
54. de Mello, A.H.; Costa, A.B.; Engel, J.D.G.; Rezin, G.T. Mitochondrial dysfunction in obesity. *Life Sci.* **2018**, *192*, 26–32. [CrossRef]
55. Sarparanta, J.; Garcia-Macia, M.; Singh, R. Autophagy and Mitochondria in Obesity and Type 2 Diabetes. *Curr. Diabetes Rev.* **2017**, *13*, 352–369. [CrossRef] [PubMed]
56. Chen, Y.; Azad, M.B.; Gibson, S.B. Superoxide is the major reactive oxygen species regulating autophagy. *Cell Death Differ.* **2009**, *16*, 1040–1052. [CrossRef]
57. Pietrocola, F.; Bravo-San Pedro, J.M. Targeting Autophagy to Counteract Obesity-Associated Oxidative Stress. *Antioxidants* **2021**, *10*, 102. [CrossRef]
58. Sreevalsan, S.; Safe, S. Reactive Oxygen Species and Colorectal Cancer. *Curr. Colorectal Cancer Rep.* **2013**, *9*, 350–357. [CrossRef] [PubMed]
59. Myant, K.B.; Cammareri, P.; McGhee, E.J.; Ridgway, R.A.; Huels, D.J.; Cordero, J.B.; Schwitalla, S.; Kalna, G.; Ogg, E.L.; Athineos, D.; et al. ROS production and NF-kappaB activation triggered by RAC1 facilitate WNT-driven intestinal stem cell proliferation and colorectal cancer initiation. *Cell Stem. Cell* **2013**, *12*, 761–773. [CrossRef]
60. Vaquero, E.C.; Edderkaoui, M.; Pandol, S.J.; Gukovsky, I.; Gukovskaya, A.S. Reactive oxygen species produced by NAD(P)H oxidase inhibit apoptosis in pancreatic cancer cells. *J. Biol. Chem.* **2004**, *279*, 34643–34654. [CrossRef]
61. Sade-Feldman, M.; Jiao, Y.J.; Chen, J.H.; Rooney, M.S.; Barzily-Rokni, M.; Eliane, J.P.; Bjorgaard, S.L.; Hammond, M.R.; Vitzthum, H.; Blackmon, S.M.; et al. Resistance to checkpoint blockade therapy through inactivation of antigen presentation. *Nat. Commun.* **2017**, *8*, 1136. [CrossRef]
62. Lee, J.H.; Shklovskaya, E.; Lim, S.Y.; Carlino, M.S.; Menzies, A.M.; Stewart, A.; Pedersen, B.; Irvine, M.; Alavi, S.; Yang, J.Y.H.; et al. Transcriptional downregulation of MHC class I and melanoma de- differentiation in resistance to PD-1 inhibition. *Nat. Commun.* **2020**, *11*, 1897. [CrossRef] [PubMed]
63. Shklovskaya, E.; Lee, J.H.; Lim, S.Y.; Stewart, A.; Pedersen, B.; Ferguson, P.; Saw, R.P.; Thompson, J.F.; Shivalingam, B.; Carlino, M.S.; et al. Tumor MHC Expression Guides First-Line Immunotherapy Selection in Melanoma. *Cancers* **2020**, *12*, 3374. [CrossRef] [PubMed]
64. Zhitomirsky, B.; Assaraf, Y.G. Lysosomes as mediators of drug resistance in cancer. *Drug Resist. Updat.* **2016**, *24*, 23–33. [CrossRef] [PubMed]
65. Zhitomirsky, B.; Assaraf, Y.G. Lysosomal accumulation of anticancer drugs triggers lysosomal exocytosis. *Oncotarget* **2017**, *8*, 45117–45132. [CrossRef]
66. Chen, D.; Zheng, Q.; Sun, L.; Ji, M.; Li, Y.; Deng, H.; Zhang, H. ORF3a of SARS-CoV-2 promotes lysosomal exocytosis-mediated viral egress. *Dev. Cell* **2021**. [CrossRef] [PubMed]
67. Challenor, S.; Tucker, D. SARS-CoV-2-induced remission of Hodgkin lymphoma. *Br. J. Haematol.* **2021**, *192*, 415. [CrossRef] [PubMed]
68. Ottaiano, A.; Scala, S.; D'Alterio, C.; Trotta, A.; Bello, A.; Rea, G.; Picone, C.; Santorsola, M.; Petrillo, A.; Nasti, G. Unexpected tumor reduction in metastatic colorectal cancer patients during SARS-CoV-2 infection. *Ther. Adv. Med. Oncol.* **2021**, *13*. [CrossRef]
69. Icenogle, T. COVID-19: Infection or Autoimmunity. *Front. Immunol.* **2020**, *11*, 2055. [CrossRef]
70. Delorme-Axford, E.; Klionsky, D.J. Highlights in the fight against COVID-19: Does autophagy play a role in SARS-CoV-2 infection? *Autophagy* **2020**, *16*, 2123–2127. [CrossRef]
71. Shojaei, S.; Suresh, M.; Klionsky, D.J.; Labouta, H.I.; Ghavami, S. Autophagy and SARS-CoV-2 infection: Apossible smart targeting of the autophagy pathway. *Virulence* **2020**, *11*, 805–810. [CrossRef]

cancers

Review

A Narrative Review of the Safety of Anti-COVID-19 Nutraceuticals for Patients with Cancer

Karlen Stade Bader-Larsen [1,†], **Elisabeth Anne Larson** [1,†], **Maria Dalamaga** [2] **and Faidon Magkos** [1,*]

1. Department of Nutrition, Exercise and Sports, University of Copenhagen, 1958 Frederiksberg, Denmark; skc639@alumni.ku.dk (K.S.B.-L.); kfg323@alumni.ku.dk (E.A.L.)
2. Department of Biological Chemistry, Medical School, National and Kapodistrian University of Athens, 11527 Athens, Greece; madalamaga@med.uoa.gr
* Correspondence: fma@nexs.ku.dk; Tel.: +45-3533-3671
† Two authors contributed equally to this work.

Simple Summary: Dietary supplement use has increased more than 35% globally since the COVID-19 outbreak. While some nutraceuticals are potentially efficacious against severe disease from COVID-19, their indiscriminate use by patients with cancer without medical supervision is concerning. The aim of this narrative review was to evaluate the data on safety of "anti-COVID-19" nutraceuticals for patients with cancer. We found that the use of vitamin C, vitamin D, and selenium supplements is likely safe and even potentially beneficial at typically recommended doses. However, caution is advised regarding the use of omega-3 fatty acids and zinc, as risks from their use may outweigh the benefits.

Abstract: Interest in dietary supplements and their efficacy in treating and preventing disease has increased greatly since the outbreak of the COVID-19 pandemic. Due to the risk of severe COVID-19 in patients with cancer, we conducted a narrative review aiming to better understand the data on the safety of the most efficacious "anti-COVID-19" nutraceuticals for patients with cancer. We conducted a PubMed database search aimed at identifying the most effective nutrients for use against COVID-19. For the identified nutraceuticals, we searched PubMed again regarding their safety for patients with cancer. Fifty-four total records (52 independent studies) were retrieved, pertaining to vitamin D, vitamin C, selenium, omega-3 fatty acids, and zinc. Vitamin D results from 23 articles indicated safe use, but two articles indicated potential harm. All 14 articles for vitamin C and five out of six articles for selenium indicated the safety of use (one study for selenium suggested harm with high-dose supplementation). Results for omega-3 fatty acids (seven articles) and zinc (one article), however, were rather mixed regarding safety. We conclude that vitamin D, vitamin C, and selenium supplements are likely safe or even beneficial at typically recommended doses; however, caution is urged with omega-3 fatty acid supplements, and zinc supplements should likely be avoided. More experimental research is needed, and nutraceutical use by patients with cancer should always be under the supervision of a healthcare team.

Keywords: cancer; nutraceuticals; supplements; COVID-19; SARS-CoV-2

1. Introduction

In December 2019, a novel virus of unknown etiology was detected in Wuhan, China [1]. The virus, which most often manifests as a severe respiratory syndrome, quickly spread from Wuhan, with cases appearing globally by 30 January 2020 [2]. It was quickly labeled by the World Health Organization as a public health outbreak of international concern and was later declared a pandemic [2,3]. This novel airborne pathogen, since named severe acute respiratory syndrome coronavirus 2 (SARS-CoV-2), causes the disease now known as COVID-19 [2]. Despite containment efforts and the introduction of a vaccine in late 2020, by November 2021, over 5 million deaths had been attributed to the virus [4].

COVID-19 has been shown to manifest heterogeneously across different patient populations. Mild cases often result in flu-like symptoms, fever, or loss of taste and smell [5]. However, in severe cases, the effects of infection are more significant, resulting in an abnormal cytokine and chemokine response that causes systemic inflammation, affecting multiple tissues and organ systems [6]. Individuals with co-morbidities such as obesity, diabetes, cardiovascular disease, and cancer have a greater tendency to elicit this cytokine storm, making infection with COVID-19 particularly dangerous for these at-risk subgroups of the population [7–11].

Accordingly, attention has focused on protecting these vulnerable individuals, as well as the general public, from infection. However, the lack of efficacious pharmacological treatments for COVID-19 has led the public to seek alternative therapies, including nutraceuticals [12,13]. Nutraceuticals are foods or substances derived from food that may have a physiological effect or protect against disease. They have received heightened interest as some may affect the severity of COVID-19. For example, several observational studies have been published describing the association between specific nutrient deficiencies and COVID-19 severity and mortality [14,15]. A review by Vassiliou et al., which examined the role of vitamin D status in predicting outcomes in critical illness, concluded that there is an association between insufficient vitamin D status and infection, severity of illness, and mortality from COVID-19 [16]. Another review by Lordan et al. found an association between zinc deficiency and increased COVID-19 complications [17]. In vivo studies have also pointed to the role of nutraceuticals in the treatment and prevention of COVID-19, including a study by Corrao et al., which demonstrated an inverse relationship between C-reactive protein (CRP), a marker of systemic inflammation, and supplementation with vitamin C, vitamin D, and zinc [18]. Furthermore, there have been several theoretical papers discussing the potential mechanistic roles of nutraceuticals and how they might target the SARS-CoV-2 virus [19–21]. For example, for probiotics, one of the proposed mechanisms is by acting as angiotensin-converting enzyme (ACE) inhibitors, preventing SARS-CoV-2 from binding to ACE receptors in gastrointestinal cells [22]. For the keto-carotenoid astaxanthin (a terpene), it has been suggested that it may play a role in regulating reactive oxygen species formation, and therefore, supplementation may inhibit oxidative stress caused by SARS-CoV-2 [23]. Additionally, immunomodulatory nutraceuticals, such as glycophosphopeptide AM3, may be beneficial as either prophylactic or adjuvant therapy for SARS-CoV-2, as they improve the efficacy of action of natural killer cells and increase the production of anti-inflammatory cytokines [24]. While the use of most of these nutraceuticals is advocated on the basis of in vitro and in vivo observations for other similar viruses (e.g., SARS-CoV and MERS-CoV), there is a growing number of observational studies and randomized controlled trials (RCTs) specifically for COVID-19 that point to the potential efficacy of nutraceuticals in the fight against this novel pathogen.

The potential use of nutraceuticals for the supportive treatment of COVID-19 is particularly relevant and promising for those who are more susceptible to both infection and a severe course of the disease. Patients with cancer, in particular, may be at high risk of severe disease and mortality from COVID-19 depending on their disease stage, treatment, and type of cancer [25]. Generally speaking, there are numerous mechanisms behind the increased risk of COVID-19 infection in these patients, including immunosuppression from cancer therapy and immunosuppression from cancer itself [26]. Chemotherapy, which limits the growth of cancer cells, also impacts the production of white blood cells, leaving patients more susceptible to infection [27]. Patients with late-stage cancer are also at increased risk of infection as bone metastases can trigger an immune response that leads to bone marrow aplasia, resulting in a reduction of white blood cells, red blood cells, and platelets, which again leaves these individuals vulnerable to worse outcomes if infected with COVID-19 [28]. Additionally, patients with cancer tend to be older and have more co-morbidities, putting them at risk of a severe course of disease with COVID-19 [26].

It is therefore not surprising that the COVID-19 pandemic also resulted in increased fear and worsened anxiety and depression associated with a cancer diagnosis [29]. As such, many individuals, immunocompromised and healthy alike, have sought out ways to improve immunity [30]. Concurrently, popular media outlets have promoted the use of a variety of dietary supplements with putative immune-boosting potential that may help against COVID-19 infection [31,32]. This has led to a major increase in dietary supplement use during the pandemic, with a roughly 35% increase in North and South America, a 40% increase in Asia, and a 38% increase in Europe [30,33]. Concerningly, only 40% of these individuals consume supplements at the recommendation of a licensed medical professional [30].

Increased supplement use during the COVID-19 pandemic, especially without appropriate medical supervision, is troubling for oncologists and other oncology specialists. Specifically, one concern relates to the potential dampening of the cytotoxicity of chemotherapy by antioxidants and other supplements. The Diet, Exercise, Lifestyle, and Cancer Prognosis (DELCaP) study, a correlative study to the phase III SWOG SO221 [34], examined supplement use in patients with breast cancer and survivorship. This study found that the use of any antioxidant supplements, before or during breast cancer treatment, was associated with an increased risk of breast cancer recurrence and that vitamin B12 use during treatment was associated with poorer survival rates and poorer disease-free survival [34]. Results such as these indicate that nutraceutical use during or around chemotherapy may not be benign.

Given the rise in oral supplement use during the COVID-19 pandemic, as well as the increased interest in the efficacy of nutraceuticals in preventing or reducing the severity of COVID-19, we conducted a narrative review focusing on the safety of the most efficacious "anti-COVID-19" oral supplements for patients with cancer. As COVID-19 is still a present threat, individuals with cancer and their providers need up-to-date, evidence-based guidance for supplement use around their respective treatments.

2. Methods

We conducted our initial literature search on 8 September 2021 focusing on the efficacy of nutraceuticals for the treatment and prevention of COVID-19. We performed the search in the PubMed database and included variations of the search terms "SARS-CoV-2" or "coronavirus" or "COVID-19" AND "supplement" or "phytonutrient" or "nutraceutical" AND "review." There were no restrictions on time period, language, or place of publication, and only review articles were included. This yielded 137 review articles after removing duplicates, from which titles and abstracts were reviewed. Sixty-seven articles were then removed for not pertaining to the research question and 25 for not being review articles, leaving 45 articles for full-text review and data extraction.

Our data extraction tool at this step focused on determining which nutraceuticals are most efficacious for the treatment or prevention of COVID-19 and included the name of the nutraceutical considered, the type of studies included in the review (e.g., in vitro, in vivo, animal or human studies), and the evidence for use against COVID-19.

For the purpose of our review, a nutraceutical was considered efficacious if our data extraction tool resulted in two or more reviews in favor of that nutraceutical's ingestion for COVID-19, either through food or supplement form, and no reviews indicating harm from use. Nutraceuticals for which there was only one review in favor were searched again in PubMed for original articles. If this secondary search yielded two or more original results in its favor, that nutraceutical was also included. This process resulted in the inclusion of the following nutraceuticals for review of the safety of single-nutrient supplements in patients with cancer: vitamin D, vitamin C, zinc, selenium, omega-3 fatty acids, and quercetin (see Supplementary Materials).

At the next step of the process, for each of the identified "anti-COVID-19" nutrients, we conducted a new PubMed search regarding safety for use in patients with cancer. The search was performed using the nutraceutical name (e.g., "vitamin D") AND "supplement" AND "cancer" AND "survivorship" or "safety" or "recurrence" or "disease progression" or "mortality" or "adverse events." Additional articles were sourced from a hand-search of related literature by the included authors. After duplicate removal, this yielded 470 articles in total across all included nutraceuticals for review.

3. Results

Out of 470 articles reviewed, 406 were excluded, leaving a total of 52 independent studies across all included nutraceuticals for data extraction (two of which included data for two nutraceuticals, resulting in a total of 54 records [35,36]). From those 52 studies, we extracted information about the authors, type of study, participants, cancer studied, nutraceutical dosing, and results. The search and selection process is graphically illustrated in Figure 1, and extracted information from the retrieved studies is shown in Tables 1–5.

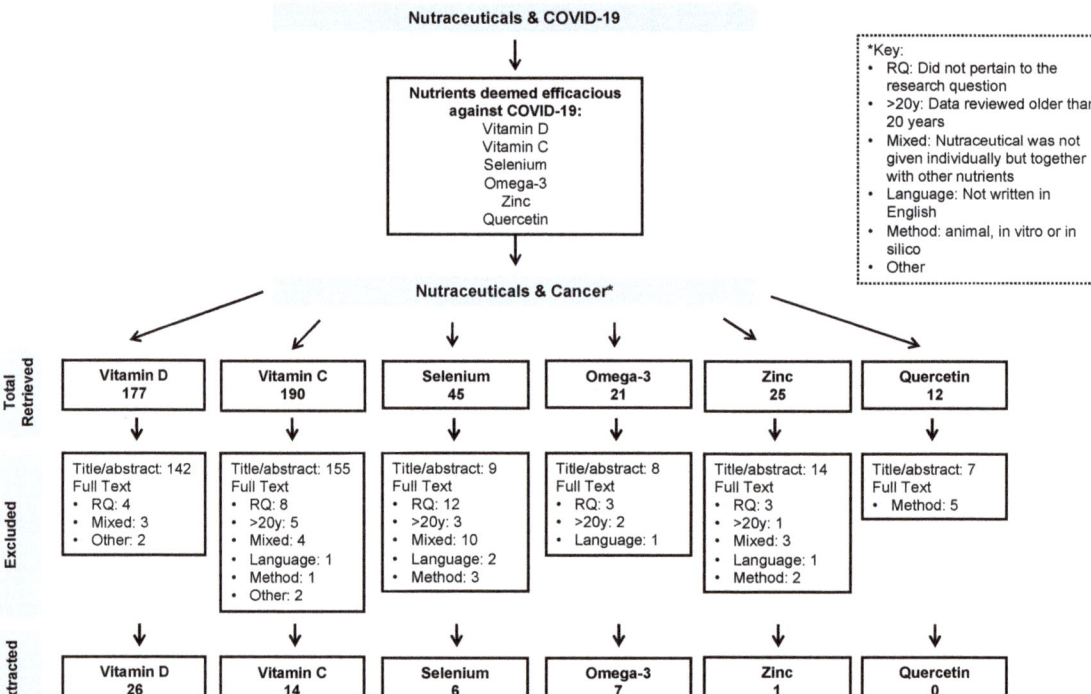

Figure 1. Search methodology and article selection process.

3.1. Vitamin D

A total of 177 unique articles were retrieved for vitamin D through our PubMed search. We reviewed titles and abstracts, resulting in 35 for full-text review. After a full-text review, 26 articles remained for data extraction (Table 1).

Of those 26 studies, 23 reported results that indicated benefit, no harm, or null effects of vitamin D supplementation for patients with cancer. Two of the studies reported results with a negative impact for patients with cancer, and one study reported mixed results.

In the studies that found that vitamin D supplements were either beneficial or not harmful for patients with cancer, nine found that supplementation had no effect on a variety of outcomes including symptom management, risk of death, and risk of recurrence [43,51,52,54,57–61].

Table 1. Safety of vitamin D supplements for patients with cancer.

Study	Type	Participants	Cancer	Dosage	Outcomes	Safety
Andersen et al., 2019 [37]	Observational	• n = 553 patients with breast cancer/survivors (193 from cohort saw naturopathic physicians specializing in oncology, 360 usual care cohort) • Age (mean ± SD) oncology cohort 53 ± 11 y; usual care cohort 55 ± 10 y • Female • BMI[1] not reported	• Breast cancer • All stages • Therapy: chemotherapy and/or radiation	• >50% reported taking <1000 IU daily	• Users reported ↑ physical function, role-physical function, social function, and role-emotional function on the SF-36 HRQOL[2] assessment subscales at baseline ($p < 0.05$) • At 6-month follow-up, users reported ↑ role-physical function, less pain, better general health, and ↑ vitality and social function ($p < 0.05$) • Users at 6-month follow-up reported ↑ social function and mental health when assessed at the 12-month follow-up ($p < 0.05$)	(+)
Bjelakovic et al., 2014 [38]	Cochrane review	• n = 50,623 • Age (range) 18–107 y • Male and female • BMI not reported	• All cancers • All stages • Therapy not specified	• Not reported	• Users had ↓ cancer mortality (RR = 0.88, 0.78–0.98, p = 0.02; 44,492 participants; 4 trials)	(+)
Campbell et al., 2021 [39]	Intervention	• n = 68 • Age (range) 59–67 y • Male • BMI not reported	• Prostate cancer • Stage 1 • Therapy not specified	• Dose titrated to achieve serum levels of 60 ng/mL • Administered periodically	• Participants with ↑ initial vitamin D levels were twice as likely to have ↓ prostate-specific antigen slope (OR = 2.04, 1.04–4.01, p = 0.04)	(+)
Chen et al., 2019 [40]	Prospective cohort study	• n = 30,899 • Age 20+ y • Male and female • n of non-users/users per BMI category, 4301/4401 (<25 kg/m²), 5119/4862 (25–30 kg/m²), 5483/4388 (≥30 kg/m²)	• All cancers • All stages • Therapy not specified	• Evaluated use as >10 mg/d from a 30-day questionnaire	• Users had ↑ risk of cancer mortality (RR = 2.11, 1.18–3.77)	(−)
Chlebowski et al., 2013 [41]	Literature review	• n ranged from 200 to >100 participants per study • Age not reported • Male and female • BMI not reported	• Breast cancer • All stages • Therapy: bisphosphonate, chemotherapy, aromatase inhibitor therapy, letrozole, zoledronic, or unspecified	• Varied based on study	• Prospective cohort studies showed no association between ↑ 25(OH)D[3] levels and ↓ breast cancer incidence • Studies of vitamin D and subsequent breast cancer recurrence were mixed • ↓ vitamin D levels associated with ↑ risk of recurrence in analyses not controlled for prognostic variables, cancer therapy, BMI, and physical activity • ↑ prevalence of ↓ vitamin D levels seen in early-stage breast cancer, but control population information is lacking • 1 RCT[4] did not demonstrate ↓ breast cancer incidence in postmenopausal women (1000 mg of calcium and 400 IU vitamin D3 daily in intervention group compared to placebo)	(+)
Chowdhury et al., 2014 [42]	Systematic review and meta-analysis	• n = 849,412 in observational studies • n = 30,716 in interventional • Age not reported • Male and female • BMI not reported	• All cancers • All stages • Therapy not specified	• Varied based on study	• Observational studies report associations of ↓ circulating 25(OH)D with ↑ risk of mortality from cancer	(+)

Table 1. *Cont.*

Study	Type	Participants	Cancer	Dosage	Outcomes	Safety
Cook et al., 2010 [43]	Meta-analysis	• Total *n* not reported • Age not reported • Sex not reported • BMI not reported	• Ovarian cancer • Stage not reported • Therapy not specified	• Varied based on study	• About half of the case-control studies reported ↓ mortality with ↑ latitude, solar radiation, or dietary intake or supplementation, and the rest had null associations • Cohort studies found no risk reduction with ↑ dietary intake or supplementation pre-diagnosis (note: vitamin D intakes were low in all studies)	(+)
Datta et al., 2012 [44]	Review	• Total *n* not reported • Age not reported • Sex not reported • BMI not reported	• Prostate cancer • All stages • Therapy: androgen deprivation therapy	• Varied based on study	• Clinical trial evidence does not show that supplementation with calcium and vitamin D prevents loss of bone mineral density during androgen deprivation therapy	(+)
Du et al., 2017 [45]	Review	• Total *n* not reported • Age not reported • Sex not reported • BMI not reported	• Gastric cancer • All stages • Therapy not specified	• Varied based on study	• Inconsistent results on efficacy • Vitamin D deficiency may ↑ the risk and mortality of gastric cancer	(+)
Grant et al., 2019 [46]	Review	• Total *n* not reported • Age not reported • Sex not reported • BMI not reported	• All cancers All stages • Therapy not specified	• Varied based on study	• Meta-analysis of 10 RCTs involving 45,197 participants found vitamin D use (variable dose and duration) was associated with 15% ↓ cancer mortality (RR = 0.85, 0.75–0.96) • Vitamin D deficiency may ↑ risk and mortality of gastric cancer • 1 RCT found women with a serum 25(OH)D concentration >40 ng/mL had 65% ↓ all-cancer incidence rate than women with values <20 ng/mL	(+)
Harvie et al., 2014 [47]	Review	• Total *n* not reported • Age not reported • Sex not reported • BMI not reported	• Prostate, hematologic cancers, melanoma, breast, colorectal, lung cancers • All stages • Therapy: 1 RCT in prostate cancer included docetaxel chemotherapy; therapy not reported in other trials	• Not reported	• 1 RCT showed positive results (longer survival time) in patients with advanced prostate cancer receiving docetaxel chemotherapy	(+)
Holm et al., 2014 [48]	Prospective cohort	• *n* = 1064 • Age not reported • Female • BMI (median) 24.7 kg/m²	• Breast cancer • Stage not reported • Therapy: hormone replacement therapy vs. no therapy pre-diagnosis	• Not reported	• Use was associated with ↑ breast cancer mortality (HR = 1.47, 1.07–2.00)	(−)
Kanellopoulou et al., 2021 [49]	Meta-analysis	• Total *n* not reported • Age not reported • Sex not reported • BMI not reported	• All cancers • All stages • Therapy not specified	• Not reported	• In breast cancer survivors, use ↓ risk of total mortality (RR = 0.85, 0.72–0.99)	(+)

Table 1. Cont.

Study	Type	Participants	Cancer	Dosage	Outcomes	Safety
Khan et al., 2017 [50]	RCT	• $n = 160$ • Age (range) 54–69 y • Female • Average group BMI (placebo/supplementation) was 29.6/29.9 kg/m^2, respectively	• Breast cancer • All stages • Therapy: chemotherapy and/or radiation	30,000 IU vitamin D3 weekly	• Scores for measures of pain intensity in BPI[5] were better in women randomized to vitamin D compared to placebo • Worsening of aromatase inhibitor-associated musculoskeletal symptoms observed in 71% of subjects randomized to placebo (plus the standard supplement of 600 IU of D3/day) vs. 40% of subjects randomized to high dose vitamin D3 plus the standard supplemental dose ($p < 0.001$) • Six months of oral vitamin D3 at 30,000 IU/week was safe in women starting an aromatase inhibitor for adjuvant treatment of breast cancer and is effective to ↑ serum 25(OH)D levels	(+)
Klapdor et al., 2012 [51]	Prospective cohort	• $n = 248$ ambulatory patients ($n = 103$ with pancreatic cancer) • Age not reported • Sex not reported • BMI not reported	• Pancreatic cancer • Stage not reported • Therapy: pancreatic enzyme drugs	• Vitamin D oral to ↑ serum levels to >30 ng/mL in group II and in the patients of group III in order to reach stable serum 25(OH)D concentrations in the normal range • Doses varied	• Oral vitamin D can be supplied without side-effects	(+)
Lewis et al., 2016 [52]	Prospective cohort	• $n = 453$ • Age (mean) 63.3 y • Male and female • BMI (mean) 28.7 kg/m^2	• Colorectal cancer • Stage II • Therapy: any	Not reported	• No association between vitamin D use and risk of recurrence or mortality • Beneficial association between use and functional assessment in colorectal cancer subscale of the FACT-C[6] ($p = 0.04$)	(+)
Madden et al., 2018 [53]	Longitudinal cohort	• $n = 5417$ • Age at diagnosis (range) 50–80 y • Female • BMI not reported	• Breast cancer • Stage I–III • Therapy: any	Categories of no use, 1–400 IU/day, and >400 IU/day	• 20% ↓ in breast cancer-specific mortality in de novo vitamin D users vs. non-users (HR = 0.80, $p = 0.048$) • 49% ↓ breast cancer-specific mortality if vitamin D initiated within 6 months of breast cancer diagnosis (HR = 0.51, $p < 0.001$)	(+)
Martinez et al., 2012 [54]	Review	• Total n not reported • Age not reported • Sex not reported • BMI not reported	• All cancers • Stage not reported • Therapy not specified	Not reported	• One RCT showed no effect of use on cancer mortality • One RCT showed no effect of use in breast or colorectal cancer incidence with vitamin D plus calcium • One RCT showed ↓ in total cancer incidence with vitamin D plus calcium vs. placebo	(+)

Table 1. *Cont.*

Study	Type	Participants	Cancer	Dosage	Outcomes	Safety
Morita et al., 2021 [55]	Post-hoc analysis of RCT	• $n = 396$ • Age (median) 66 y • Male and female • BMI (median) 21.9 kg/m^2	• Digestive tract • Stage I–III • Therapy: post-curative surgery with complete tumor resection	• 200 IU/day vs. placebo, until relapse or death	• In lowest PD-L1 [7] quintile, vitamin D upregulated serum PD-L1 levels ($p = 0.0008$); no change with placebo • In the highest quintile, vitamin D downregulated serum PD-L1 levels ($p = 0.0001$); no change with placebo • A significant effect of vitamin D on death, compared with placebo, only in the highest PD-L1 quintile (HR = 0.34, 0.12–0.92); not observed in other quintiles • Significant effect of vitamin D on death or relapse, compared with placebo, only in the highest PD-L1 quintile (HR = 0.37, 0.15–0.89)	(+/−)
Mulpur et al., 2015 [56]	Cohort	• $n = 470$ • Age (median) 59 y • Male and female • BMI not reported	• Glioblastoma • High grade • Therapy: standard of care treatment involving surgery, chemotherapy, and radiation therapy	• Not reported	• Vitamin D use associated with ↓ age-adjusted mortality (HR = 0.68, $p = 0.019$) and after multivariate adjustment (HR = 0.72, $p = 0.043$) • Results for vitamin D attenuated when the reference category confined to non-alternative medicine users in a multivariate model	(+)
Poole et al., 2013 [35]	Cohort	• $n = 12,019$ • Age (mean) 56.8 y • Female • Frequency of BMI < 25 kg/m^2, 25–30 kg/m^2, and ≥30 kg/m^2 was roughly 50%, 30%, and 20%, respectively	• Breast cancer • Excluded in situ or stage IV • Therapy: varied—chemotherapy, radiation, or hormone therapy present in cohort	• Not reported	• Vitamin D use was associated with ↓ risk of recurrence in ER+ [8] (HR = 0.64) but not in ER− tumors (HR = 1.25) • Stratified by joint ER/PR status, vitamin D was only associated with ↓ risk of recurrence in ER+/PR+ [9] and ER+/PR− tumors, but not ER−/PR+ or ER−/PR− tumors ($p = 0.002$ for interaction)	(+)
Saquib et al., 2011 [57]	Cohort derived from RCT	• $n = 3081$ • Age (mean) 53 y • Female • 24% of users and 36% of non-users had obesity	• Breast cancer • Operable invasive stage I (≥1 cm), II, or IIIA • Therapy: none (study done in survivors)	• 6 µg/day total intake of vitamin D in those who took supplements	• No significant findings related to all-cause mortality	(+)
Sarre et al., 2016 [58]	Cohort from men participating in the third round of the FinRSPC [10] randomized screening study	• $n = 12,740$ • Ages: 63, 67, or 71 y • Males • BMI not reported	• Prostate cancer • Stage not reported • Therapy not specified	• Not reported	• Vitamin D use had no association with prostate cancer incidence, high-grade/metastatic cancers, or death	(+)
Wang et al., 2016 [59]	Longitudinal observational	• $n = 303$ • Age of users and non-users (means) 62 and 65 y, respectively • Predominately male • BMI (mean) 21 kg/m^2	• Esophageal cancer • Roughly 65% stage 0/I/II, 35% stage III/IV, 44% with lymph node involvement • Therapy: esophagectomy and some with postoperative chemotherapy and/or radiotherapy	• 200–400 IU/day for 1 year	• Associations between use and QOL [11], including global health, physical functioning, social functioning, fatigue, and appetite loss measured by QLQ-C30 [12] • Users more likely to have improved disease-free survival ($p = 0.030$) • No association of use with overall survival	(+)

Table 1. *Cont.*

Study	Type	Participants	Cancer	Dosage	Outcomes	Safety
Zhang et al., 2019 [60]	Meta-analysis of RCTs	• $n = 77,653$ from 9 studies • Age (range) 20–84 y • Male and female • BMI not reported	• All cancers • Staging not reported • Therapy not specified	Varied across 9 studies	• No significant effect on cancer incidence or mortality	(+)
Zirpoli et al., 2017 [61]	Cohort	• $n = 922$ • Age not reported • Female • BMI not reported	• Breast cancer • Stage I-III breast cancer (node-positive (pN1-3) • Any primary tumor ≥ 2 cm, or any tumor ≥ 1 cm if estrogen receptor negative/progesterone receptor negative or hormone receptor positive with 21-gene recurrence score ≥ 26 • Therapy: paclitaxel (1/week for 12 weeks or every other week)	Not reported	• No improvement in peripheral neuropathy Fact-NTX[13] or CTCAE[14] scores	(+)

Abbreviations used: [1] Body Mass Index, [2] Short Form Health-Related Quality of Life, [3] 25-hydroxy vitamin D, [4] Randomized Controlled Trial, [5] Brief Pain Index, [6] Functional Assessment of Cancer Therapy—Colorectal, [7] Programed death ligand 1, [8] Estrogen Receptor, [9] Progesterone Receptor, [10] Finnish Randomized Study for Screening of Prostate Cancer, [11] Quality of Life, [12] Quality of Life Questionnaire-Core Questionnaire, [13] Functional Assessment of Cancer Therapy-Neurotoxicity, [14] Common Terminology Criteria for Adverse Events. The last column indicates the overall direction of the effects of vitamin D supplementation on safety: (+) no risks to health; (−) some risks to health outcomes; (+/−) mixed risk profile. Relative risks (RR) and odds/hazard ratios (OR/HR) are shown as means with 95% confidence intervals.

Table 2. Safety of vitamin C supplements for patients with cancer.

Study	Type	Participants	Cancer	Dosage	Outcomes	Safety
Ambrosone et al., 2020 [34]	Correlative analysis from SWOG S0221	• $n = 1134$ • Age (mean) progression free 50.9 y • Age (mean) with progression 52.8 y • Female • BMI [1] (mean) progression free 29.1 kg/m^2 • BMI (mean) with progression 30.1 kg/m^2	• Breast cancer • Stage not available, most node negative • Randomized to treatment of cyclophosphamide, doxorubicin, and paclitaxel	• Not reported	• No association with use of vitamin C before and during treatment and recurrence (HR = 1.36, 0.87–2.13) • No association with vitamin C and overall survival	(+)
Bjelakovic et al., 2008 [62]	Systematic review	• n not reported • Age not reported • Male and female • BMI not reported	• Gastrointestinal cancer • Stage not reported • Therapy not specified	• Dose ranged 120–2000 mg/day depending on the trial	• Vitamin C supplement use (RR = 0.97, 0.77–1.23) did not influence mortality • Combination vitamin C with beta-carotene, vitamin E, and selenium did not influence mortality compared to placebo	(+)
Greenlee et al., 2012 [63]	Cohort	• $n = 2264$ • Age (range) 18–79 y • Female • BMI not reported • Majority had BMI < 25 kg/m^2	• Breast cancer • Stage I–IIIA • Therapy completed	• Categories of no use, occasional use (<1–5 days/week), and frequent use (6–7 days/week) • No details on dose	• Frequent use of vitamin C associated with ↓ risk of breast cancer recurrence (HR = 0.73, 0.55–0.97)	(+)
Harris et al., 2013 [64]	Cohort	• $n = 3405$ • Age (mean) at dx^2 = 65 y • Female • Mean BMI = 25 kg/m^2	• Breast cancer • All stages • All therapies	• ≈1000 mg/day	• No association between vitamin C supplement use and breast cancer-specific mortality (HR = 1.06, 0.52–2.17)	(+)
Harris et al., 2014 [65]	Meta-analysis	• n not reported • Age not reported • Female • BMI not reported	• Breast cancer • Stage not reported • All therapies	• Various	• Post-diagnosis usage reduced breast cancer-specific mortality (RR = 0.85, 0.74–0.99)	(+)
Jacobs et al., 2002 [66]	Cohort	• $n = 942,993$ • Age 30+ y • Male and female • BMI not reported	• Stomach cancer • Stage not reported • Therapy not specified	• Not reported	• Regular vitamin C use tended to ↓ risk of stomach cancer mortality (RR = 0.83, 0.68–1.01) • ↓ risk only in participants using vitamin C for a relatively short duration of time (RR = 0.68, 0.51–0.91 for <10 years use; RR = 1.00 0.73–1.38 for ≥10 years use)	(+)
Jacobs et al., 2002 [67]	Cohort	• $n = 991,552$ • Age not reported • Male and female • BMI not reported	• Bladder cancer • Stage not reported • All therapies	• Not reported	• Regular vitamin C supplement use (≥15 times per month) not associated with bladder cancer mortality	(+)
Kanellopoulo et al., 2020 [49]	Meta-analysis	• n not reported • Age 18+ y • Male and female • BMI not reported	• All cancers • Stage 0–IV • All therapies	• Not reported	• In breast cancer survivors, vitamin C supplement use associated with ↓ total mortality • Vitamin C supplement use associated with ↓ breast cancer recurrence (RR = 0.76)	(+)

Table 2. Cont.

Study	Type	Participants	Cancer	Dosage	Outcomes	Safety
Lin et al., 2009 [68]	RCT[3]	• $n = 7627$ • Age (mean) 60.4 y • Female • BMI (mean) 30 kg/m² in Vitamin C group	• Any cancer • No dx at baseline • Therapy: none	500 mg/day	• No effects of use of any antioxidant on cancer incidence. • Vitamin C vs. placebo, no difference in mortality	(+)
Messerer et al., 2008 [69]	Cohort	• $n = 38,994$ • Age (range) 45–79 y • Male • BMI not reported	• All cancers • No cancer at baseline • Therapy: none	Estimated 1000 mg/day	• No association between use of any dietary supplementation and all-cause mortality, cancer, or CVD[4] mortality	(+)
Nechuta et al., 2011 [70]	Cohort	• $n = 4877$ • Age (range) 20–75 y • Female • BMI not reported	• Breast cancer • Stage I–IV • All therapies	Majority consumed <400 mg/day supplement	• Use of vitamin C for >3 months had a 44% ↓ in risk of mortality and 38% ↓ in risk of recurrence	(+)
Pocobelli et al., 2009 [71]	Cohort	• $n = 77,719$ • Age 50–76 y • Male and female • BMI not reported	• All cancers • All stages • Therapy not specified	Varied	• Vitamin C use associated with ↓ risk of cancer mortality, but no dose-response trend	(+)
Poole et al., 2013 [35]	Cohort	• $n = 12,019$ • Age (mean) 56.8 y • Female • Frequency of BMI was roughly 50% <25 kg/m², 30% 25–29.9 kg/m², 20% above 30 kg/m²	• Breast cancer • Excluded in situ or stage IV • Therapy: varied—chemotherapy, radiation, or hormone therapy	Not reported	• Vitamin C use associated with ↓ risk of death (RR = 0.81) • Use of antioxidant supplements (multivitamins, vitamin C or E) not associated with recurrence	(+)
Zirpoli et al., 2017 [61]	Cohort	• $n = 922$ • Age not reported • Female • BMI not reported	• Breast cancer • Stage I–III (node-positive (pN1–3) • Any primary tumor ≥ 2 cm, or any tumor ≥ 1 cm estrogen receptor negative/progesterone receptor negative or hormone receptor positive with 21-gene recurrence score ≥ 26) • Therapy-Paclitaxel (1x/week for 12 weeks or every other week)	Not reported	• Use of vitamin C, folic acid, calcium, iron, or fish oil before diagnosis was not associated with CTCAE[5] grade 3 or 4 neurotoxicity	(+)

Abbreviations used: [1] Body Mass Index, [2] diagnosis, [3] Randomized Control Trial, [4] Cardiovascular disease, [5] Common Terminology Criteria for Adverse Events. The last column indicates the overall direction of the effects of vitamin C supplementation on safety: (+) no risks to health; (−) some risks to health outcomes; (+/−) mixed risk profile. Relative risks (RR) and odds/hazard ratios (OR/HR) are shown as means with 95% confidence intervals.

Table 3. Safety of selenium supplements for patients with cancer.

Study	Type	Participants	Cancer	Dosage	Outcomes	Safety
Bjelakovic et al., 2008 [62]	Systematic review of RCTs [1]	• n = 211,818 participants total in 20 RCTs • Age (mean) 56.5 y (range 15–84 y) • Male (59%) and female • BMI [2] not reported	• Gastrointestinal cancer • All stages • Therapy not specified	Not reported	• Selenium use (singly or with other antioxidants) significantly ↓ mortality (RR = 0.90, 0.83–0.98), effect attenuated when high-risk trials excluded	(+)
Jenkins et al., 2020 [72]	Systematic review/meta-analysis of RCTs	• n not reported • Age not reported • Male and female • BMI not reported	• All cancers • All stages (and mortality) • Therapy not specified	Not reported	• Selenium supplement use, singly or with other antioxidants, was not associated with cancer incidence or cancer mortality	(+)
Jiang L et al., 2010 [73]	Meta-analysis of RCTs	• n = 165,056 participants across 9 RCTs • Age not reported • Male • BMI not reported	• Prostate cancer • All stages • Therapy not specified	Not reported	• Mortality among patients with prostate cancer did not significantly differ by selenium supplementation (RR = 2.98, 0.12–73.2) • Incidence/mortality of prostate cancer did not ↓ with selenium supplement intake	(+)
Kenfield et al., 2015 [74]	Prospective cohort study	• n = 4459 • Age (mean) 68.9 +/− 7.2 y at diagnosis • Male • BMI (mean) 25.8 kg/m²	• Prostate cancer • Not metastatic at diagnosis • Therapy: radical prostatectomy, EBRT [3] or brachytherapy, hormones, watchful waiting, or other	1–24 µg/day, 25–139 µg/day or 140+ µg/day of selenium supplement	• No ↑ risk of prostate cancer mortality in 1–24 µg/day and 25–139 µg/day selenium supplementation • ↑ risk of prostate cancer mortality in 140+ µg/day selenium supplementation (RR = 2.60, 1.44–4.70) vs. those not taking supplement	(+/−)
Muecke R et al., 2010 [75]	RCT	• n = 81 • Age (mean) 64.3 ± 10.1 y; (range) 31–80 • Female • BMI not reported	• Cervical and uterine cancer • All stages • Therapy: radiation therapy	• Radiation therapy days = 500 µg of selenium • Other days = 300 µg of selenium • 17 mg of sodium selenite given cumulatively over average treatment period of 38 days	• In 10 years of follow-up, no difference in disease-free survival between selenium group and control (p = 0.65) • No difference in 10-year overall survival rate in selenium group vs. control (p = 0.09)	(+)
Samuels et al., 2014 [76]	Review	• Total n not reported • Age not reported • Sex not reported • BMI not reported	• Breast cancer • All stages • Therapy in 1 RCT: standard combined decongestion therapy	• 1 RCT— 1st week = 1000 µg/d, 2nd week = 300 µg/d, final weeks = 100 µg/d for 3 total months • 1 cohort = 350 µg/m² daily for 4–6 weeks	• 1 RCT: 179 post-mastectomy patients with secondary lymphoedema. Selenium supplement use ↓ in edema volumes • 1 cohort: 48 patients with post-radiation lymphoedema (12 patients also had breast cancer). 83.3% of those with cancer had ↓ in edema with supplementation	(+)

Abbreviations used: [1] Randomized Controlled Trial, [2] Body Mass Index, [3] External Beam Radiation Therapy. The last column indicates the overall direction of the effects of selenium supplementation on safety: (+) no risks to health; (−) some risks to health outcomes; (+/−) mixed risk profile. Relative risks (RR) and odds/hazard ratios (OR/HR) are shown as means with 95% confidence intervals.

Table 4. Safety of omega-3 fatty acid supplements for patients with cancer.

Study	Type	Participants	Cancer	Dosage	Outcomes	Safety
Campbell et al., 2021 [39]	Intervention	• $n = 68$ • Age (range) 59.3–66.9 y • Male • BMI[1] not reported	• Prostate cancer • Stage 1 (very low or low risk) • Therapy not specified	• 720 mg (3/day)	• Relationship between prostate-specific antigen slope and initial total omega-3 levels were not statistically significant ($r = 0.05$; $p = 0.792$) • Similarly not significant for initial omega-6:3 ratio ($r = -0.1$; $p = 0.95$), final omega-3 levels ($r = 0.16$; $p = 0.531$), and final omega-6:3 ratio ($r = -0.28$; $p = 0.282$) • Study cohort had no pathologic or clinical progression and no serious side effects from omega-3 supplement use	(+)
Klassen et al., 2020 [77]	Review article	• $n = 140$ participants across studies • Age not reported • Male and female • BMI not reported	• Breast and gastrointestinal cancers • All stages • Therapy: chemotherapy or otherwise not specified	• Varied across studies	• All study results support safety/tolerability of omega-3 supplement during chemotherapy • Evidence supporting benefits for omega-3 supplement in breast and gastrointestinal cancer is weak	(+)
Miyata et al., 2017 [78]	RCT[2]	• $n = 61$ patients • Age (range) 56.1–72.7 y • 52 male, 9 female • BMI: Omega-3 group (mean) 21.8 +/− 10 kg/m^2, placebo group (mean) 20.8 +/− 7.1 kg/m^2	• Esophageal cancer • All stages • Therapy: neoadjuvant chemotherapy	• 900 mg/day omega-3 in intervention group and 250 mg/day in comparison group • Both groups had enteral nutrition supplement provided 3 days before initiation of chemotherapy to day 12 of chemotherapy	• No difference in incidence of grade 3/4 neutropenia between both groups (77.4% in intervention vs. 83.3% in comparison $p = 0.561$) or frequency (93.5 in intervention vs. 86% in comparison, $p = 0.363$) • Omega-3 enteral nutrition support ↓ frequency of chemotherapy-induced mucosal toxicities and prevented increase in the aspartate amino transferase and alanine amino transferase levels	(+)
Mulpur et al., 2015 [56]	Longitudinal cohort	• $n = 106$ • Age (range) 18–84 y • Male and female • BMI not reported	• Glioblastoma • All stages • Therapy: surgery, chemotherapy, radiation	• Not reported	• No effect of omega-3 supplementation on mortality	(+)
Shen et al., 2018 [79]	Exploratory analysis of RCT	• $n = 249$ • Age (median) 59 y • Females • 56% = BMI < 30 • 44% = BMI ≥ 30	• Breast cancer • Stages I–III • Therapy: Aromatase-inhibitor therapy	• 3.3 g/day (560 mg EPA[3] plus DHA[4] acid in a 40:20 ratio) omega-3 in intervention group and placebo (soybean-corn oil blend) in comparison group for 24 weeks	• Omega-3 supplement use associated with ↓ BPI[5] worst pain scores vs. placebo (4.36 vs. 5.70, $p = 0.02$) in patients with obesity • No difference in scores between treatment arms (5.27 vs. 4.58, $p = 0.28$; $p = 0.05$) in patients who weren't obese • Omega-3 supplement use in patients with obesity was associated with ↓ BPI average pain and pain interference scores vs. placebo ($p = 0.005$)	(+)
Sorensen et al., 2020 [80]	RCT	• $n = 148$ • Age (mean) 68.3 +/− 11.3 y • Males and female • BMI not reported	• Colorectal cancer • All stages • Therapy: surgery	• Intervention group, 2.0 g EPA and 1.0 g DHA per day • No EPA/DHA for control group	• No difference in 5-year survival for intervention group vs. control ($p = 0.193$) • Adjusted for age/disease stage/therapy, omega-3 supplement associated with ↑ mortality (HR = 1.73, 1.06–2.83; $p = 0.029$)	(−)

Table 4. *Cont.*

Study	Type	Participants	Cancer	Dosage	Outcomes	Safety
Vernieri et al., 2018 [81]	Review	• Total n not reported • Age not reported • Male and female • BMI not reported	• All cancers • All stages • Therapy not specified	• Not reported	• Omega-3 supplement was tolerable with antitumor activity in 2 prospective trials for patients with advanced lung and breast cancer • Preclinical study reported that the 16:4 (n-3) omega-3 in commercial fish oils impedes tumor-directed cytotoxicity of platinum compounds. Warns against indiscriminate fish oil supplementation	(+/−)

Abbreviations used: [1] Body Mass Index, [2] Randomized Controlled Trial, [3] Eicosapentanoic acid, [4] Docosahaxaenoic acid, [5] Brief Pain Inventory. The last column indicates the overall direction of the effects of Omega-3 supplementation on safety: (+) no risks to health; (−) some risks to health outcomes; (+/−) mixed risk profile. Relative risks (RR) and odds/hazard ratios (OR/HR) are shown as means with 95% confidence intervals.

Table 5. Safety of zinc supplements for patients with cancer.

Study	Type	Participants	Cancer	Dosage	Outcomes	Safety
De Sousa Melo et al., 2021 [82]	Narrative review	• n not reported • Age not indicated • Male and female • BMI[1] not reported	• Head and neck cancer • All stages • Therapy: various	• Varied	• Zinc sulfate supplementation ↓ severity of mucositis, delayed its onset • 25 mg/day ↓ incidence and duration of oral mucositis • May induce nausea and vomiting, should not be taken on empty stomach	(+/−)

Abbreviations used: [1] Body Mass Index. The last column indicates the overall direction of the effects of Zinc supplementation on safety: (+) no risks to health; (−) some risks to health outcomes; (+/−) mixed risk profile. Relative risks (RR) and odds/hazard ratios (OR/HR) are shown as means with 95% confidence intervals.

Three of the studies found that vitamin D was associated with better quality-of-life outcomes, including better scores on the cancer quality-of-life questionnaire (QLQ-C30) for physical functioning, social functioning, fatigue, and appetite, and better scores on the colorectal cancer subscale of the Functional Assessment of Cancer Therapy-Colorectal (FACT-C) tool [37,52,59]. Beyond quality-of-life measures, four studies reported a decrease in cancer mortality in those who took vitamin D supplements, and two showed a decrease in overall mortality [38,43,46,49,53,56]. One study found a lower risk of breast cancer recurrence in those who were supplemented with vitamin D post-diagnosis, but only among estrogen receptor (ER)-positive tumors and not among ER-negative tumors (HR = 0.64, 95% CI: 0.47–0.87 and HR = 1.25, 95% CI: 0.78–1.98; respectively) [35].

In the two studies that found vitamin D supplementation was harmful in patients with cancer, one found a positive association between vitamin D supplement use above 10 μg/day and cancer mortality (RR = 2.11, 95% CI: 1.18–3.77) [40], and the other found that vitamin D supplementation increased the risk of breast cancer mortality (HR = 1.47, 95% CI: 1.07–2.00) [48].

One RCT found mixed results for vitamin D supplementation with 200 IU/day in patients with digestive-tract cancer, post-curative surgery [55]. The study found that the effect of supplementation depended on the levels of serum Programmed Death Ligand 1 (PD-L1), a regulatory molecule expressed in T cells with immunosuppressive function [55]. Since PD-L1 is associated with a poorer cancer prognosis in various types of cancer (gastric cancer, small cell lung cancer, pancreatic cancer, breast cancer) [83–86], for those patients in the lowest PD-L1 concentration quintile, vitamin D supplementation seemed to have a detrimental effect by upregulating serum PD-L1 levels; however, for those in the highest quintile, vitamin D was beneficial and downregulated serum PD-L1 levels [55,87].

3.2. Vitamin C

A total of 190 unique articles were retrieved for vitamin C through our PubMed search. We reviewed titles and abstracts, resulting in 35 for full-text review. After a full-text review, 14 articles remained for data extraction (Table 2).

Of those 14 studies, all provided results in the direction of benefit, no harm, or null effects of vitamin C supplementation in patients with cancer. Six of the fourteen studies found no association between the use of vitamin C supplements and adverse cancer-related events, including recurrence, survival, overall mortality, and cancer-specific mortality [34,62,64,67–69]. Additionally, a study on chemotherapy-induced peripheral neuropathy found no significant effect of pre-treatment vitamin C supplementation on neurotoxicity [61]. Three studies found that vitamin C intake was associated with decreased overall mortality, three found a decreased risk of cancer-specific mortality, and three found a decreased risk of recurrence [35,63,65,66,70,71]. None of the studies reported an increased risk to health from the use of vitamin C supplements.

3.3. Selenium

A total of 45 unique articles were retrieved for selenium through our PubMed search. We reviewed titles and abstracts, resulting in 28 for full-text review. After a full-text review, six articles remained for data extraction (Table 3).

Five of these six papers showed no harmful effects of selenium supplementation in patients with cancer and included two meta-analyses [72,73], two reviews [62,76], and one RCT [75]. Three articles did not find a beneficial effect on the incidence or progression of gastrointestinal cancer [62], prostate cancer [73], or cervical and uterine cancer [75], but found selenium supplementation was not otherwise harmful. Beneficial effects were highlighted in a review that addressed an association between selenium supplementation and decreased edema volumes and incidence of skin infection in patients with breast cancer in an RCT of 179 post-mastectomy patients with secondary lymphedema, as well as decreased edema volumes in 10 out of 12 patients with breast cancer included in a 48-participant cohort study [76].

A meta-analysis of RCTs by Jenkins et al. concluded that selenium taken independently (i.e., not as a multivitamin or mixed with other supplements) was not associated with cancer mortality [72]. However, a prospective cohort study within the review found that high-dose selenium supplementation (≥ 140 μg/day) may be associated with a greater risk of prostate cancer mortality [72].

3.4. Omega-3 Fatty Acids

A total of 21 unique articles were retrieved for omega-3 fatty acids through our search. We reviewed titles and abstracts, resulting in 17 for full-text review. After a full-text review, seven articles remained for data extraction (Table 4).

In five of these seven studies, there were no adverse effects of supplementation. One study found that supplementation with omega-3 fatty acids decreased aromatase-inhibitor-related pain in patients with breast cancer and obesity [79]. Additionally, omega-3 supplementation showed promising antitumor activity in two prospective trials of patients with advanced lung and breast cancer, as reviewed by Vernieri et al. [81]. The same review, however, highlighted a pre-clinical study that reported that the 16:4 omega-3 (hexadeca-4,7,10,13-tetraenoic) fatty acid supplement, commonly found in commercial fish oils, may be unsafe for patients with cancer as it can hinder tumor-directed cytotoxicity of platinum compounds used in cancer treatments [81].

Furthermore, an RCT pointed towards an increased mortality rate 5 years after patients with colorectal cancer (from a country with traditionally high fish intake) took omega-3 supplements in the 7 days before and after colorectal resection surgery [80].

3.5. Zinc

A total of 25 unique articles were retrieved for zinc through our PubMed search. We reviewed titles and abstracts, resulting in 11 for full-text review. After a full-text review, only one article remained for data extraction (Table 5).

The study found that zinc supplementation reduced the duration and severity of oral mucositis in patients with head and neck cancer but sometimes caused gastrointestinal distress, which suggests that zinc supplements should not be taken on an empty stomach [88].

3.6. Quercetin

A total of 12 unique articles were retrieved for quercetin through our PubMed search. We reviewed titles and abstracts, resulting in five for full-text review. After a full-text review, one was removed for being conducted in animals, and the remaining four were review articles that did not include human studies; therefore, no articles qualified for further consideration.

4. Discussion

This narrative review aimed to synthesize the currently available literature regarding the safety of the most efficacious "anti-COVID-19" nutraceuticals for patients with cancer. Our findings reveal heterogeneous results, with safety largely depending on the type of nutraceutical or supplement consumed, the dose consumed, and the type of cancer studied. Across nutraceuticals, our results were heavily based on observational studies. Taking the potential risk of confounding into consideration, clear conclusions could not be drawn, further emphasizing the need for caution from healthcare providers.

Vitamin D may decrease CRP, which has been implicated in the cytokine storm seen in severe cases of COVID-19 infection [18]. We identified an overwhelming majority of studies with results that point in favor of vitamin D use in patients with cancer, with positive effects seen in quality-of-life measures, mortality, recurrence, and pain indexes. However, the mechanism between vitamin D and these positive cancer-related outcomes was not always well characterized. Anderson et al. documented improved quality-of-life measures in an observational cohort of patients with breast cancer, but ultimately noted that it was unclear whether the supplement itself was responsible or whether participants who took vitamin D were in general more optimistic or more likely to take other actions towards improving their overall health and mood [37]. Similarly, Bjelakovic et al. reported decreased cancer mortality from vitamin D3 supplementation (RR = 0.88, 95% CI: 0.78–0.98) but noted the lack of RCTs made it hard to draw robust conclusions [38].

Only two studies point to an increased risk of vitamin D intake in patients with cancer; one noted this was observed only among those who were not deficient in vitamin D [40], and the other noted that the association of vitamin D supplementation with higher breast cancer mortality needed further exploration, as there was no clear mechanism behind this observation [48]. Given that the majority of evidence is in support of vitamin D use, oncologists can likely safely allow their patients to continue supplementation at typically recommended doses (600 IU/day).

Vitamin C, similar to vitamin D, may contribute to a decrease in the pro-inflammatory cytokines, which are a hallmark of severe COVID-19 infection [18]. The evidence for vitamin C also strongly points in the direction of supplementation being safe, or perhaps even beneficial, for patients with cancer. In fact, none of the included articles found an indication of harm. Given that there has been concern that the use of antioxidants, including vitamin C, may negatively impact the effect of chemotherapeutic agents, these results are encouraging [70]. Nevertheless, we urge caution as the studies are, by and large, observational in nature, which stresses the need for additional clinical trials [49]. At the present state of knowledge, supplementation with vitamin C at typically recommended doses (75–90 mg/day) is likely not harmful and could conceivably confer benefit.

Selenium may reduce the severity of COVID-19 infection by impeding viral entry into the cytoplasm and has promising results in patients with cancer [89]. All but one out of six studies addressing selenium supplementation demonstrated no adverse effects in patients with cancer. However, the type of cancer (i.e., prostate, uterine, cervical, gastrointestinal) and outcome of interest varied greatly across studies. One prospective cohort study in patients with prostate cancer noted that selenium supplementation might be associated with a higher risk of mortality if intake is high ($\geq$140 µg/day) [72]. Given these results, it is likely that selenium use is safe for patients with cancer, though high-dose supplementation should be avoided (typically recommended doses: 40–70 mg/day).

Omega-3 fatty acids may play a role in decreasing the severity of COVID-19 infection by inhibiting cellular viral entry, suppressing the production of pro-inflammatory cytokines, and increasing the phagocytic capacity of the innate immune system [20]. Out of seven identified articles for omega-3 fatty acids, five found their use to be safe, though estimates of efficacy varied [39,77]. The seven articles addressed safety in a variety of different cancers, including skin cancer, prostate cancer, gastrointestinal cancer, breast cancer, esophageal cancer, glioblastoma, and colorectal cancer. Two studies evaluated the long-term effects of supplementation with omega-3 fatty acids. The first, a longitudinal cohort study, did not find an association between mortality and supplementation in glioblastoma patients [56]. In contrast, the other, an RCT, pointed towards an increased mortality rate after five years of intake in patients with colorectal cancer who supplemented one week before and one week after colorectal resection surgery [80]. Additionally, one review specifically warned against the indiscriminate use of fish oil supplements, which may be unsafe for patients with cancer if they contain hexadeca-4,7,10,13-tetraenoic acid; this omega-3 fatty acid can dampen the tumor-directed cytotoxicity of platinum compounds used to treat some cancers [81]. Based on this evidence, caution should be used as far as omega-3 fatty acid supplements are concerned. At the very least, scrutiny of the exact fatty acid composition of the supplement together with frequent patient monitoring is warranted.

For zinc, which may counteract inflammation associated with tumor necrosis factor-α in COVID-19 infection [90], results did not universally show harm-free supplementation. Although one study indicated a reduced incidence of oral mucositis with supplementation in patients with head and neck cancer, the same study also cited potential gastrointestinal distress at the same dosage [88]. Given the lack of a sufficiently large body of evidence on this nutraceutical, with only one study being relevant, it is hard to draw any conclusions. That said, at present, it is probably prudent to advise patients with cancer against supplementation with zinc.

While this review thoroughly and systematically assessed the literature regarding the safety of these supplements for patients with cancer, our conclusions are not without limitations. The heterogeneity of results may in part be due to our inclusion of all stages and types of cancer, as well as our inclusion of all treatment types and clinical settings. It is possible that a narrower scope would have revealed more homogenous results due to the vast differences in the biology of various cancers. However, at the current state of knowledge, there is not enough information for a cancer type-specific assessment. Additionally, our review did not consider in detail possible toxicity issues resulting from supra-supplementation but rather evaluated safety at typically recommended doses. Lastly, due to the relatively recent onset of the COVID-19 pandemic, there are limited clinical trials on the efficacy of nutraceuticals for SARS-CoV-2. As a result, data on only a limited number of nutraceuticals could be identified. As more research becomes available, it is possible that more nutraceuticals will be deemed efficacious, and an updated safety review may become necessary.

5. Conclusions

Patients with cancer are one of several co-morbid populations who are at increased risk of a severe course of disease if infected with COVID-19. While a number of nutraceuticals have attracted interest due to their potential "anti-COVID-19" activity, there is concern about the safety of their usage in patients with cancer due to the potential interactions with their treatment regimen and possible associations with an increased risk of recurrence, cancer incidence, or even death.

This review highlights the heterogeneity of results regarding the safety of nutraceuticals for patients with cancer. It is conceivable that a large part of this heterogeneity is due to different types and stages of cancer, different treatments, and different clinical settings among the identified studies. Our findings indicate that vitamin D, vitamin C, and selenium supplementation are likely safe at normal doses (i.e., the dosages typically recommended for the general population). However, caution should be used with omega-3 fatty acid supplementation due to a conflict in the results between two long-term studies and a paucity of data overall. Similarly, zinc supplementation should probably be avoided due to a lack of relevant studies and because the currently available evidence indicates potential for harm or discomfort in patients with cancer.

Overall, this work emphasizes a sizeable gap in the literature surrounding the safety of nutraceuticals in patients with cancer and underscores the potential danger of liberal use of supplements by this high-risk group. Furthermore, this review provides important and immediately relevant clinical guidance for cancer care practitioners during an ongoing public health crisis. It is important to note that any supplement intake by patients with cancer should be discussed with their healthcare team so their providers may more accurately monitor their health and assess potential risks. Lastly, though early evidence indicates a potential benefit of some nutraceuticals against COVID-19, and thus potentially to high-risk cancer populations, we do not recommend supplementation as a substitute for regular medical care and a balanced diet.

Supplementary Materials: The following are available online at https://www.mdpi.com/article/10.3390/cancers13236094/s1, Table S1. References supporting nutraceutical use against COVID-19.

Author Contributions: K.S.B.-L. and E.A.L. contributed equally to the work reported. They were both involved in study conceptualization, data extraction, analysis, methodology, visualization, and writing the original draft. M.D. was involved in reviewing and editing the manuscript. F.M. was involved in study conceptualization, data extraction, methodology, supervision, visualization, and writing—review and editing. All authors have read and agreed to the published version of the manuscript.

Funding: This research did not receive any specific grant from funding agencies in the public, commercial, or not-for-profit sectors.

Conflicts of Interest: The authors declare no conflict of interest.

References

1. WHO. *WHO-Convened Global Study of Origins of SARS-CoV-2: China Part*; Online; World Health Organization: Geneva, Switzerland, 2021.
2. WHO. Timeline: WHO's COVID-19 Response. Available online: https://www.who.int/emergencies/diseases/novel-coronavirus-2019/interactive-timeline (accessed on 1 November 2021).
3. WHO. Novel Coronavirus (2019-nCoV): Situation Report 10. Available online: https://www.who.int/docs/default-source/coronaviruse/situation-reports/20200130-sitrep-10-ncov.pdf?sfvrsn=d0b2e480_2 (accessed on 1 November 2021).
4. WHO. WHO Coronavirus (COVID-19) Dashboard. Available online: https://covid19.who.int/ (accessed on 1 November 2021).
5. CDC. Symptoms of COVID-19. Available online: https://www.cdc.gov/coronavirus/2019-ncov/symptoms-testing/symptoms.html (accessed on 1 November 2021).
6. Song, P.; Li, W.; Xie, J.; Hou, Y.; You, C. Cytokine storm induced by SARS-CoV-2. *Clin. Chim. Acta* **2020**, *509*, 280–287. [CrossRef]
7. Di Salvo, E.; Di Gioacchino, M.; Tonacci, A.; Casciaro, M.; Gangemi, S. Alarmins, COVID-19 and comorbidities. *Ann. Med.* **2021**, *53*, 777–785. [CrossRef] [PubMed]
8. Ejaz, H.; Alsrhani, A.; Zafar, A.; Javed, H.; Junaid, K.; Abdalla, A.E.; Abosalif, K.O.A.; Ahmed, Z.; Younas, S. COVID-19 and comorbidities: Deleterious impact on infected patients. *J. Infect. Public Health* **2020**, *13*, 1833–1839. [CrossRef]
9. Liang, W.; Guan, W.; Chen, R.; Wang, W.; Li, J.; Xu, K.; Li, C.; Ai, Q.; Lu, W.; Liang, H.; et al. Cancer patients in SARS-CoV-2 infection: A nationwide analysis in China. *Lancet Oncol.* **2020**, *21*, 335–337. [CrossRef]
10. Miyashita, H.; Mikami, T.; Chopra, N.; Yamada, T.; Chernyavsky, S.; Rizk, D.; Cruz, C. Do patients with cancer have a poorer prognosis of COVID-19? An experience in New York City. *Ann. Oncol.* **2020**, *31*, 1088–1089. [CrossRef] [PubMed]
11. Dalamaga, M.; Christodoulatos, G.S.; Karampela, I.; Vallianou, N.; Apovian, C.M. Understanding the Co-Epidemic of Obesity and COVID-19: Current Evidence, Comparison with Previous Epidemics, Mechanisms, and Preventive and Therapeutic Perspectives. *Curr. Obes. Rep.* **2021**, *10*, 214–243. [CrossRef]
12. Lin, M.; Dong, H.Y.; Xie, H.Z.; Li, Y.M.; Jia, L. Why do we lack a specific magic anti-COVID-19 drug? Analyses and solutions. *Drug Discov. Today* **2021**, *26*, 631–636. [CrossRef]
13. Gunalan, E.; Cebioglu, I.K.; Conak, O. The Popularity of the Biologically-Based Therapies During Coronavirus Pandemic Among the Google Users in the USA, UK, Germany, Italy and France. *Complement. Ther. Med.* **2021**, *58*, 102682. [CrossRef]
14. Pereira, M.; Dantas Damascena, A.; Galvao Azevedo, L.M.; de Almeida Oliveira, T.; da Mota Santana, J. Vitamin D deficiency aggravates COVID-19: Systematic review and meta-analysis. *Crit. Rev. Food Sci. Nutr.* **2020**, 1–9. [CrossRef] [PubMed]
15. Moghaddam, A.; Heller, R.A.; Sun, Q.; Seelig, J.; Cherkezov, A.; Seibert, L.; Hackler, J.; Seemann, P.; Diegmann, J.; Pilz, M.; et al. Selenium Deficiency Is Associated with Mortality Risk from COVID-19. *Nutrients* **2020**, *12*, 2098. [CrossRef]
16. Vassiliou, A.G.; Jahaj, E.; Orfanos, S.E.; Dimopoulou, I.; Kotanidou, A. Vitamin D in infectious complications in critically ill patients with or without COVID-19. *Metab. Open* **2021**, *11*, 100106. [CrossRef] [PubMed]
17. Lordan, R.; Rando, H.M.; Consortium, C.-R.; Greene, C.S. Dietary Supplements and Nutraceuticals under Investigation for COVID-19 Prevention and Treatment. *mSystems* **2021**, *6*, e00122-21. [CrossRef] [PubMed]
18. Corrao, S.; Mallaci Bocchio, R.; Lo Monaco, M.; Natoli, G.; Cavezzi, A.; Troiani, E.; Argano, C. Does Evidence Exist to Blunt Inflammatory Response by Nutraceutical Supplementation during COVID-19 Pandemic? An Overview of Systematic Reviews of Vitamin D, Vitamin C, Melatonin, and Zinc. *Nutrients* **2021**, *13*, 1261. [CrossRef]
19. Shakoor, H.; Feehan, J.; Al Dhaheri, A.S.; Ali, H.I.; Platat, C.; Ismail, L.C.; Apostolopoulos, V.; Stojanovska, L. Immune-boosting role of vitamins D, C, E, zinc, selenium and omega-3 fatty acids: Could they help against COVID-19? *Maturitas* **2021**, *143*, 1–9. [CrossRef] [PubMed]
20. Hathaway, D.; Pandav, K.; Patel, M.; Riva-Moscoso, A.; Singh, B.M.; Patel, A.; Min, Z.C.; Singh-Makkar, S.; Sana, M.K.; Sanchez-Dopazo, R.; et al. Omega 3 Fatty Acids and COVID-19: A Comprehensive Review. *Infect. Chemother.* **2020**, *52*, 478–495. [CrossRef]
21. Carr, A.C.; Rowe, S. The Emerging Role of Vitamin C in the Prevention and Treatment of COVID-19. *Nutrients* **2020**, *12*, 3286. [CrossRef]
22. Heidari, Z.; Tajbakhsh, A.; Gheibi-Hayat, S.M.; Moattari, A.; Razban, V.; Berenjian, A.; Savardashtaki, A.; Negahdaripour, M. Probiotics/ prebiotics in viral respiratory infections: Implication for emerging pathogens. *Recent Pat. Biotechnol.* **2021**, *15*, 112–136. [CrossRef]
23. Talukdar, J.; Bhadra, B.; Dattaroy, T.; Nagle, V.; Dasgupta, S. Potential of natural astaxanthin in alleviating the risk of cytokine storm in COVID-19. *Biomed. Pharmacother.* **2020**, *132*, 110886. [CrossRef]
24. Fernandez-Lazaro, D.; Fernandez-Lazaro, C.I.; Mielgo-Ayuso, J.; Adams, D.P.; Garcia Hernandez, J.L.; Gonzalez-Bernal, J.; Gonzalez-Gross, M. Glycophosphopeptical AM3 Food Supplement: A Potential Adjuvant in the Treatment and Vaccination of SARS-CoV-2. *Front. Immunol.* **2021**, *12*, 698672. [CrossRef] [PubMed]
25. Johannesen, T.B.; Smeland, S.; Aaserud, S.; Buanes, E.A.; Skog, A.; Ursin, G.; Helland, A. COVID-19 in Cancer Patients, Risk Factors for Disease and Adverse Outcome, a Population-Based Study from Norway. *Front. Oncol.* **2021**, *11*, 652535. [CrossRef]

26. Kuderer, N.M.; Choueiri, T.K.; Shah, D.P.; Shyr, Y.; Rubinstein, S.M.; Rivera, D.R.; Shete, S.; Hsu, C.Y.; Desai, A.; de Lima Lopes, G., Jr.; et al. Clinical impact of COVID-19 on patients with cancer (CCC19): A cohort study. *Lancet* **2020**, *395*, 1907–1918. [CrossRef]
27. Pathania, A.S.; Prathipati, P.; Abdul, B.A.; Chava, S.; Katta, S.S.; Gupta, S.C.; Gangula, P.R.; Pandey, M.K.; Durden, D.L.; Byrareddy, S.N.; et al. COVID-19 and Cancer Comorbidity: Therapeutic Opportunities and Challenges. *Theranostics* **2021**, *11*, 731–753. [CrossRef]
28. Wu, M.Y.; Li, C.J.; Yiang, G.T.; Cheng, Y.L.; Tsai, A.P.; Hou, Y.T.; Ho, Y.C.; Hou, M.F.; Chu, P.Y. Molecular Regulation of Bone Metastasis Pathogenesis. *Cell Physiol. Biochem.* **2018**, *46*, 1423–1438. [CrossRef]
29. Bandinelli, L.; Ornell, F.; von Diemen, L.; Kessler, F.H.P. The Sum of Fears in Cancer Patients Inside the Context of the COVID-19. *Front. Psychiatry* **2021**, *12*, 557834. [CrossRef] [PubMed]
30. Hamulka, J.; Jeruszka-Bielak, M.; Gornicka, M.; Drywien, M.E.; Zielinska-Pukos, M.A. Dietary Supplements during COVID-19 Outbreak. Results of Google Trends Analysis Supported by PLifeCOVID-19 Online Studies. *Nutrients* **2020**, *13*, 54. [CrossRef]
31. 15 Best Supplements to Boost Your Immune System Right Now. Available online: https://www.healthline.com/nutrition/immune-boosting-supplements (accessed on 4 October 2021).
32. 20 Vitamins and Supplements to Boost Immune Health for COVID-19. Available online: https://www.medicinenet.com/covid_19_supplements/article.htm (accessed on 1 November 2021).
33. Aysin, E.; Urhan, M. Dramatic Increase in Dietary Supplement Use during COVID-19. *Curr. Dev. Nutr.* **2021**, *5*, 207. [CrossRef]
34. Ambrosone, C.B.; Zirpoli, G.R.; Hutson, A.D.; McCann, W.E.; McCann, S.E.; Barlow, W.E.; Kelly, K.M.; Cannioto, R.; Sucheston-Campbell, L.E.; Hershman, D.L.; et al. Dietary Supplement Use During Chemotherapy and Survival Outcomes of Patients with Breast Cancer Enrolled in a Cooperative Group Clinical Trial (SWOG S0221). *J. Clin. Oncol.* **2020**, *38*, 804–814. [CrossRef] [PubMed]
35. Poole, E.M.; Shu, X.; Caan, B.J.; Flatt, S.W.; Holmes, M.D.; Lu, W.; Kwan, M.L.; Nechuta, S.J.; Pierce, J.P.; Chen, W.Y. Postdiagnosis supplement use and breast cancer prognosis in the after Breast Cancer Pooling Project. *Breast Cancer Res. Treat.* **2013**, *139*, 529–537. [CrossRef]
36. Bjelakovic, G.; Nikolova, D.; Simonetti, R.G.; Gluud, C. Antioxidant supplements for preventing gastrointestinal cancers. *Cochrane Database Syst. Rev.* **2008**, CD004183. [CrossRef]
37. Andersen, M.R.; Sweet, E.; Hager, S.; Gaul, M.; Dowd, F.; Standish, L.J. Effects of Vitamin D Use on Health-Related Quality of Life of Breast Cancer Patients in Early Survivorship. *Integr. Cancer Ther.* **2019**, *18*, 1534735418822056. [CrossRef]
38. Bjelakovic, G.; Gluud, L.L.; Nikolova, D.; Whitfield, K.; Wetterslev, J.; Simonetti, R.G.; Bjelakovic, M.; Gluud, C. Vitamin D supplementation for prevention of mortality in adults. *Cochrane Database Syst. Rev.* **2014**, CD007470. [CrossRef]
39. Campbell, R.A.; Li, J.; Malone, L.; Levy, D.A. Correlative Analysis of Vitamin D and Omega-3 Fatty Acid Intake in Men on Active Surveillance for Prostate Cancer. *Urology* **2021**, *155*, 110–116. [CrossRef] [PubMed]
40. Chen, F.; Du, M.; Blumberg, J.B.; Ho Chui, K.K.; Ruan, M.; Rogers, G.; Shan, Z.; Zeng, L.; Zhang, F.F. Association Among Dietary Supplement Use, Nutrient Intake, and Mortality Among U.S. Adults: A Cohort Study. *Ann. Intern. Med.* **2019**, *170*, 604–613. [CrossRef]
41. Chlebowski, R.T. Vitamin D and breast cancer incidence and outcome. *Anticancer Agents Med. Chem.* **2013**, *13*, 98–106. [CrossRef]
42. Chowdhury, R.; Kunutsor, S.; Vitezova, A.; Oliver-Williams, C.; Chowdhury, S.; Kiefte-de-Jong, J.C.; Khan, H.; Baena, C.P.; Prabhakaran, D.; Hoshen, M.B.; et al. Vitamin D and risk of cause specific death: Systematic review and meta-analysis of observational cohort and randomised intervention studies. *BMJ* **2014**, *348*, g1903. [CrossRef]
43. Cook, L.S.; Neilson, H.K.; Lorenzetti, D.L.; Lee, R.C. A systematic literature review of vitamin D and ovarian cancer. *Am. J. Obstet. Gynecol.* **2010**, *203*, 70.e1–70.e8. [CrossRef]
44. Datta, M.; Schwartz, G.G. Calcium and vitamin D supplementation during androgen deprivation therapy for prostate cancer: A critical review. *Oncologist* **2012**, *17*, 1171–1179. [CrossRef] [PubMed]
45. Du, C.; Yang, S.; Zhao, X.; Dong, H. Pathogenic roles of alterations in vitamin D and vitamin D receptor in gastric tumorigenesis. *Oncotarget* **2017**, *8*, 29474–29486. [CrossRef] [PubMed]
46. Grant, W.B.; Boucher, B.J. A Review of the Potential Benefits of Increasing Vitamin D Status in Mongolian Adults through Food Fortification and Vitamin D Supplementation. *Nutrients* **2019**, *11*, 2452. [CrossRef]
47. Harvie, M. Nutritional supplements and cancer: Potential benefits and proven harms. *Am. Soc. Clin. Oncol. Educ. Book* **2014**, *34*, e478–e486. [CrossRef]
48. Holm, M.; Olsen, A.; Kroman, N.; Tjonneland, A. Lifestyle influences on the association between pre-diagnostic hormone replacement therapy and breast cancer prognosis—Results from The Danish 'Diet, Cancer and Health' prospective cohort. *Maturitas* **2014**, *79*, 442–448. [CrossRef] [PubMed]
49. Kanellopoulou, A.; Riza, E.; Samoli, E.; Benetou, V. Dietary Supplement Use after Cancer Diagnosis in Relation to Total Mortality, Cancer Mortality and Recurrence: A Systematic Review and Meta-Analysis. *Nutr. Cancer* **2021**, *73*, 16–30. [CrossRef] [PubMed]
50. Khan, Q.J.; Kimler, B.F.; Reddy, P.S.; Sharma, P.; Klemp, J.R.; Nydegger, J.L.; Yeh, H.W.; Fabian, C.J. Randomized trial of vitamin D3 to prevent worsening of musculoskeletal symptoms in women with breast cancer receiving adjuvant letrozole. The VITAL trial. *Breast Cancer Res. Treat.* **2017**, *166*, 491–500. [CrossRef]
51. Klapdor, S.; Richter, E.; Klapdor, R. Vitamin D status and per-oral vitamin D supplementation in patients suffering from chronic pancreatitis and pancreatic cancer disease. *Anticancer Res.* **2012**, *32*, 1991–1998. [PubMed]

52. Lewis, C.; Xun, P.; He, K. Vitamin D supplementation and quality of life following diagnosis in stage II colorectal cancer patients: A 24-month prospective study. *Support. Care Cancer* **2016**, *24*, 1655–1661. [CrossRef] [PubMed]
53. Madden, J.M.; Murphy, L.; Zgaga, L.; Bennett, K. De novo vitamin D supplement use post-diagnosis is associated with breast cancer survival. *Breast Cancer Res. Treat.* **2018**, *172*, 179–190. [CrossRef] [PubMed]
54. Martinez, M.E.; Jacobs, E.T.; Baron, J.A.; Marshall, J.R.; Byers, T. Dietary supplements and cancer prevention: Balancing potential benefits against proven harms. *J. Natl. Cancer Inst.* **2012**, *104*, 732–739. [CrossRef]
55. Morita, M.; Okuyama, M.; Akutsu, T.; Ohdaira, H.; Suzuki, Y.; Urashima, M. Vitamin D Supplementation Regulates Postoperative Serum Levels of PD-L1 in Patients with Digestive Tract Cancer and Improves Survivals in the Highest Quintile of PD-L1: A Post Hoc Analysis of the AMATERASU Randomized Controlled Trial. *Nutrients* **2021**, *13*, 1687. [CrossRef] [PubMed]
56. Mulpur, B.H.; Nabors, L.B.; Thompson, R.C.; Olson, J.J.; LaRocca, R.V.; Thompson, Z.; Egan, K.M. Complementary therapy and survival in glioblastoma. *Neurooncol. Pract.* **2015**, *2*, 122–126. [CrossRef]
57. Saquib, J.; Rock, C.L.; Natarajan, L.; Saquib, N.; Newman, V.A.; Patterson, R.E.; Thomson, C.A.; Al-Delaimy, W.K.; Pierce, J.P. Dietary intake, supplement use, and survival among women diagnosed with early-stage breast cancer. *Nutr. Cancer* **2011**, *63*, 327–333. [CrossRef]
58. Sarre, S.; Maattanen, L.; Tammela, T.L.; Auvinen, A.; Murtola, T.J. Postscreening follow-up of the Finnish Prostate Cancer Screening Trial on putative prostate cancer risk factors: Vitamin and mineral use, male pattern baldness, pubertal development and non-steroidal anti-inflammatory drug use. *Scand. J. Urol.* **2016**, *50*, 267–273. [CrossRef] [PubMed]
59. Wang, L.; Wang, C.; Wang, J.; Huang, X.; Cheng, Y. Longitudinal, observational study on associations between postoperative nutritional vitamin D supplementation and clinical outcomes in esophageal cancer patients undergoing esophagectomy. *Sci. Rep.* **2016**, *6*, 38962. [CrossRef] [PubMed]
60. Zhang, X.; Niu, W. Meta-analysis of randomized controlled trials on vitamin D supplement and cancer incidence and mortality. *Biosci. Rep.* **2019**, *39*, BSR20190369. [CrossRef] [PubMed]
61. Zirpoli, G.R.; McCann, S.E.; Sucheston-Campbell, L.E.; Hershman, D.L.; Ciupak, G.; Davis, W.; Unger, J.M.; Moore, H.C.F.; Stewart, J.A.; Isaacs, C.; et al. Supplement Use and Chemotherapy-Induced Peripheral Neuropathy in a Cooperative Group Trial (S0221): The DELCaP Study. *J. Natl. Cancer Inst.* **2017**, *109*, djx098. [CrossRef]
62. Bjelakovic, G.; Nikolova, D.; Simonetti, R.G.; Gluud, C. Systematic review: Primary and secondary prevention of gastrointestinal cancers with antioxidant supplements. *Aliment. Pharmacol. Ther.* **2008**, *28*, 689–703. [CrossRef]
63. Greenlee, H.; Kwan, M.L.; Kushi, L.H.; Song, J.; Castillo, A.; Weltzien, E.; Quesenberry, C.P., Jr.; Caan, B.J. Antioxidant supplement use after breast cancer diagnosis and mortality in the Life After Cancer Epidemiology (LACE) cohort. *Cancer* **2012**, *118*, 2048–2058. [CrossRef]
64. Harris, H.R.; Bergkvist, L.; Wolk, A. Vitamin C intake and breast cancer mortality in a cohort of Swedish women. *Br. J. Cancer* **2013**, *109*, 257–264. [CrossRef]
65. Harris, H.R.; Orsini, N.; Wolk, A. Vitamin C and survival among women with breast cancer: A meta-analysis. *Eur. J. Cancer* **2014**, *50*, 1223–1231. [CrossRef]
66. Jacobs, E.J.; Connell, C.J.; McCullough, M.L.; Chao, A.; Jonas, C.R.; Rodriguez, C.; Calle, E.E.; Thun, M.J. Vitamin C, vitamin E, and multivitamin supplement use and stomach cancer mortality in the Cancer Prevention Study II cohort. *Cancer Epidemiol. Biomark. Prev.* **2002**, *11*, 35–41.
67. Jacobs, E.J.; Henion, A.K.; Briggs, P.J.; Connell, C.J.; McCullough, M.L.; Jonas, C.R.; Rodriguez, C.; Calle, E.E.; Thun, M.J. Vitamin C and vitamin E supplement use and bladder cancer mortality in a large cohort of US men and women. *Am. J. Epidemiol.* **2002**, *156*, 1002–1010. [CrossRef]
68. Lin, J.; Cook, N.R.; Albert, C.; Zaharris, E.; Gaziano, J.M.; Van Denburgh, M.; Buring, J.E.; Manson, J.E. Vitamins C and E and beta carotene supplementation and cancer risk: A randomized controlled trial. *J. Natl. Cancer Inst.* **2009**, *101*, 14–23. [CrossRef] [PubMed]
69. Messerer, M.; Hakansson, N.; Wolk, A.; Akesson, A. Dietary supplement use and mortality in a cohort of Swedish men. *Br. J. Nutr.* **2008**, *99*, 626–631. [CrossRef]
70. Nechuta, S.; Lu, W.; Chen, Z.; Zheng, Y.; Gu, K.; Cai, H.; Zheng, W.; Shu, X.O. Vitamin supplement use during breast cancer treatment and survival: A prospective cohort study. *Cancer. Epidemiol. Biomark. Prev.* **2011**, *20*, 262–271. [CrossRef] [PubMed]
71. Pocobelli, G.; Peters, U.; Kristal, A.R.; White, E. Use of supplements of multivitamins, vitamin C, and vitamin E in relation to mortality. *Am. J. Epidemiol.* **2009**, *170*, 472–483. [CrossRef]
72. Jenkins, D.J.A.; Kitts, D.; Giovannucci, E.L.; Sahye-Pudaruth, S.; Paquette, M.; Blanco Mejia, S.; Patel, D.; Kavanagh, M.; Tsirakis, T.; Kendall, C.W.C.; et al. Selenium, antioxidants, cardiovascular disease, and all-cause mortality: A systematic review and meta-analysis of randomized controlled trials. *Am. J. Clin. Nutr.* **2020**, *112*, 1642–1652. [CrossRef]
73. Jiang, L.; Yang, K.H.; Tian, J.H.; Guan, Q.L.; Yao, N.; Cao, N.; Mi, D.H.; Wu, J.; Ma, B.; Yang, S.H. Efficacy of antioxidant vitamins and selenium supplement in prostate cancer prevention: A meta-analysis of randomized controlled trials. *Nutr. Cancer* **2010**, *62*, 719–727. [CrossRef] [PubMed]
74. Kenfield, S.A.; Van Blarigan, E.L.; DuPre, N.; Stampfer, M.J.; Giovannucci, E.L.; Chan, J.M. Selenium supplementation and prostate cancer mortality. *J. Natl. Cancer Inst.* **2015**, *107*, 360. [CrossRef] [PubMed]

75. Muecke, R.; Schomburg, L.; Glatzel, M.; Berndt-Skorka, R.; Baaske, D.; Reichl, B.; Buentzel, J.; Kundt, G.; Prott, F.J.; Devries, A.; et al. Multicenter, phase 3 trial comparing selenium supplementation with observation in gynecologic radiation oncology. *Int. J. Radiat. Oncol. Biol. Phys.* **2010**, *78*, 828–835. [CrossRef] [PubMed]
76. Samuels, N.; Schiff, E.; Ben-Arye, E. Non-herbal nutritional supplements for symptom relief in adjuvant breast cancer: Creating a doctor-patient dialogue. *BMJ Support. Palliat. Care* **2014**, *4*, e1. [CrossRef]
77. Klassen, P.; Cervantes, M.; Mazurak, V.C. N-3 fatty acids during chemotherapy: Toward a higher level of evidence for clinical application. *Curr. Opin. Clin. Nutr. Metab. Care* **2020**, *23*, 82–88. [CrossRef]
78. Miyata, H.; Yano, M.; Yasuda, T.; Yamasaki, M.; Murakami, K.; Makino, T.; Nishiki, K.; Sugimura, K.; Motoori, M.; Shiraishi, O.; et al. Randomized study of the clinical effects of omega-3 fatty acid-containing enteral nutrition support during neoadjuvant chemotherapy on chemotherapy-related toxicity in patients with esophageal cancer. *Nutrition* **2017**, *33*, 204–210. [CrossRef]
79. Shen, S.; Unger, J.M.; Crew, K.D.; Till, C.; Greenlee, H.; Gralow, J.; Dakhil, S.R.; Minasian, L.M.; Wade, J.L.; Fisch, M.J.; et al. Omega-3 fatty acid use for obese breast cancer patients with aromatase inhibitor-related arthralgia (SWOG S0927). *Breast Cancer Res. Treat.* **2018**, *172*, 603–610. [CrossRef]
80. Sorensen, L.S.; Rasmussen, S.L.; Calder, P.C.; Yilmaz, M.N.; Schmidt, E.B.; Thorlacius-Ussing, O. Long-term outcomes after perioperative treatment with omega-3 fatty acid supplements in colorectal cancer. *BJS Open* **2020**, *4*, 678–684. [CrossRef] [PubMed]
81. Vernieri, C.; Nichetti, F.; Raimondi, A.; Pusceddu, S.; Platania, M.; Berrino, F.; de Braud, F. Diet and supplements in cancer prevention and treatment: Clinical evidences and future perspectives. *Crit. Rev. Oncol. Hematol.* **2018**, *123*, 57–73. [CrossRef]
82. De Sousa, R.A.L.; Improta-Caria, A.C.; Aras-Junior, R.; de Oliveira, E.M.; Soci, U.P.R.; Cassilhas, R.C. Physical exercise effects on the brain during COVID-19 pandemic: Links between mental and cardiovascular health. *Neurol. Sci.* **2021**, *42*, 1325–1334. [CrossRef]
83. Wang, C.; Zhu, H.; Zhou, Y.; Mao, F.; Lin, Y.; Pan, B.; Zhang, X.; Xu, Q.; Huang, X.; Sun, Q. Prognostic Value of PD-L1 in Breast Cancer: A Meta-Analysis. *Breast J.* **2017**, *23*, 436–443. [CrossRef]
84. Gu, L.; Chen, M.; Guo, D.; Zhu, H.; Zhang, W.; Pan, J.; Zhong, X.; Li, X.; Qian, H.; Wang, X. PD-L1 and gastric cancer prognosis: A systematic review and meta-analysis. *PLoS ONE* **2017**, *12*, e0182692. [CrossRef] [PubMed]
85. Vrankar, M.; Zwitter, M.; Kern, I.; Stanic, K. PD-L1 expression can be regarded as prognostic factor for survival of non-small cell lung cancer patients after chemoradiotherapy. *Neoplasma* **2018**, *65*, 140–146. [CrossRef] [PubMed]
86. Hu, Y.; Chen, W.; Yan, Z.; Ma, J.; Zhu, F.; Huo, J. Prognostic value of PD-L1 expression in patients with pancreatic cancer: A PRISMA-compliant meta-analysis. *Medicine* **2019**, *98*, e14006. [CrossRef] [PubMed]
87. Hudson, K.; Cross, N.; Jordan-Mahy, N.; Leyland, R. The Extrinsic and Intrinsic Roles of PD-L1 and Its Receptor PD-1: Implications for Immunotherapy Treatment. *Front. Immunol.* **2020**, *11*, 568931. [CrossRef]
88. de Sousa Melo, A.; de Lima Dantas, J.B.; Medrado, A.; Lima, H.R.; Martins, G.B.; Carrera, M. Nutritional supplements in the management of oral mucositis in patients with head and neck cancer: Narrative literary review. *Clin. Nutr. ESPEN* **2021**, *43*, 31–38. [CrossRef] [PubMed]
89. Kieliszek, M.; Lipinski, B. Selenium supplementation in the prevention of coronavirus infections (COVID-19). *Med. Hypotheses* **2020**, *143*, 109878. [CrossRef] [PubMed]
90. Pal, A.; Squitti, R.; Picozza, M.; Pawar, A.; Rongioletti, M.; Dutta, A.K.; Sahoo, S.; Goswami, K.; Sharma, P.; Prasad, R. Zinc and COVID-19: Basis of Current Clinical Trials. *Biol. Trace Elem. Res.* **2021**, *199*, 2882–2892. [CrossRef] [PubMed]

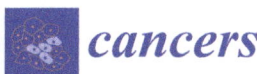

Review

Cancer Patients and the COVID-19 Vaccines: Considerations and Challenges

Muna Almasri [1], Khalifa Bshesh [1], Wafa Khan [1], Malik Mushannen [1], Mohammad A. Salameh [1,2], Ameena Shafiq [1,3], Ahamed Lazim Vattoth [1], Nadine Elkassas [4] and Dalia Zakaria [5,*]

1. Division of Medical Education, Weill Cornell Medicine-Qatar, Qatar Foundation, Education City, Doha 24144, Qatar
2. Department of Obstetrics and Gynecology, Mayo Clinic, Rochester, MN 55902, USA
3. Neurological Institute, University Hospitals Cleveland Medical Center, Cleveland, OH 44106, USA
4. Peninsula Medical School, University of Plymouth, Plymouth PL4 8AA, UK
5. Division of Premedical Education, Weill Cornell Medicine-Qatar, Qatar Foundation, Education City, Doha 24144, Qatar
* Correspondence: dez2003@qatar-med.cornell.edu

Simple Summary: Coronavirus disease 2019 (COVID-19) is the greatest present-day public and global health challenge, and patients with cancer are especially vulnerable, emphasizing the importance of vaccination. However, little is known about the effects of cancer and treatment on vaccine effectiveness and its safety. The aim of this review is to explore current literature regarding the immune response rate and safety profile of COVID-19 vaccination in patients with solid and hematologic cancers and those receiving various forms of treatment. Immune response rates were described to be lower amongst cancer patients, especially those with hematologic cancers, and those receiving chemotherapy, radiotherapy, or immunosuppressants. Nevertheless, sufficient immune response was still generated in many patients, and vaccination was overall described to be safe and well-tolerated, therefore supporting vaccine encouragement.

Abstract: Few guidelines exist for COVID-19 vaccination amongst cancer patients, fostering uncertainty regarding the immunogenicity, safety, and effects of cancer therapies on vaccination, which this review aims to address. A literature review was conducted to include the latest articles covering the immunogenicity and safety of COVID-19 vaccination in patients with solid and hematologic cancers receiving various treatments. Lower seropositivity following vaccination was associated with malignancy (compared to the general population), and hematologic malignancy (compared to solid cancers). Patients receiving active cancer therapy (unspecified), chemotherapy, radiotherapy, and immunosuppressants generally demonstrated lower seropositivity compared to healthy controls; though checkpoint inhibition, endocrine therapy, and cyclin dependent kinase inhibition did not appear to affect seropositivity. Vaccination appeared safe and well-tolerated in patients with current or past cancer and those undergoing treatment. Adverse events were comparable to the general population, but inflammatory lymphadenopathy following vaccination was commonly reported and may be mistaken for malignant etiology. Additionally, radiation recall phenomenon was sporadically reported in patients who had received radiotherapy. Overall, while seropositivity rates were decreased, cancer patients showed capacity to generate safe and effective immune responses to COVID-19 vaccination, thus vaccination should be encouraged and hesitancy should be addressed in this population.

Keywords: cancer; cancer therapies; COVID-19; vaccination; immunogenicity; safety; vaccine hesitancy

1. Introduction

The novel coronavirus disease 2019 (COVID-19) has affected millions of lives around the world and has become the largest public and global health challenge of our time.

Citation: Almasri, M.; Bshesh, K.; Khan, W.; Mushannen, M.; Salameh, M.A.; Shafiq, A.; Vattoth, A.L.; Elkassas, N.; Zakaria, D. Cancer Patients and the COVID-19 Vaccines: Considerations and Challenges. *Cancers* **2022**, *14*, 5630. https://doi.org/10.3390/cancers14225630

Academic Editors: Maria Dalamaga, Narjes Nasiri-Ansari and Nikolaos Spyrou

Received: 5 September 2022
Accepted: 25 October 2022
Published: 16 November 2022

Publisher's Note: MDPI stays neutral with regard to jurisdictional claims in published maps and institutional affiliations.

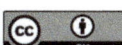

Copyright: © 2022 by the authors. Licensee MDPI, Basel, Switzerland. This article is an open access article distributed under the terms and conditions of the Creative Commons Attribution (CC BY) license (https://creativecommons.org/licenses/by/4.0/).

Several studies and clinical observations in patient populations around the world have shown that individuals with advanced age and co-morbid conditions have a higher rate of morbidity and mortality from severe acute respiratory syndrome coronavirus 2 (SARS-CoV-2) infection.

Cancer Patients and COVID-19

Patients with cancer have demonstrated higher infection rates from COVID-19, increased morbidity, more severe progression of disease, prolonged hospital stays, and increased risk of severe clinical events, as compared to those without cancer [1,2]. Furthermore, cancer patients may face increased contact with COVID-19 infected patients due to regular exposure to the hospital setting for anti-cancer treatment [2]. Combined, these factors place an urgent need for protection against COVID-19 amongst the cancer population. Worldwide, cancer societies have insisted that patients with cancer be considered a high-priority population for COVID-19 vaccination, despite the exclusion of patients with an active cancer status from clinical trials [3,4]. In particular, it has been suggested that patients with later-stage cancer are even more susceptible to SARS-CoV-2 [2]. Furthermore, cancer survivors have also demonstrated increased severity of COVID-19 symptoms, suggesting an incomplete recovery of immune surveillance methods and weakened defense system [2].

A few mechanisms have been hypothesized to explain why cancer patients are increasingly susceptible to higher infection rates and more severe disease. Patients with cancer, especially hematological cancers, commonly have a dysregulated immune system either caused by the cancer itself or the treatment they receive [5]. In cancer patients, the immune suppressive M2 macrophages are activated which inadvertently allows for tumor progression. This immunosuppression also disrupts the antiviral immune response, weakening the host's defense against infections such as COVID-19. Additionally, the receptor that SARS-CoV-2 interacts with to infect host cells is the angiotensin-converting enzyme 2 (ACE2) receptor [6]. Studies have reported that ACE2 expression is increased in certain cancers, including lung cancer, which may contribute to the increased susceptibility [7]. Another link may involve the host transmembrane serine protease 2 (TMPRSS2), which is required by SARS-CoV-2 to release its viral RNA. As the protease is androgen-regulated, upregulation of the protease is seen in androgen-dependent cancers such as prostate cancer. One study showed that prostate cancer patients that were treated with androgen deprivation therapy (ADT) had significantly reduced COVID-19 infection rates as compared to patients without ADT [8]. This may indicate that upregulation of TMPRSS2 plays a role in the pathogenicity for certain cancers. Figure 1 summarizes the reasons behind the importance of vaccinating cancer patients against COVID-19, as well as the attributed mechanisms to this population's vulnerability to the disease.

Though the extent of benefit from vaccination in this population is not fully delineated, accumulating data supports that COVID-19 vaccines are safe and demonstrate efficacy in cancer patients [9], which this review explores further. This narrative review aims to summarize the latest available information regarding the immunogenicity and safety of COVID-19 vaccines in cancer patients of different types (e.g., solid versus hematological) receiving different cancer treatments (e.g., chemotherapy, radiotherapy) in hopes of communicating an optimal strategy to better manage the health of this vulnerable population. The COVID-19 vaccines mentioned in this review span the mRNA vaccines (Pfizer, New York, NY, USA, Moderna, Cambridge, MA, USA), viral vectored vaccines (AstraZeneca, Cambridge, UK, Johnson & Johnson/Janssen, Beerse, Belgium), and inactivated vaccines (Sinopharm, Beijing, China).

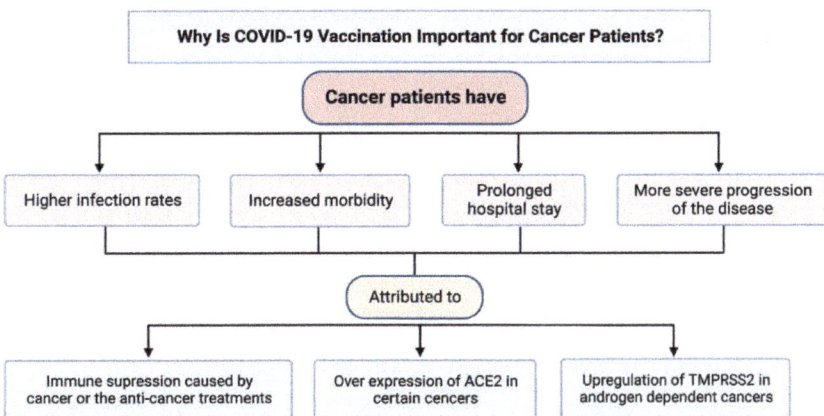

Figure 1. Reasons supporting the importance of COVID-19 vaccination in cancer patients, and mechanisms attributed to cancer patients' increased susceptibility, severity, and morbidity from COVID-19 disease.

2. Immunogenicity of the COVID-19 Vaccines in Solid and Hematologic Cancer Patients

In general, some studies reported lower immunogenicity in the cancer patients as compared to healthy controls. For example, Palaia et al., reported that there was no significant difference in the mean antibody titer one month after the second dose of Pfizer vaccination in 44 cancer patients as compared to the controls [10]. However, a significantly lower titer was reported three months after the second dose in cancer patients as compared to the healthy controls. Similarly, a study by Yasin et al., reported a significantly lower seropositivity rate in 661/776 (85.2%) of cancer patients compared to 697/715 (97.5%) of the control group after the second dose of the Sinovac vaccine [1]. Another study conducted by Ligumsky et al., reported that 287/326 (88%) of cancer patients had significantly lower immunoglobulin G (IgG) titer following the second dose of the Pfizer vaccine (median IgG titer 931 AU/mL) as compared to 159/164 (96.95%) of the healthy controls (median IgG of 2817 AU/mL) [9].

When comparing patients with solid malignancies to healthy controls, median neutralizing antibody titers were found to be similar between solid cancer patients and controls ($p = 0.566$), indicating comparable protection in seropositive people who mounted an immune response to vaccination [11]. On the other hand, a study conducted by Massarweh et al., found that patients with primary brain tumors had an 88.2% seroconversion rate following the Pfizer vaccine, though these patients demonstrated significantly lower IgG titers than controls ($p = 0.002$) [12].

Fendler and colleagues conducted a longitudinal prospective cohort study entitled *COVID-19 antiviral response in a pan-tumor immune monitoring study (CAPTURE)*. This study analyzed 585 patients, of which 76% had solid malignancies and 24% had hematological malignancies. Amongst these patients, 74% received two doses of the AstraZeneca vaccine, and 26% received two doses of the Pfizer vaccine [13]. The CAPTURE study found that most solid cancer patients developed durable humoral responses to SARS-CoV-2 infection or vaccination, with a seroconversion rate of 44% after the first dose and 85% after the second dose. Additionally, when the immunogenicity was compared in patients with solid or hematologic malignancy (HM), Fendler et al., described a reduced neutralizing antibody response in HM compared to solid cancer patients or controls [13]. Interestingly, Singer et al., reported that antibody titers against the SARS-CoV-2 spike (S) protein were significantly higher in solid cancer patients over HM indicating that the type of cancer may also affect the immunogenicity [14]. Furthermore, Agha et al., reported that 31/67 (46.3%) of patients with HM such as B-cell chronic lymphocytic leukemia (CLL), lymphomas, or multiple myeloma (MM) did not produce antibodies to COVID-19 messenger RNA (mRNA) vaccination [15]. In fact, patients with CLL were significantly less likely to respond to vaccination compared to other hematologic malignancies (23.1% vs. 61.1%; $p = 0.01$) [15]. Additionally, the United Kingdom's prospective observational study evaluating COVID-19 vaccine responses in individuals with lymphoma (PROSECO) documented that 52% of patients with B-cell lymphoma undergoing active cancer treatment who received two vaccine doses had undetectable humoral response, though 70% of patients with indolent B-cell lymphoma showed increased antibody response after a booster dose [16]. Patients with hematological malignancies demonstrating a lower immune response as compared to solid tumors is, in part, because the disease process in hematological malignancies such as acute lymphoma, leukemia, and multiple myeloma is widespread and invasive and is particularly disruptive to the immune system [17]. In addition, treatments for hematological malignancies in general are more immunosuppressive, often leading to myelosuppression and lymphodepletion [17].

The above studies have shown evidence of lower seropositivity in cancer patients as compared to healthy controls and lower seropositivity in patients with hematologic malignancies as compared to those with solid cancers. However, in addition to the implication of the disease itself, cancer treatment affects the immunogenic response to vaccine which has been reported in numerous studies. The next sections summarize the findings of the studies that compared the seropositivity of cancer patients who received specific types of treatments with healthy controls or compared the seropositivity in those who received different types of treatments.

2.1. Lower Seropositivity in Patients Receiving Active Therapy Compared with Healthy Controls or Patients Not Receiving Active Therapy

Unlike the long-term anti-cancer treatments which are used to maintain remittance, active treatments are used to cure cancer, such as chemotherapy, radiotherapy, and others. This section reports the findings of the studies that mainly compared seropositivity in patients receiving active treatments with control groups, without specifying the individual effects of the different treatments. Nelli et al., reported that the median IgG titer in cancer patients without active treatment (control group) was more than twofold of that in cancer patients undergoing active treatment (exposed group) prior to receiving the second dose of either the Pfizer or Moderna vaccine. The median IgG titer 8 weeks after receiving the second dose in the control group had an approximately 15-fold increase compared to the exposed group [18]. A study conducted by Cavanna et al., showed that out of a total 257 cancer patients (85.2% on active treatments), 195 (75.88%) were seropositive 15–42 days after the second dose of the Pfizer or Moderna vaccine in comparison to 100% seropositivity in the healthy control group. Additionally, the median IgG titer in patients (118 AU/mL) was significantly lower than that in the control group (380.5 AU/mL) ($p < 0.001$) [19]. Furthermore, out of 195 seropositive cancer patients, 36 received no treatment, 84 received chemotherapy, 15 received immunotherapies, 26 received biological therapy, 24 received a combination of chemotherapy and biological therapy, and 10 received a combination of chemotherapy and immunotherapy [19]. Cavanna et al., reported in their second study that, following the second dose of either the Pfizer or the Moderna vaccine, 75/115 cancer patients (65.22%) were seropositive in comparison to 100% in the control group [20]. Furthermore, patients with HM yielded the lowest seroconversion rate (42.86% seroconverted vs. 70.21% of patients with solid tumor, $p = 0.02$). The differences in seroconversion were insignificant between patients who received active cancer therapy as compared to patients who did not (64.00% versus 73.33%). Furthermore, no significant difference was observed between the different individual treatments (chemotherapy 63.64%, immunotherapy 52.94%, biologic therapy 76.92%, hormone therapy 75.00%, and no treatment 73.33%) [20]. Overall, these studies support both decreased seropositivity rates as well as decreased antibody concentrations in patients receiving active cancer therapy compared to healthy controls, but no difference compared to cancer patients not receiving active therapy.

The next sections discuss the effect of specific types of treatments on the seropositivity of cancer patients after receiving different COVID-19 vaccines.

2.2. Lower Seropositivity in Cancer Patients Receiving Chemotherapy Compared to Healthy Controls or Patients Receiving Other Treatments

Chemotherapy consists of cytotoxic drugs that can disrupt the process of mitosis in cell division or cause deoxyribonucleic acid (DNA) damage. However, the susceptibility of cancer cells to these drugs can vary greatly. Such drugs induce stress or damage to the cells, enough to induce apoptosis [21]. Most therapeutic agents are delivered intravenously, but some are given orally, and both provide systemic therapy. Combination chemotherapy is a type of administration strategy which utilizes multiple different drugs to decrease the risk of developing resistance and allows for reducing the doses and consequently lowering toxicity [22]. However, these drugs lack the ability to distinguish between cancerous and healthy body cells, therefore resulting in adverse side effects due to damage of healthy, rapidly dividing cells in the bone marrow, hair follicles, and digestive tract [23].

Chemotherapy has been implicated in altering the immunogenic response to the vaccine. In fact, some studies present it as a main player in the reduced immunogenicity in cancer patients. Comparing chemotherapy to other treatment modalities produces useful conclusions but results can be variable. For example, Figueiredo et al., found that the effect of chemotherapy was less pronounced as compared to immunotherapy [24]. On the contrary, a study by Grinshpun et al., found that immunotherapy was associated with higher mean antibody levels compared to chemotherapy in 172 cancer patients who received two doses of the Pfizer vaccine ($p = 0.0017$) [25]. With regards to other treatment modalities, Ariamanesh et al., looked at 364 patients with cancer of which 131 were receiving chemotherapy. Chemotherapy treatment was associated with lower rates of seroconversion (83.5%) compared to radiotherapy or hormonal therapy (97%) [26]. Likewise, the study by Yasin et al., showed that the seropositivity rates were 78.6% in the active chemotherapy group, 85.7% in the immunotherapy group, 86.0% in the targeted therapies group, 87.1% in the hormone therapy group, and 91.1% in those receiving no active treatment where chemotherapy was found to be significantly associated with lower seropositivity ($p < 0.001$) [1]. The findings of Agbarya et al., also supported the impaired seropositivity in cancer patients who received chemotherapy. They looked at 140 patients with solid malignancies and 215 controls and found the odds ratio (OR) for negative serology in cancer patients to be 7.35 times compared to controls after adjusting for age and gender [27]. However, it was notable that negative serology was found only in chemotherapy treated patients and not in the other treatments, such as immunotherapy [27]. The case-control study conducted by Addeo et al., reported significantly lower antibody titers after two doses of the Pfizer or Moderna vaccine in patients receiving chemotherapy compared to those only under clinical surveillance [28]. Similar results were obtained by Funakoshi et al., who reported significantly lower median antibody titer for the 24 cancer patients receiving chemotherapy (0.161, 95% confidence interval (CI) [0.07–0.857]) after the second dose of the Pfizer vaccine as compared to 12 healthy controls (0.644, 95% CI [0.259–1.498]) ($p < 0.0001$) [29]. Likewise, Palaia et al., found that cancer patients who were receiving active chemotherapy treatment had lower median antibody titer one month and three months after the second dose as compared to those who were not receiving active chemotherapy [10]. Interestingly, the specific effect of the chemotherapy treatment and its extent varies depending on the drug at hand. A study by Ruggeri et al., looked at the rates of seroconversion with the Pfizer vaccine at the time of and just before the second dose, and then 8 weeks later [30]. It found that alkylating agents and tyrosine kinase (TK) inhibitors caused a significant reduction in IgG titers after the first dose of the vaccine and before the second dose. This effect was mitigated after the second dose. On the other hand, mammalian target of rapamycin (mTOR) inhibitors caused reductions in IgG titers after both doses at 8 weeks [30].

Overall, the above-mentioned studies consistently demonstrated significantly lower seropositivity and antibody titers amongst cancer patients receiving chemotherapy, including alkylating agents, TK inhibitors, and mTOR inhibitors, compared to healthy controls.

2.3. Effect of Radiotherapy on the Immunogenicity of COVID-19 Vaccines in Cancer Patients

Radiotherapy aims to treat cancer locally by using ionizing radiation, decreasing the chances of undesired damage in healthy body tissues, and thus reducing side effects. Despite local treatment, dosage of radiation must be limited as some nearby healthy cells are also destroyed during the process, resulting in adverse side effects such as fatigue and nausea [23].

Radiotherapy has also been associated with decreased seropositivity following vaccination. A subset of the Cancer, COVID-19 and Vaccination (CANVAX) prospective cohort study included 33 patients who had received thoracic radiotherapy, the majority of which had non-small cell lung cancer (NSCLC) or small cell lung cancer (SCLC) [31]. Of these patients, 14 had received stereotactic body, palliative, or definitive radiotherapy, 13 had received chemotherapy, and 9 had potentially immunosuppressive medical conditions; 79% of patients received radiotherapy prior to vaccination with either the Moderna, Pfizer, or AstraZeneca vaccine. This analysis found that antibody concentrations against the spike protein were significantly lower in the 33 patients treated with thoracic radiotherapy compared to vaccinated healthy controls ($p = 0.01$) [31]. However, though lower antibody concentrations were noted between patients with thoracic malignancies who received radiotherapy versus those who did not, the difference was not statistically significant ($p = 0.07$) [31]. Moreover, amongst patients receiving radiotherapy, those with immunosuppressive conditions (including those receiving chemotherapy) were found to have significantly lower antibody concentrations; 44% of patients with immunosuppressive conditions had antibody levels < 100 U/mL, compared to 13% without ($p = 0.04$) [31]. Overall, this study supported the notion that cancer patients receiving radiotherapy demonstrate significantly lower seropositivity compared to healthy controls, but an insignificant difference compared to patients with malignancy not treated with radiotherapy.

2.4. Effect of Checkpoint Inhibitors on the Immunogenicity of COVID-19 Vaccines in Cancer Patients

Immunotherapy involves stimulating the immune system to fight cancer cells. There are several types of immunotherapies, including the checkpoint inhibitor therapy (CPI). The immune system checkpoints are vital for regulation, and some reduce the action of T-cells. CPI therapy consists of drugs which block these checkpoints and allow T-cells to continue attacking the cancer cells [32]. Current drugs target molecules such as programmed cell death protein 1 (PD-1), and programmed death ligand-1 (PD-L1) which play a role in T-cell regulation [33,34].

Immunotherapies with immune amplifying effects have been associated with an adjusted response to the vaccine. Figueiredo and others found a significant drop in the four-to-six month antibody level of those with solid tumors receiving immune CPI therapy compared to those receiving other treatment modalities, including chemotherapy ($p = 0.004$) [24]. Notably, the reduction in antibody levels was more pronounced in those who received the vaccine after starting the CPI therapy compared to those who received it before CPI therapy [24]. On the contrary, the study by Naranbhai found that those receiving immune checkpoint (ICP) modulators tended to have a higher neutralization [35]. Ma et al., recruited 545 cancer patients who received either progression cell death-1 blockers (PD-1B), COVID-19 vaccination, or both in three matched cohorts and compared them with a non-cancer control group of 206 participants. Seropositivity was detected in 68.1%, 71.3%, and 80.5% of the vaccinated cancer patients who received PD-1B, who did not receive PD-1B, or the healthy control subjects respectively [36]. The study concluded that patients with cancer tolerated the COVID-19 vaccines well and that the PD-1B treatment did not affect the seroconversion rate following vaccination. However, the seroconversion rate was generally lower in the cancer patients as compared to the healthy control participants [36]. Similarly, Funakoshi et al., reported that the median antibody titer for the 17 cancer patients receiving ICP treatment was significantly lower after the second dose of the Pfizer vaccine (0.241, 95% CI [0.063–1.205]) as compared the 12 healthy controls (to 0.644, 95% CI [0.259–1.498]) (p = 0.0024) [29]. Another study by Lasagna et al., looked at 88 patients treated with PD-L1 inhibitors and assessed their response to the Pfizer vaccine at three weeks. It found that recipients of this treatment were able to illicit a robust T-cell (CD4 and CD8) response to the vaccine, demonstrating the vaccine's ability to include both types of adaptive responses [37]. A continuation study of the same cohort found significantly waning immunity at 6 months, particularly for those who were SARS-CoV-2 naïve [38]. These studies indicate that while seroconversion rate was generally unaffected, the antibody titers were significantly decreased in patients receiving immunomodulating therapy, though adaptive T-cell responses amongst this patient population remained intact.

2.5. Lower Seropositivity in Cancer Patients Receiving Immunosuppressives Compared to Healthy Controls or Patients Receiving Other Treatments

Immunosuppressive drugs are given to reduce the activity of the immune system [39]. It is also important to note that immunosuppression can also be a result of cytotoxic drugs used in chemotherapy, as they mainly target cells that rapidly divide, including T-cells [40]. Deliberate immunosuppression is vital for preventing body rejection after organ transplants, which is common amongst cancer patients. These drugs are also given when treating graft-versus-host disease (GvHD) following bone marrow transplants [41]. Certain types of immunotherapies may lead to immunosuppression such as the anti-CD20 treatments which block the B cells and the chimeric antigen receptor (CAR) T-cells. The CAR T-cell method is the genetic modification of T-cell receptor proteins which allows for antigen binding and T-cell activation via a single receptor. For cancer therapy, these T-cells can be engineered to recognize specific antigens found on tumor cells only. This is done by the extraction of the T-cells from patients, genetic modification, then reintroduction into the body. The CAR T-cells then become cytotoxic once they attach to the tumor cells [42]. Derivation of T-cells can be from either the patient's blood or a healthy donor [43].

Several studies demonstrated reduced immunogenicity in response to the vaccine in the setting of immunomodulating therapy. One frequently reported treatment is anti-CD20, which blocks a B-cell surface protein involved in B-cell activation and hence alters immune response. Addeo and others looked at 131 cancer patients, four of which received anti-CD20 treatment and found that none of the latter developed a humoral response to the vaccine [28]. Another study conducted by Thakkar et al., looked at 200 cancer patients with solid or hematologic cancers in New York City and found that those with HM had an 85% rate of seroconversion after receiving two doses of the Pfizer or Moderna vaccine or one dose of the Johnson & Johnson/Janssen adenoviral vaccine. This rate was reduced to 70% if the patients were receiving anti-CD20 therapy (p = 0.0001) [44]. Other immunosuppressive therapies that were associated with reduced immunity include stem cell transplantation with seroconversion rate of 73% (p = 0.0002), and CAR-T cell therapy with zero of the three patients who received it seroconverting (p = 0.0002) [44]. Further, a paper by Shapiro and colleagues examined the efficacy of the Pfizer or Moderna booster dose in 88 cancer patients. This study noted significantly lower seroconversion rates amongst patients receiving anti-CD20 therapy in the last 3.9 months. Of the 88 patients, 32 were seronegative prior to the booster, and fourteen (44%) remained seronegative following the booster, including two patients undergoing CAR T-cell therapy and two receiving stem cell transplants; 18/32 seroconverted following the booster (p = 0.000062) [45]. Similar results were obtained by Peeters et al., who conducted a multicohort study, whose results revealed extremely low antibody response in HM patients receiving rituximab [46]. Furthermore, the PROSECO study revealed that 60% of fully vaccinated patients demonstrated undetectable antibodies within 12 months of receiving anti-CD20 therapy [16].

Regarding corticosteroid therapy, a study by Nelli et al., found that amongst 311 patients who received two doses of the Pfizer vaccine, receiving initial corticosteroid therapy was associated with reduced IgG response ($p = 0.005$) [47]. Similarly, Naranbhai et al., looked at the response of 656 patients who received two doses of Pfizer or Moderna, or one dose of the Johnson & Johnson/Janssen vaccine and found that patients currently on steroid therapy had lower antibody titers ($p = 0.003$) [35].

Daratumumab, a CD38 inhibitor, was associated with a similar decrease in immunogenicity. By targeting CD38 on plasma cells, daratumumab thus depletes antibody production and reduces vaccine immunogenicity, potentially explaining this finding. In patients with multiple myeloma, active treatment with proteasome inhibitor-based or Imids-based had a higher likelihood of response to Pfizer vaccine than treatment which included daratumumab (92.9% vs. 50%; $p = 0.003$) [48].

In summary, various modalities of immunosuppressive cancer treatment, including anti-CD20 agents, corticosteroids, and CD38 inhibitors, are associated with significantly lower seroconversion rates as well as immunogenicity, likely due to the mechanism of action of immunosuppressives.

2.6. Effect of Other Treatments on the Immunogenicity of COVID-19 Vaccines in Cancer Patients

2.6.1. Endocrine Therapy

The main function of hormonal therapies is to block or change certain hormone systems to slow down the growth of specific cancers. For example, hormonal therapy is used to treat estrogen receptor positive breast cancer [49].

Referring to the study conducted by Addeo and colleagues, of 131 patients, 15% received endocrine therapy prior to vaccination with Pfizer or Moderna. Some 94% of patients receiving endocrine therapy were seropositive after dose one, and 100% demonstrated seropositivity after dose two, with excellent median antibody titers (>2500 U/mL). Overall, it was found that endocrine therapy had no discernable impact on seropositivity at a minimum of three weeks post-vaccination series, with similar outcomes to patients receiving no therapy [28].

2.6.2. Cyclin Dependent Kinase Inhibitors

A prospective study conducted by Cortés et al., found that amongst 26 patients being treated with cyclin dependent kinase inhibitors (CDKi), rates of humoral response in patients treated with CDK4/6i were similar to healthcare worker (HCW) controls [50]. Some 100% of the CDK4/6i cohort showed positive serology after the first and second doses, with no significant difference in anti-S IgG levels. However, there was a significantly lower cellular response in CDK4/6i recipients compared to HCW; the anti-S CD4 response was found to be 59.7% and 91.7% amongst CDK4/6i and HCW cohorts, respectively ($p = 0.001$), and the anti-S CD8 response was 55.6% and 94.4% amongst CDK4/6i and HCW cohorts, respectively ($p < 0.001$) [50]. There was no known predictive factor for poor cellular response amongst patient characteristics. Though seropositivity and humoral response were seemingly unaffected by CDK4/6i, the difference in cellular response was thought to be due to CDK4/6i induced neutropenia via reversible bone marrow suppression by cell cycle arrest [50].

2.6.3. Stem Cell Transplants

Khan and colleagues conducted a prospective, observational longitudinal cross-sectional study of 453 cancer patients undergoing treatment or who received stem cell transplantation (SCT). Within this population, 114 patients received SCT [51]. Patients receiving allogeneic SCT, autologous SCT, or CAR T-cell therapy demonstrated adequate levels of anti-S titers (>100 U/mL) at one and three months following the second dose of either the Moderna, Pfizer, or Johnson & Johnson/Janssen vaccine; the geometric mean titer amongst the SCT group was 325.35 (95% CI [149.93–706.01]) after one month, and increased to 454.36 (95% CI [237.48–869.32]) after three months [51]. Anti-S titers > 100 U/mL or higher are associated with protection and thus higher vaccine effectiveness [51].

2.6.4. Combination Treatment with Chemotherapy and Immunotherapy

Combining treatments was reported to intensify the anti-cancer effect compared to receiving individual therapies. A study by Massarweh et al., looked at 102 patients with cancer and their seroconversion in response to two doses of the Pfizer vaccine. Multivariate analysis of the cohort found that the only variable significantly associated with lower IgG values was combination treatment with both chemotherapy and immunotherapy, compared to chemotherapy or immunotherapy alone ($p = 0.001$) [52]. However, though Grinshpun et al., found the seroconversion rate amongst patients receiving immunotherapy plus chemotherapy to be lower (10/12, 83.3%) than those receiving immunotherapy alone (32/34, 94.1%), this difference was not significant [25].

2.7. *Effect of the Number of the COVID-19 Vaccine Doses on the Seropositivity of the Cancer Patients*

The study by Monin et al., followed individuals who received the Pfizer vaccine and showed that a single dose of 30 μg failed to induce seroconversion in most patients with cancer. However, the same dose induced T-cell responses in a majority of healthy controls and solid cancer patients even though many of them were seronegative [4]. This should support prioritizing the cancer patients to receive an early (day 21) second dose of the Pfizer vaccine. Other studies reported that cancer patients were seropositive after receiving the second dose of different types of vaccines, including those who were on active cancer treatments. For example, Goshen-Lago et al., demonstrated seropositivity in 25/86 cancer patients (29%) with a median titer of 42.3 compared with 220/261 (84%) in controls ($p < 0.001$), who had a median titer of 72.0 following the first dose. However, the rates increased to 187/218 patients (86%) following the second dose of the Pfizer vaccine. Of the 187 seropositive cancer patients following the second dose, 55% received chemotherapy, 38% received immunotherapy and 37% received biological agents [53]. Similarly, following the second dose of inactivated Sinopharm vaccine, 102/119 (85.7%) cancer patients were SARS-CoV-2 anti-spike IgG positive, 65 of which received endocrine therapy, trastuzumab, 18 received chemotherapy and 19 received radiotherapy. Furthermore, 104/119 (87.4%) were SARS-CoV2 anti-receptor binding domain (RBD) IgG (neutralizing antibody) positive, 66 of which received endocrine therapy, trastuzumab, 19 received chemotherapy and 19 received radiotherapy [54]. Additionally, despite postulated lower immunogenicity amongst patients with solid malignancy, antibody titers were found to increase following the second dose of the COVID-19 vaccine, highlighting the need for a third. For example, Trontzas et al., found that in patients with thoracic cancer (93.1% lung cancer, including NSCLC, SCLC, and pleural malignant mesothelioma), a second dose of the Pfizer, Moderna, or AstraZeneca vaccine given in patients with thoracic cancer increased antibody response [55]. Similarly, the serologic response rate amongst cancer patients increased from 14.2% after the first dose to 86% after the booster dose. Following the booster dose, 73.8% of the non-responders were receiving active chemotherapy and 40.5% were reported to receive targeted therapy [56]. When compared to controls, the serological response rate for cancer patients was lower at different time points [56].

3. Safety of the COVID-19 Vaccines on the Cancer Patients

Several new trials have reported that COVID-19 vaccines have shown similar safety profiles in cancer patients as compared to the general population. The most common local and systemic side effects were pain at injection site, myalgia, and fatigue [17]. These were mostly mild to moderate in severity in the general population and cancer patients [17]. The following sections describe the reported side effects post-COVID-19 vaccination in cancer patients.

3.1. Safety of the COVID-19 Vaccines in Cancer Patients with Different Treatments

Shulman et al., reported 1753 individuals who had received both doses of the Pfizer vaccine, out of which 570 had no cancer, 1183 had a history of cancer, and 211 were on active treatment. Treatment methods included surgery, radiation, chemotherapy, immunotherapy, hormone therapy, and targeted therapy. Rates of adverse events (AE) following vaccination were similar in both patients with and without cancer (73.3% vs. 72.5%; $p = 0.71$) [57]. The most common adverse event was local pain at the injection site, but these rates did not differ between patient category nor dose number. Patients with cancer and receiving therapy were significantly less likely to report pain at the injection following the first dose compared to patients with cancer not receiving therapy (30% vs. 41.4%; $p = 0.002$) [57]. Muscle pain after the first dose was significantly more common in patients with cancer compared to those without (16.5% vs. 11.9%; $p = 0.012$), but they had it for significantly shorter duration (mean 2.2 vs. 3.0 days; $p = 0.04$) [57]. The onset of symptoms was similar for both groups of cancer patients [57]. Another study conducted by Kian et al., revealed no significant difference between treatment protocol and development on the side effects of the Pfizer vaccine on cancer patients who received different types of anti-cancer treatments including chemotherapy, radiotherapy, immunotherapy, biological therapy, hormonal therapy, or who had a combination of two therapies. The overall incidence of side effects following either dose was 31%, similar to that reported in the safety data from the phase III trial (27%) [58].

In patients with urologic cancers, Kawaguchi et al., reported 214 patients, of which 180 received the AstraZeneca vaccine (2 patients received one dose, 178 received two doses). The patients were on different treatments where 36 patients received ICP inhibitors, 17 received systemic chemotherapy, 24 received molecular targeted therapy, 140 received hormonal therapy, and 6 patients received intravesical infusion therapy. Furthermore, bone modifying agents (BMA) were used in 28 patients, denosumab in 18, and zoledronic acid in 10 patients. Of the 180 vaccinated patients, 69 (38.3%) reported adverse events [59]. The study found that in their population, the incidence of adverse events was significantly higher in females than males (72.7% vs. 36.1%; $p = 0.015$) [59]. Of these, only one patient had to postpone therapy due to adverse reaction of immune checkpoint inhibitors, and only one due to adverse effects of the vaccine. Overall, the vaccine was found to be safe in urologic cancer patients receiving different types of therapy [59].

Furthermore, of 373 cancer patients at a London oncology center, 281 (75.4%) received mRNA (Pfizer or Moderna) vaccines, 88 (23.6%) received the adenoviral (Johnson & Johnson/Janssen) vaccine, and 4 (1.1%) received an unknown vaccine. Only four had received the second dose and three of them experienced new adverse events, including worsening pre-existing grade 1 pruritus, grade 2 transaminitis, and grade 2 hypercortisolism, all of which were not seen in other groups. These patients were on different types of anti-cancer treatments where 23.6% received hormonal therapy, 36.2% received parenteral chemotherapy and 15.3% received immunotherapy. It was found that patients receiving immunotherapy within 6 months of vaccination appear to be at lower risk of developing adverse events (OR 0.495, 95% CI [0.256–0.958]; $p = 0.0037$) [60]. Other negative independent predictors for developing vaccine-related systemic adverse events include: male gender (OR 0.632, 95% CI [0.400–0.999]; $p = 0.049$), presence of metastatic cancer (OR 0.548, 95% CI [0.347–0.867]; $p = 0.010$), receiving chemotherapy within 28 days of vaccination (OR 0.373, 95% CI [0.221–0.629]; $p < 0.001$) or receiving the Pfizer vaccine (OR 0.452, 95% CI [0.274–0.747]; $p = 0.002$) [60].

3.2. Safety of the COVID-19 Vaccines in Cancer Patients Receiving Radiotherapy

In patients receiving radiotherapy, Soyfer et al., reported two patients who developed acute skin reactions in previously irradiated areas after receiving the second dose of Pfizer vaccine. Both reactions were diagnosed as radiation recall phenomenon (RRP), which is an uncommon inflammatory skin reaction in areas previously receiving radiation therapy (RT). One case was treated with topical steroids and painkillers until resolved, and the other required no intervention and self-resolved [61]. Similarly, Marples et al., reported three cases of breast cancer female patients (62, 69 and 56 years old, respectively) who received radiotherapy and developed AstraZeneca vaccine induced RRP. The first case had left breast cancer and underwent bilateral mastectomy with reconstruction. Three days following her first dose of the AstraZeneca vaccine, she began having swelling, erythema, and pain in her left breast. She had no fever or systemic symptoms. She received a four-week course of steroids and received the second dose afterward without issues. The second case received adjuvant radiotherapy following left breast cancer treated with lumpectomy and sentinel node biopsy. She had fever, muscle aches, and lethargy three days after receiving the AstraZeneca vaccine, followed by pain and erythema in the left breast with left axillary pain. She was treated conservatively after ruling out collection or other serious issues, diagnosed with RRP, and never received the second dose. The third case had therapeutic reduction mammoplasty and sentinel node biopsy for multifocal lobular carcinoma of the right breast followed by whole breast radiotherapy. She had flu-like symptoms after receiving the AstraZeneca vaccine, and three days later experienced a warm, pruritic, and heavy sensation in her right breast, in a similar area to her radiation therapy. She received two days of antibiotics from her general practitioner, ruled out collection with ultrasound, and was diagnosed with RRP by her breast surgeon [62].

Scoccianti and colleagues evaluated overall tolerance to the Moderna vaccine with a cohort study involving 153 patients who had received either postoperative, definitive, palliative, or stereotactic ablative radiotherapy. Of this cohort, 33% of patients had no adverse events after the first dose, 38% had no AE after the second dose, and 20% had no AE after the first and second doses. It was concluded that overall, tolerance was not worse in radiotherapy patients compared to controls [63].

3.3. Safety of the COVID-19 Vaccines in Cancer Patients Receiving Immune Checkpoint Inhibitors

According to Waissengrin et al., of a total of 170 patients on immune checkpoint inhibitors, 134 patients received two vaccine doses, three patients received only one dose, and 33 did not receive the Pfizer vaccine at all. The most common side-effect after the first dose was localized pain at the site of injection (21%). Systemic side-effects included fatigue in five (4%), headache in three (2%), muscle pain in three (2%), and chills in one (1%) patient. More local and systemic side effects occurred following the second dose. The local adverse events include pain at injection site in 85 (63%), local rash in three (2%), and local swelling in twelve (9%) patients. The systemic side effects included muscle pain in 46 (34%), fatigue in 45 (34%), headache in 22 (16%), fever in 14 (10%), chills in 14 (10%), GI complications in 14 (10%), and flu-like symptoms in 3 (2.2%) patients [64]. None of the reported side effects required hospitalization or special intervention, and no immune-related AE were observed. Of note, patients were all matched by sex and birth year to compare the side effects; there was only a significantly higher rate of muscle pain in the immune checkpoint group compared to healthy controls following the second dose of the vaccine ($p = 0.024$) [64].

Strobel et al., reported 89 patients receiving immune checkpoint inhibitors. Four patients received one vaccine dose (one Johnson & Johnson/Janssen, 1 AstraZeneca, and 2 Pfizer) while 85 patients received two doses of an mRNA vaccine (76 Pfizer, 2 Moderna), AstraZeneca (8 patients) and mixed AstraZeneca and Pfizer (2 patients). Overall, they found that the rate of general side effects was lower than that seen in preliminary data from the vaccination studies [65].

Mei et al., compared 1518 vaccinated cancer patients (288 with one dose, 1134 with two doses, 96 with three doses) receiving camrelizumab alone or in conjunction with other therapies to unvaccinated patients. Compared with matched unvaccinated patients, a statistically greater percentage of vaccinated patients had mild AE ≤ 2 (33.8% vs. 19.8%; $p < 0.001$) following camrelizumab treatment [66].

One case report published by Au et al., described a 58-year-old male on anti-PD-1 monotherapy for metastatic colorectal cancer complicated by neurological and endocrine immune-related adverse events which required stopping and restarting the immunotherapy treatment. He finished his course of ICP therapy and received the first dose of the Pfizer vaccine 27 days later. Five days later, he presented with myalgia, diarrhea, fever, as well as elevated inflammatory markers, LDH, and thrombocytopenia. He was started on methylprednisolone for suspected cytokine release syndrome (CRS), and his symptoms resolved within seven days of treatment and was successfully restarted on the anti-PD-1 treatment. The vaccine was more likely to be the cause of CRS because the median time to CRS following immune checkpoint therapy is four weeks from initiation, and this patient began treatment 22 months prior [67].

Overall, the rates of AE varied across studies in cancer and non-cancer populations, however, reassuringly, reported AE tended to be mild, despite one isolated case of cytokine release syndrome following vaccination.

3.4. Lymphadenopathy Post-COVID-19 Vaccination in Cancer Patients

Lymphadenopathy signifies any inconsistency or abnormality in the lymph nodes; this abnormality can refer to the size, firmness, or number of lymph nodes in a given area of the body [68]. These lymphadenopathies can be a consequence of infections, including bacterial, viral, and parasitic causes. Recent studies have shown that unilateral lymphadenopathy has a great association with vaccines, such as the influenza vaccine, HPV vaccine, and BCG vaccine [69]. Post-vaccination lymphadenopathy may be falsely attributed to an oncological process in individuals who have been diagnosed with cancer, in remission, or at an increased risk of developing malignancies. As such, the possibility of post-vaccination lymphadenopathy must be considered in individuals who receive COVID-19 vaccinations, especially in patients with underlying or increased risk of oncological disorders [70]. Hypermetabolic lymphadenopathy refers to an abnormal lymph node which has an increased rate of metabolism, and this process can be visualized using an F-18 fluorodeoxyglucose positron emission tomography-computed tomography (FDG-PET-CT) scan. This scan utilizes radiotracers to map lesions that are metabolically active throughout the body, and FDG-PET-CT of the entire body is a component of the examination of cancer patients to evaluate progression of disease. However, FDG uptake is not unique to oncological disorders and can be seen in inflammatory or infectious conditions, which might be a consequence of vaccination [71].

Bshesh et al., reported 6022 cases of lymphadenopathy amongst COVID-19 vaccination recipients, of which 693 had confirmed malignancies [68]. All subjects in the studies conducted by Cohen et al., Eifer et al., and Bernstine et al., had underlying oncological disorders and were assessed for lymphadenopathy using FDG-PET-CT or other PET-CT tracers; relatively high rates of FDG-PET-CT positivity was reported amongst the cohorts [71–73]. Several studies have revealed that cancer patients had FDG-PET-CT hypermetabolic axillary lymph nodes and a focal hypermetabolic region in the ipsilateral deltoid muscle after Pfizer vaccination [71,73].

Cohen et al., reported that it may be difficult to distinguish between benign and malignant hyperactivity in lymph nodes, especially when vaccination was conducted on the same side, as the tumor is expected to undergo nodal drainage. Hence, the recommendation was made that patients with breast cancer, axillary lymphoma, and malignancy of the upper limb should not undergo vaccination in the arm that has a lymph node with expected nodal drainage of a tumor [72]. Placke et al., identified a further 8 patients with underlying melanoma or Meckel cell carcinoma who were misdiagnosed with lymph node metastases and underwent lymph node excision after COVID-19 vaccination [74]. The studies reiterate the notion that physicians must be aware of the possibility of post-vaccination lymphadenopathy when making diagnoses and management plans in patients with oncological disorders or complaints of a newly arising lymph node abnormality [75]. Studies reported that lymphadenopathy after COVID-19 vaccination should be considered reactive at first glance, due to stimulation of the immune system. If the patient has pre-existing unilateral cancer, vaccination should be given on the contralateral arm whenever feasible. Lymph nodes that are persistently enlarged several weeks later can be investigated for an underlying malignancy using fast, cost-effective methods such as fine needle aspiration [76]. In the context of breast cancer surgery, studies have recommended scheduling COVID-19 vaccination at least a week prior to surgery so that symptoms such as fever can be accurately attributed to a vaccination side effect rather than from surgery [77]. Moreover, vaccination is recommended at the contralateral side to the affected breast or the anterolateral thigh. Vaccination could also be done once the patient is recovered, one to two weeks after surgery. Ultimately, COVID-19 vaccination- induced reactive lymphadenopathy could possibly mask side effects of breast cancer surgery and the timing of vaccination should be modified accordingly [77]. If FDG-PET-CT is required urgently for cancer disease staging or treatment initiation, it is recommended that it should be attempted to be done prior to vaccination if possible. If the indication for FDG is not urgent, it is advised to delay or reschedule the scan. From clinical experiences from routine vaccinations, vaccine-induced lymphadenopathy typically arises within seven days of vaccination and resolves in twelve to fourteen days [78,79]. However, there have been reported instances of COVID-19 vaccine-related nodal FDG uptake up to four to six weeks after vaccination. Therefore, it is suggested that in patients with a cancer that is expected to be difficult to interpret with FDG after vaccination, the FDG-PET-CT scans should be delayed for at least two weeks unless there is a clinical indication which requires oncological imaging to be done sooner. More ideally, if oncological imaging is not urgent whatsoever, the FDG-PET-CT should be delayed for four to six weeks to circumvent possible confounding findings [80]. Becker et al., provides a set of recommendations for radiological management of post-vaccination adenopathy. They recommend observing for at least six weeks for resolution before referring for diagnostic imaging evaluation or biopsy of the nodes [81]. Moreover, if the cause of adenopathy is overwhelmingly likely to be due to recent vaccination than an underlying neoplasm, an expectant management strategy without default follow-up imaging is suggested. Imaging follow-up with ultrasound to assure resolution of adenopathy is recommended in high-risk patients such as one with ipsilateral breast cancer [81].

Lehman et al., recommends that vaccinations should not be delayed, and that vaccination history should be provided to the radiologist when they are interpreting imaging findings. In the context of known recent COVID-19 vaccination, the authors suggest that ipsilateral axillary lymphadenopathy can be managed clinically as there is a low pretest probability of malignant lymphadenopathy [82]. Lane et al., also suggests a conservative approach, but also recognizes that false nodal biopsy might be inevitable in certain breast cancer patients. To reduce false positive nodal findings post-vaccination, the history of COVID-19 vaccinations, number of doses and dates, as well as site and side of injection should be strictly documented at time of vaccine administration [83].

Locklin and Woodard state that mammographic findings such as trabecular and skin thickening, as well as increased echogenicity on ultrasound, can be visualized with edema secondary to poor lymphatic drainage or capillary leak, and should be kept in consideration as a potential etiology for breast edema after recent COVID-19 vaccination. They suggest that much like evaluations for suspected mastitis, imaging should be conducted for a short period to ensure resolution for patients with ipsilateral vaccinations histories. Inflammatory breast cancer can closely resemble inflammation and infection, and careful observation of resolution is important to not neglect cancer [84]. Chung et al., states that cortical thickness and its morphology on ultrasound are most helpful in distinguishing between malignancy or a benign reactive post-vaccination lymph node in the context of breast cancer. A cortical thickness threshold of 5.4 mm showed greatest specificity and accuracy for differentiating between benign and malignant processes. Moreover, completely hypoechoic nodes with no visible hila were observed in only malignant nodes [85]. Adin et al., reports a case of a patient with bilateral lymphadenopathy, one due to an ipsilateral breast malignancy and the contralateral one due to recent COVID-19 vaccination. The malignant node demonstrated asymmetric cortical thickening and marked cortical enhancement compared to the reactive node, further supporting Chung et al.'s findings [86]. Granata et al., identified that lymphangitis is also a possible consequence of COVID-19 vaccination. This must be considered with possible lymphadenopathies, to avoid alarmism in patients and physicians alike. Having knowledge of such a possibility allows for avoidance of economic waste via the utilization of several radiological studies in the hunt for a tumor that is likely not there [87].

4. Hesitancy/Acceptance of the COVID-19 Vaccination among Cancer Patients

The lower immunogenicity in cancer patients has been responsible for higher rates of infection in patients with cancer as well as higher risk of developing serious complication and death. The inadequate serological response can be attributed to malignancy-related immune dysregulation as well as a greater likelihood of co-morbid conditions in patients with cancer. In addition, cancer treatments contribute to immune suppression making it difficult to confer adequate immunity against many infections including COVID-19. As a result, patients with cancer are considered high risk and have been given priority in most vaccine rollout programs. However, hesitancy of receiving the COVID-19 vaccines among cancer patients has been widely reported.

4.1. Major Reasons for COVID-19 Vaccination Hesitancy

Studies from several countries explored the rate of vaccine acceptance among cancer patients and the reasons behind their hesitancy. With the initial rollout of vaccines, hesitancy among cancer patient was higher than the public. Similarly, in a cross-sectional study of 111 cancer patients from a Lebanese institution, 14.4% refused to get the vaccine while 30.6% were hesitant [88]. The main reason for refusal was the patient's belief that vaccines were incompatible with their disease or treatment while hesitant patients wanted more information about the risk of vaccination in cancer patients and its efficacy [88]. Cross-sectional surveys done in Poland, Mexico, Bosnia and Herzegovina, Hong Kong, and Germany all revealed considerable rates of vaccine hesitancy in cancer patients, with vaccine acceptance rates of 58.8% out of 644 patients, 66% of 540 breast cancer patients, 41.8% of 364 cancer patients, 17.9% of 660 cancer patients and 62% of 101 patients respectively [89–93]. The studies reported the reasons for hesitancy/rejection, some of which were similar to the reasons for vaccination hesitancy among the public. For example, some patients were skeptical of how rapidly the vaccines were developed, with major concerns of the side effects post-vaccination. Others believed that their natural immunity could provide enough protection against COVID-19. However, some concerns were unique to cancer patients. Since the main clinical trials excluded immunocompromised patients including cancer patients, there was a concern of the applicability of the reported safety and efficacy of the vaccines in cancer patients. Additionally, concerns regarding the effect of cancer treatments on the vaccine's safety and its possible interaction with cancer treatments were expressed. In one study that included 767 cancer patients, there were 447 unvaccinated individuals among them, of which 52% reported their preference to end cancer treatment before receiving the vaccine [3]. Patients from another study were most concerned that vaccine-related adverse events would worsen current anti-cancer therapy side effects (29%) and that there is not enough information regarding the safety of the COVID-19 vaccine in cancer patients undergoing oncological therapy (27%) [93].

4.2. Significantly Associated Factors with Vaccine Hesitancy/Acceptance

Several studies investigated factors that were associated with increased vaccine hesitancy. Mistrust in the health care system (OR 8.79, 95% CI [4.26–18.15]), noncompliance with prior influenza immunization (OR 2.27, 95% CI [1.57–3.29]), and low educational attainment (OR 1.84, 95% CI [1.17–2.89]) were all associated with increased vaccine hesitancy [90]. Higher education was also associated with increased vaccine acceptance ($p = 0.0056$) [89]. Interestingly, patients who routinely received the influenza vaccine were much more accepting of COVID vaccination, with 91.6% acceptance (14,905/16,269) compared to the 45.9% (2083/4545) acceptance prevalence among those who did not routinely receive an influenza vaccine ($p < 0.001$) [94]. In a separate study of 200 Tunisian cancer patients, the willingness to receive influenza vaccine was significantly associated with COVID-19 vaccine acceptance (OR = 3.9, 95% CI [1.6–9.3]; $p = 0.002$) [95]. These studies suggest that a general distrust in vaccines or a lack of appreciation of the severity of COVID-19 infections may contribute to the vaccine hesitancy expressed among cancer patients. A general distrust in the country's healthcare system and its ability to effectively rollout a vaccination program has also been associated with vaccine hesitancy [96]. A study conducted in China that included 744 breast cancer survivors revealed that vaccine hesitancy or refusal was expressed by over 73% of the respondents [97]. The primary reason for hesitancy or refusal in 46% of patients was the lack of knowledge about the safety of the vaccines for cancer patients. Factors associated with vaccine hesitancy/refusal included current endocrine or targeted therapy (OR 1.52, 95% CI [1.03–2.24]) and no notification from communities or units (OR 2.46, 95% CI [1.69–3.59]). This demonstrated that many cancer patients were unaware of the effect of COVID-19 vaccines on cancer treatments and preferred to avoid the risk of any possible complications. Similarly, in a separate study, current endocrine or targeted therapy was associated with increased vaccine hesitancy (OR 1.52, 95% CI [1.03–2.24]) [97].

4.3. How to Combat Vaccination Hesitancy among Cancer Patients?

Current guidelines indicate that COVID-19 vaccines are safe and recommended in the majority of cancer patients, including patients undergoing therapy, with few exceptions. Better education and dissemination of information to patients with cancer is needed to combat vaccine hesitancy. Several ways to combat vaccine hesitancy have been suggested, the most prominent being the increased advocacy by oncologists and primary physicians. Patients indicated that they are most likely to listen to their oncologists regarding recommendations of vaccination. In a German survey of 425 cancer patients, around 85% of participants claimed to trust their attending physician's recommendations regarding the COVID-19 vaccines [98]. Similarly, Villarreal-Garza et al., reported that 64.5% of the hesitant patients would consider receiving the vaccine if recommended by their oncologists [90]. Marijanović et al., conveyed that the majority of participants (82.4%) stated recommendation by their oncologist could influence their decision about vaccination [91]. One study in Korea showed that the initial rate of vaccine acceptance was 61% of the 1001 cancer patients surveyed. The rate increased to 91% of participants who received their attending physician's recommendation for vaccination [99]. Results from several other studies further support the notion that recommendations coming from a patient's oncologist would be well received by cancer patients [97,100]. Therefore, it is imperative that all oncological providers are well informed of the most accurate and up-to-date recommendations regarding vaccination and to start discussions with their patients to address their concerns. Figure 2 summarizes the reasons behind, and factors associated with vaccination hesitancy or acceptance among cancer patients compiled from the above-mentioned studies and the suggested ways to combat such hesitancy.

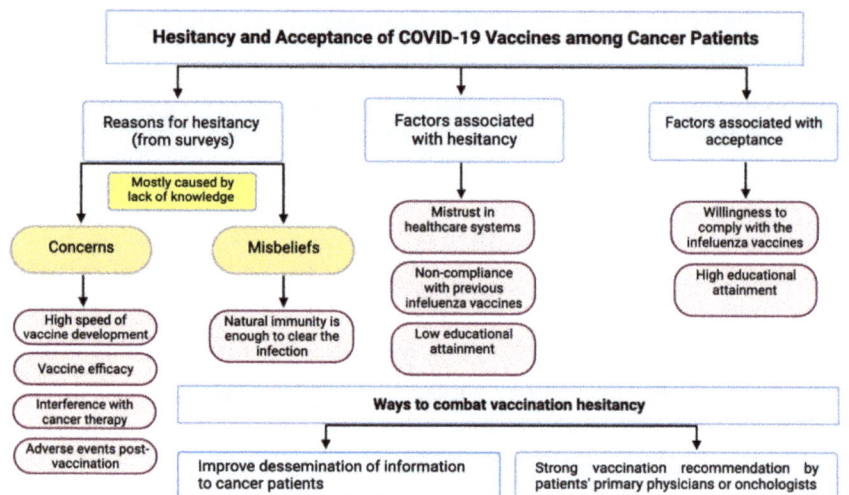

Figure 2. Reasons for and factors associated with vaccination hesitancy or acceptance among cancer patients compiled from studies which conducted surveys in different countries and the suggested ways to combat such hesitancy.

5. Ongoing Clinical Trials and Future Challenges

As of date, fifteen interventional/clinical trials that explore the immunogenicity and safety of COVID-19 vaccines in cancer patients are listed on ClinicalTrials.gov [101]. These studies, outlined with their identifiers in Table 1, take place worldwide across Europe, Asia, North America, and Australia. The listed trials include participants with both hematologic & solid malignancies; a few of the trials focus on immunocompromised patients, including transplant recipients, patients with human immunodeficiency virus (HIV), or patients with malignancy or autoimmune disease receiving chemotherapy, radiotherapy, anti-PD-1 therapy, anti-PD-L1 therapy, or anti-CD20 therapy. Three of the trials have published results which demonstrated lower seropositivity rates in cancer populations compared to healthy controls, but highlight the ability for cancer patients to achieve seroconversion and an increase in anti-SARS-CoV-2 antibody following a third booster dose of the vaccine [1,102,103]. As most of these trials are still ongoing, shortcomings have not yet been clearly identified, but the finalized trials indicated a need for studies with larger sample sizes to determine the effective vaccine type and dosage appropriate for cancer patients, with the aim to provide protection against COVID-19 without disrupting cancer therapy [1].

Table 1. Current Clinical Trials Investigating COVID-19 Vaccination in Patients with Cancer or Immunocompromised States.

Study Title & ClinicalTrials.gov Identifier	Country	Study Phase	Primary Outcome Measures	Study Participants & Inclusion Criteria	Intervention & Model	Results
Evaluation of the Effect and Side Effect Profile of COVID-19 Vaccine in Cancer Patients Identifier: NCT04771559 [1,101]	Turkey	Complete	COVID-19 antibody titers. Time frame: 1 month	N = 1500 Patient group: Individuals aged 18+ diagnosed with cancer, who had received two doses of the COVID-19 vaccine Control group: Individuals aged 18+ with no history of cancer, who had received two doses of the COVID-19 vaccine	Intervention: COVID-19 antibody test. Non-randomized, parallel assignment	Seropositivity rates at one month: Patient group: 85.2% Control group: 97.5% ($p < 0.001$) Lower seropositivity in cancer patients associated with chemotherapy and age 60+ ($p < 0.001$)
Immune Response to the COVID-19 Vaccine Identifier: NCT04936997 [101,102]	USA	Early Phase 1	Immune response to 2nd COVID-19 vaccination booster (3rd vaccine) in patients with solid malignancies on immunosuppressive therapy Time frame: 3 months	N = 20 Patient group: Individuals aged 18+ with active solid tumor malignancy on active chemotherapy, who had received two doses of the Pfizer COVID-19 vaccine	Intervention: SARS-COV2 Pfizer Vaccine Single group assignment	80% (16/20) of participants demonstrated a median threefold increase in antibody response one week following a third dose of the Pfizer vaccine. No improvement was noted in T-cell responses. Adverse events were mild in nature.
Impact of the Immune System on Response to Anti-Coronavirus Disease 19 (COVID-19) Vaccine in Allogeneic Stem Cell Recipients (Covid Vaccin Allo) Identifier: NCT04951323 [101]	Belgium	Phase 3	Quantification of anti-SARS-CoV-2 IgG antibodies after vaccination in allogenic stem cell recipients Time frame: 49 days following first injection	Estimated N = 50 Patient group: Individuals aged 18+ who had undergone allogeneic hematopoietic stem cell transplantation 3 months to 5 months prior. Patients were excluded if they had active malignant disease at the time of inclusion	Intervention: Anti-COVID19 mRNA-based vaccine (BNT162b2, Comirnaty®, commercialized by Pfizer) Single group assignment	N/A

Table 1. Cont.

Study Title & ClinicalTrials.gov Identifier	Country	Study Phase	Primary Outcome Measures	Study Participants & Inclusion Criteria	Intervention & Model	Results
Safety and Immunogenicity of COVID-19 Vaccination in Patients With Cancer Identifier: NCT05018078 [101]	China	N/A	Primary Outcome 1: Safety of the COVID-19 vaccine, monitoring the occurrence of adverse effects Time frame: Within 2 months following the first vaccine dose Primary Outcome 2: Immunogenicity of the COVID-19 vaccine, measuring antibody titers against SARS-CoV-2 Time frame: Within 2 months following the first vaccine dose	Estimated N = 300 Patient group: Individuals aged 18+, with a cancer diagnosis including hepatocellular carcinoma, breast cancer, lung cancer, esophageal cancer, gastric cancer or colorectal cancer. Individuals must have local or systemic anti-cancer therapies previously or currently; in stable condition according to the treatment guidelines with an Eastern Cooperative Oncology Group (ECOG) score below 2. Additionally, patients must have normal or basically normal multi-organ function, without contraindications to vaccination	Intervention: Coronavirus vaccine Single group assignment	N/A
A Trial of the Safety and Immunogenicity of the COVID-19 Vaccine (mRNA-1273) in Participants With Hematologic Malignancies and Various Regimens of Immunosuppression, and in Participants With Solid Tumors on PD1/PDL1 Inhibitor Therapy, Including Booster Doses of Vaccine Identifier: NCT04847050 [101]	USA	Phase 2	Primary Outcome 1: Safety and reactogenicity of the mRNA-1273 vaccine, soliciting local and systemic adverse reactions 7 days after each injection, and unsolicited adverse events up to 28 days post-injection Time frame: 14 months Primary Outcome 2: Immunogenicity of the mRNA-1273 vaccine in patients with a hematological malignancy and are immunosuppressed due to their disease, and/or receiving PD-1/PDL-1 inhibitor for treatment of a solid tumor. Measured titers of specific binding antibody (bAb) on day 1, 29, 36, 57, 209, and 394 Time frame: 14 months	Estimated N = 220 Patient group: Individuals aged 18+ with either: - Solid tumor diagnosis, receiving PD1/PDL1 inhibitor treatment, - Diagnosis of acute leukemia (myeloid (AML) or lymphoid (ALL) or other); multiple myeloma; Waldenstrom macroglobulinemia, or - Diagnosis of lymphoma, including chronic lymphocytic leukemia Individuals must demonstrate adequate organ and bone marrow function on laboratory assessment within 4 weeks of vaccine administration	Intervention: mRNA-1273 injection. Non-randomized, parallel assignment	N/A

Table 1. *Cont.*

Study Title & ClinicalTrials.gov Identifier	Country	Study Phase	Primary Outcome Measures	Study Participants & Inclusion Criteria	Intervention & Model	Results
The Immune Reaction Upon COVID-19 Vaccination in the Belgian Cancer Population. Identifier: NCT05033158 [101]	Belgium	N/A	Immune response measuring quantification of anti-SARS-CoV-2 IgG antibodies (against full Spike, S1, S2, RBD, and N proteins) 4 weeks after first vaccine administration Time frame: 4 months	Estimated N = 3000 Patient group: Individuals aged 18+ with oncological or hematological malignancy, or a history of it, with a life expectancy >3 months	Intervention: Blood sampling Single group assignment	N/A
SARS-CoV-2 Vaccine (COH04S1) Versus Emergency Use Authorization SARS-COV-2 Vaccine for the Treatment of COVID-19 in Patients With Blood Cancer Identifier: NCT04977024 [101]	USA	Phase 2	Biological response, based on at least a 3-fold increase in anti-SARS-CoV-2 antibodies or interferon gamma levels Time frame: At 28 days post the second vaccine injection	Estimated N = 240 Patient group: Individuals aged 18+ with hematologic malignancy and an ECOG score of 2 or less. They must have received either allogenic or autologous hematopoietic cell transplant, or cellular therapy (chimeric antigen receptor [CAR] T-cell) therapy and be at least 3 months post treatment infusion	Interventions: COVID-19 Vaccine, Diagnostic Laboratory Biomarker Analysis, and Synthetic MVA-based SARS-CoV-2 Vaccine COH04S1 Randomized. parallel assignment	N/A
Safety and Immunogenicity of Prime-boost Vaccination of SARS-CoV-2 in Patients With Cancer Identifier: NCT05273541 [101]	China	Phase 1 Phase 2	Primary Outcome 1: Determining the safety of the prime-boost vaccine, measuring the occurrence of adverse effects post-vaccination Time frame: Within 1 week after the prime-boost vaccination Primary Outcome 2: Determining immunogenicity by titers of anti-SARS-CoV-2 antibodies Time frame: Within 3 months after the prime-boost vaccination	Estimated N = 100 Patient group: Individuals aged 18+, with a cancer diagnosis including hepatocellular carcinoma, breast cancer, lung cancer, esophageal cancer, gastric cancer or colorectal cancer. Individuals must have local or systemic anti-cancer therapies previously or currently, in stable condition according to the treatment guidelines with an ECOG score below 2. Additionally, patients must have normal or basically normal multi-organ function, without contraindications to vaccination.	Intervention: Coronavirus vaccination Single group assignment	N/A

Table 1. *Cont.*

Study Title & ClinicalTrials.gov Identifier	Country	Study Phase	Primary Outcome Measures	Study Participants & Inclusion Criteria	Intervention & Model	Results
Study Evaluating SARS-CoV-2 (COVID-19) Humoral Response After BNT162b2 Vaccine in Immunocompromised Adults Compared to Healthy Adults Identifier: NCT04952766 [101]	France	Phase 4	Protective humoral response post-vaccination, measuring the proportion of immunocompromised individuals with neutralizing activity against the "Wuhan" stain of SARS-CoV-2, as compared to healthy subjects Time frame: 2 months	N = 196 Adult volunteers belonging to one of the following groups: Immunocompromised group (~15 participants per subgroup): - Kidney transplant - Extracorporeal dialysis - Solid cancer, receiving chemotherapy and/or radiotherapy - Myeloma, receiving chemotherapy - Hematologic malignancy, receiving chemotherapy - Diseases treated with anti-CD20 (or, patients not treated at the time of vaccination, but will be immediately after) - Multiple sclerosis, receiving anti-CD20 (or, patients not treated at the time of vaccination, but will be immediately after) - Common variable immune deficiency, or other causes of severe hypogammaglobulinemia requiring chronic treatment with polyvalent immunoglobulin - Malignant tumor, receiving anti-PD1 or anti-PDL1 therapy - HIV - Complicated type 2 diabetes (with micro and/or macroangiopathy) Non-immunocompromised group: vaccinated with either Comirnaty TM or AstraZeneca's Vaxzevria TM for the first dose	Intervention: Biological samples Single group assignment	N/A

Table 1. *Cont.*

Study Title & ClinicalTrials.gov Identifier	Country	Study Phase	Primary Outcome Measures	Study Participants & Inclusion Criteria	Intervention & Model	Results
COVID-19 VAX Booster Dosing in Patients With Hematologic Malignancies Identifier: NCT05028374 [101]	USA	Phase 2	Seroconversion rates of anti-SARS-CoV-2 antibody following a booster dose of the Moderna mRNA COVID-19 vaccine Time frame: 28 (±3 days) following booster dose	N = 119 Patient group: Individuals aged 18+ who have been previously diagnosed with multiple myeloma (MM)/amyloid light-chain amyloidosis, or other hematologic malignancy. They must have previously received any one of the available COVID-19 vaccines between 4–36 months prior to study enrollment, with anti-SARS-CoV-2 IgG titers less than 1.0 unit, or between 1.0–1.99 units. If patients are currently receiving potentially immunosuppressive cancer therapy, a two-week interruption before and after the booster dose of the vaccine is encouraged, but not required (at physician discretion)	Intervention: A single "booster" dose of the Moderna mRNA COVID-19 vaccine Single group assignment	N/A
Booster Dose Trial Identifier: NCT05016622 [101]	USA	Phase 2	Rates of seroconversion for SARS-CoV-2 anti-spike antibody Time frame: 4 weeks after booster dose	Estimated N = 100 Patient group: Individuals aged 18+ with a known diagnosis of any malignancy (either active or post completion of therapy), with negative SARS-CoV-2 spike IgG at least 14 days post-2nd dose of an mRNA-based COVID-19 vaccine, or 28 days after a single dose of the adenovirus-based Johnson & Johnson vaccine	Intervention: BNT162b2 vaccine Single group assignment	N/A

Table 1. *Cont.*

Study Title & ClinicalTrials.gov Identifier	Country	Study Phase	Primary Outcome Measures	Study Participants & Inclusion Criteria	Intervention & Model	Results
Passive Antibodies Against COVID-19 With EVUSHELD in Vaccine Non-responsive CLL Identifier: NCT05465876 [101]	Canada	Phase 2	Conferring passive immunity to CLL patients, measuring the proportion of participants with anti-spike antibodies after EVUSHELD administration Time frame: 12 months	Estimated N = 200 Patient group: Individuals aged 18+ with a diagnosis of CLL, who are either treatment-naïve, post-treatment, or on-treatment for CLL, and an ECOG score between 0–2. They must have received at least two doses of the Pfizer, Moderna, or AstraZeneca COVID-19 vaccines between 28 days-18 months prior to enrollment, demonstrating absent or suboptimal response. Participants must weigh at least 40 kg, have adequate organ function laboratory values, and have a life expectancy >6 months	Intervention: EVUSHELD Single group assignment	N/A
Bringing Optimised COVID-19 Vaccine Schedules To ImmunoCompromised Populations (BOOST-IC): an Adaptive Randomised Controlled Clinical Trial Identifier: NCT05556720 [101]	Australia	Phase 3	Measuring the geometric mean concentration (GMC) of anti-spike SARS-CoV-2 IgG antibody Time frame: 28 days after completion of vaccination trials	Estimated N = 960 Patient group: Individuals aged 16+ who have completed 3-5 doses of an Australian Therapeutic Goods Administration approved COVID-19 vaccine (Pfizer, Moderna, AstraZeneca, or Novavax). Patients must be in one of the following populations: - HIV infection, - Current recipient of a solid organ transplant, including kidney, pancreas, liver, malignancy episodes of severe rejection, requiring T- or B-cell depletion in the past 3 months, or - Undergoing chemotherapy, immunotherapy, and/or targeted therapy, or completed said therapies within the past 2 years in treatment of CLL, MM, or non-Hodgkin lymphoma	Interventions: BNT162b2, mRNA-1273, or NVX-COV2373 Randomized, parallel assignment	N/A

Table 1. *Cont.*

Study Title & ClinicalTrials.gov Identifier	Country	Study Phase	Primary Outcome Measures	Study Participants & Inclusion Criteria	Intervention & Model	Results
Anti-COVID-19 Vaccine in Children With Acute Leukemia and Their Siblings Identifier: NCT04969601 [101]	France	Phase 1 Phase 2	Primary Objective 1: Dose limiting toxicity, determined by the presence of grade ≥3 adverse events within 7 days following vaccine injection, that are deemed to be related to the vaccine Time frame: Within 7 days from first dose Primary Objective 2: Four-times or higher increase in the anti-spike IgG titer, AND positive anti-spike neutralizing test, indicating significant seroconversion Time frame: At 2 months from first dose	Estimated N = 150 Patient group: Individuals aged 1–15 years, with either: - Acute lymphoblastic leukemia (ALL), undergoing chemotherapy (within 2 weeks from the last injection) or for whom the last chemotherapy treatment was less than/equal to 12 months, or - Acute myeloid leukemia (AML) within 12 months from the end of treatment Control group: Healthy siblings aged 1–15 years, living in the same household as the child with ALL/AML more than 50% of the time	Intervention: Vaccine COMIRNATY® (BNT162b2) Single group assignment	N/A
Safety, Efficacy of BNT162b2 mRNA Vaccine in CLL Identifier: NCT04862806 [101,103]	Israel	Complete	Primary Objective 1: Change in the number of participants with adverse events related to the BNT162b2 mRNA vaccine, assessed by a questionnaire with answers reported on a scale of 0–5 Time frame: 2–6 weeks after 2nd vaccination, 3 months after 2nd vaccination, 6 months after 2nd vaccination Primary Objective 2: Antibody persistence following the 3rd dose of the BNT162b2 mRNA vaccine in seronegative patients with chronic lymphocytic leukemia Time frame: 6 months	Estimated N = 1000 Patient group: Individuals aged 18+ with a diagnosis of CLL, who have received two 30-µg doses of BNT162b2 3 weeks apart	Intervention: COVID-19 serology Single group assignment	Of patients with CLL who failed to demonstrate a seropositive response following two doses of the BNT162b2 vaccine, nearly one fourth responded to a third dose of the vaccine. However, antibody responses were lower in patients undergoing active treatment, and patients with recent exposure (<12 months prior) to anti-CD20 therapy

Abbreviations: COVID-19, coronavirus disease 2019; USA, United States of America; SARS-CoV-2, severe acute respiratory syndrome coronavirus 2; IgG, immunoglobulin G; mRNA, messenger RNA; BNT162b2 and COMIRNATY, Pfizer BioNTech COVID-19 Vaccine; ECOG, Eastern Cooperative Oncology Group; mRNA-1273, Moderna COVID-19 Vaccine; PD-1, Programmed cell death protein 1; PD-L1, Programmed death-ligand 1; bAb, binding antibody; ALL, acute lymphoblastic leukemia; S1, spike protein subunit 1; S2, spike protein subunit 2; RBD, receptor-binding domain; COH04S1, City of Hope-developed COVID-19 vaccine; CAR T-cell, chimeric antigen receptor T-cell; MVA, modified vaccinia Ankara; CD-20, B-lymphocyte antigen CD20; HIV, human immunodeficiency virus; MM, multiple myeloma; EVUSHELD, tixagevimab and cilgavimab; CLL, chronic lymphocytic leukemia; GMC, geometric mean concentration; NVX-COV2373, Novavax COVID-19 Vaccine.

6. Discussion

The initial clinical trials for COVID-19 vaccines did not provide data for cancer patients. Despite this, not many large-scale trials studying the efficacy of COVID-19 vaccines in cancer patients exist, though smaller trials around the world have provided some evidence. Cancer patients were found to have significantly diminished serological response after the first dose of the COVID-19 vaccine, but the second dose indicated an increased immune response but was still reduced when compared to healthy controls [17]. Antibody titers were lower in patients with hematological malignancies as compared to solid tumors [17]. Furthermore, chemotoxic treatments showed a diminishing effect on the serological antibodies [17,28]. Immunotherapy such anti-CD20 therapy and targeted therapies like tyrosine kinase inhibitors also resulted in a drop in serological response. Both chemotherapy and immunotherapy showed a positive correlation between time lapsed after treatment and serological response. Patients receiving only CPI were found to have higher titers of antibodies when compared to other combinations of treatments [52]. Data are still lacking on the difference of immunogenicity in cancer patient between different vaccines as most clinical trials did not assess or include cancer patients. For instance, cancer patients with immunodeficiency, as well as those receiving radiotherapy and chemotherapy were not allowed to be part of the Phase III clinical trial of Pfizer's COVID-19 vaccine due to concerns about immunosuppression [104]. Overall, even though the immunological response is not as robust in cancer patients, most trials still report a long-term seropositivity of 70–88% [52]. Figure 3 summarizes the effect of different factors on the immunogenicity of COVID-19 vaccines in cancer patients including the different types of anti-cancer therapy.

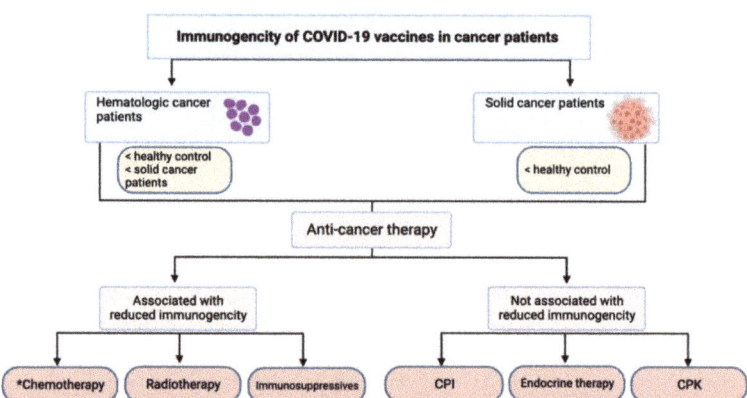

Figure 3. Immunogenicity of COVID-19 vaccines in cancer patients with hematologic or solid cancers and the effect of different types of anti-cancer therapy on the immunogenicity. Immunogenicity was measured in most of the studies by rates of seropositivity and/or antibody titers. * Only chemotherapy was reported to reduce both rates of seropositivity and antibody titers.

Cancer treatments impair immunogenicity through different modes of actions. Cytotoxic chemotherapies interfere with DNA replication and synthesis and can disrupt the proliferation of lymphocytes during immune activation. Similarly, targeted therapies like anti-CD20 agents, tyrosine kinase inhibitors, and CAR T-cell therapy can severely deplete peripheral B-cell populations and affect various cytokine pathways needed to respond to vaccine introduced antigens [17]. An exception to this includes immune check-point inhibitors, a form of immunotherapy that enhances the immune system to detect and target cancerous cells. This could explain why cancer patients being treated with immunotherapy alone have a higher serological response than those on other combinations of treatments.

Several new trials have reported that COVID-19 vaccines have shown similar safety profiles in cancer patients as compared to the general population. The most common local and systemic side effects were pain at injection site, myalgia, and fatigue [17]. These were mostly mild to moderate in severity in both the general population and patients with cancer [17]. Notably, lymphadenopathy being an expected side effect of the Pfizer vaccine may alarm cancer patients as they may attribute swollen lymph nodes to malignancy [105]. No difference in adverse events was observed between hematological or solid malignancies or between patients undergoing cancer treatment and those who were treatment-naïve [4,17,103].

Immune-related adverse events, although rare, are still observed in the general population. However, in cancer patients these immune-related adverse events might be triggered by immune dysregulation caused by the underlying disease pathophysiology of malignancy as well as the effects of different treatments. One group of treatments that has posed a particular concern are CPI, which are being increasingly used to treat cancer patients [106]. These agents activate the immune system by targeting pathways that regulate programmed cell death (PD-1 and cytotoxic T-lymphocyte-associated protein 4 (CTLA-4) in T-cells [107]. This immune activation can, on the one hand, enhance the immunogenicity of COVID-19 vaccines and can, on the other hand, lead to uncontrolled immune activation, triggering an "inflammatory storm" in response to vaccine components [107]. No increased incidence of immune-related adverse events have been observed in cancer patients being treated with CPI [108]. However, vaccine administration to patients on combined CPI therapy (anti-PD-1, anti-PD-L1 and anti-CTLA-4) causes some concern due to the possible risk of immune-related adverse events [109]. It was suggested that myelitis may occur due to interleukin-6 (IL-6) and interleukin-17 (IL-17) running an inflammatory response leading to cytokine storm [110]. One example is atezolizumab, a monoclonal antibody which binds to tumor cells expressing PD-L1; this inhibits binding with T-cell expressed PD-1 and B7.1 receptors, allowing activation and proliferation of T-cells and enhanced function and memory cell formation to fight the tumor. Vaccine -induced causes of inflammation are less known, with active antigens in the vaccine or other constituents such as adjuvants causing inflammation. Some could also have an autoimmune reaction in the presence or absence of molecular mimicry [110]. Au et al., suggested that immune checkpoint therapy blocks PD-1, allowing for T-cell proliferation, causing patients to have an increased baseline of activated T-cells. When the vaccine was given, this tipped the immune system to CRS. However, S-reactive T-cells were not detected in the periphery, making this less likely. However, the T-cells associated with CRS could reside in tissue or lymph nodes, making them undetectable in blood [67]. Mei et al., speculated that giving the COVID-19 vaccine and anti-PD1 therapy within close temporal proximity of each other may enhance co-stimulatory and reduce co-inhibitory regulation, accounting for the increase in mild AEs in vaccinated patients. Additionally, they also speculated that this increase in immune response allows for the chemotherapy to work more effectively, consistent with their finding of vaccinated patients having higher disease control rates [66].

7. Conclusions and Recommendations

This review focused on the immunogenicity and safety of COVID-19 vaccination among cancer patients, as well as vaccine hesitancy. Malignancy was described to lower seropositivity rates, most notably in patients with hematologic malignancies compared to those with solid cancers. While active cancer therapy in general showed significantly lower seroconversion rates, specific cancer therapies associated with decreased vaccine immunogenicity included chemotherapy, radiotherapy, and immunosuppressives, as compared to healthy controls. Chemotherapy specifically showed lower seropositivity and antibody titers compared to cancer patients receiving other treatments. On the other hand, CPI, endocrine therapy, and CDK inhibitors were not found to affect seropositivity. Many effects of therapy on immunogenicity are not well described but are likely to be secondary to a medication mechanism of action.

COVID-19 vaccination amongst individuals with cancer is well-tolerated and generally safe, with similar rates of adverse events in patients without cancer, with a history of cancer, or those receiving active treatment compared to healthy controls. Though rare, radiation recall phenomenon was reported in those receiving radiotherapy, and higher rates of muscle pain was noted in patients receiving CPI. Post-vaccination lymphadenopathy was a common adverse event that may be mistaken for malignancy despite being of inflammatory origin. Despite the overall safety profile, vaccine hesitancy remains due to lack of knowledge regarding compatibility with disease, risks, efficacy, side effects, and concerns about interactions with cancer therapies. A lack of information regarding vaccine safety among this population, as well as a lack of appreciation for the severity of COVID-19 infections further contribute to hesitancy. Factors associated with increased hesitancy include mistrust in the healthcare system, non-compliance with prior influenza immunization, and low educational attainment; increased acceptance was seen among patients with higher education and those willing to routinely receive the influenza vaccine.

Despite the reported lower immunogenicity of the COVID-19 vaccines in cancer patients receiving certain types of anti-cancer treatments as compared to healthy controls or to cancer patients receiving other types of treatments, booster doses were noted to statistically increase seroconversion rates amongst various cancer types and treatments, and therefore were recommended for cancer patients. Furthermore, neither cancer nor cancer therapy were viewed as contraindications to COVID-19 vaccination in the reviewed studies. Regarding lymphadenopathy, it is recommended that vaccination is not delayed, and that vaccination history is provided to the radiologist if a patient is scanned for concerning lymphadenopathy. To reduce false positive nodal findings post-vaccination, the history of COVID-19 vaccinations, number of doses and dates, as well as site and side of injection should be strictly documented at time of vaccine administration. As it may be difficult to distinguish between benign and malignant hyperactivity in lymph nodes, it is recommended that patients with breast cancer, axillary lymphoma, and malignancy of the upper limb should not undergo vaccination in the arm that has a lymph node with expected nodal drainage of a tumor. Vaccine hesitancy can be combatted with better education and dissemination of information to cancer patients, and patients generally demonstrated more compliance when primary physicians and oncologists recommended the vaccine and provided sufficient information.

Author Contributions: Conceptualization, D.Z.; writing—original draft preparation, M.A., (K.B., W.K., M.M., M.A.S., A.S. and A.L.V. equally contributed), N.E. and D.Z.; figures, N.E.; writing—review & editing, M.A.; visualization, M.A. and D.Z.; supervision, D.Z.; project administration, D.Z. All authors have read and agreed to the published version of the manuscript.

Funding: This research received no external funding.

Acknowledgments: We thank Weill Cornell Medicine-Qatar for its support. We also would like to thank Zain Burney, Cleveland Clinic, for his valuable suggestions. The publication of this article was funded by the Weill Cornell Medicine—Qatar Health Sciences Library.

Conflicts of Interest: The authors declare no conflict of interest.

References

1. Yasin, A.I.; Aydin, S.G.; Sümbül, B.; Koral, L.; Simşek, M.; Geredeli, Ç.; Öztürk, A.; Perkin, P.; Demirtaş, D.; Erdemoglu, E.; et al. Efficacy and Safety Profile of COVID-19 Vaccine in Cancer Patients: A Prospective, Multicenter Cohort Study. *Futur. Oncol.* **2022**, *18*, 1235–1244. [CrossRef] [PubMed]
2. Liu, C.; Zhao, Y.; Okwan-Duodu, D.; Basho, R.; Cui, X. COVID-19 in Cancer Patients: Risk, Clinical Features, and Management. *Cancer Biol. Med.* **2020**, *17*, 519–527. [CrossRef] [PubMed]
3. Matovina Brko, G.; Popovic, M.; Jovic, M.; Radic, J.; Bodlovic Kladar, M.; Nikolic, I.; Vidovic, V.; Kolarov Bjelobrk, I.; Kukic, B.; Salma, S.; et al. COVID-19 Vaccines and Cancer Patients: Acceptance, Attitudes and Safety. *JBUON* **2021**, *26*, 2188–2195.
4. Monin, L.; Laing, A.G.; Muñoz-Ruiz, M.; McKenzie, D.R.; del Molino del Barrio, I.; Alaguthurai, T.; Domingo-Vila, C.; Hayday, T.S.; Graham, C.; Seow, J.; et al. Safety and Immunogenicity of One versus Two Doses of the COVID-19 Vaccine BNT162b2 for Patients with Cancer: Interim Analysis of a Prospective Observational Study. *Lancet Oncol.* **2021**, *22*, 765–778. [CrossRef]
5. Sinha, S.; Kundu, C.N. Cancer and COVID-19: Why Are Cancer Patients More Susceptible to COVID-19? *Med. Oncol.* **2021**, *38*, 101. [CrossRef]

6. Wu, F.; Zhao, S.; Yu, B.; Chen, Y.M.; Wang, W.; Song, Z.G.; Hu, Y.; Tao, Z.W.; Tian, J.H.; Pei, Y.Y.; et al. A New Coronavirus Associated with Human Respiratory Disease in China. *Nature* **2020**, *579*, 265. [CrossRef]
7. Smith, J.C.; Sausville, E.L.; Girish, V.; Yuan, M.L.; Vasudevan, A.; John, K.M.; Sheltzer, J.M. Cigarette Smoke Exposure and Inflammatory Signaling Increase the Expression of the SARS-CoV-2 Receptor ACE2 in the Respiratory Tract. *Dev. Cell* **2020**, *53*, 514–529.e3. [CrossRef]
8. Sica, A.; Colombo, M.P.; Trama, A.; Horn, L.; Garassino, M.C.; Torri, V. Immunometabolic Status of COVID-19 Cancer Patients. *Physiol. Rev.* **2020**, *100*, 1839. [CrossRef]
9. Ligumsky, H.; Safadi, E.; Etan, T.; Vaknin, N.; Waller, M.; Croll, A.; Nikolaevski-Berlin, A.; Greenberg, I.; Halperin, T.; Wasserman, A.; et al. Immunogenicity and Safety of the BNT162b2 MRNA COVID-19 Vaccine Among Actively Treated Cancer Patients. *JNCI J. Natl. Cancer Inst.* **2022**, *114*, 203–209. [CrossRef]
10. Palaia, I.; Caruso, G.; Di Donato, V.; Vestri, A.; Napoli, A.; Perniola, G.; Casinelli, M.; Alunni Fegatelli, D.; Campagna, R.; Tomao, F.; et al. Pfizer-BioNTech COVID-19 Vaccine in Gynecologic Oncology Patients: A Prospective Cohort Study. *Vaccines* **2021**, *10*, 12. [CrossRef]
11. Margalit, O.; Shacham-Shmueli, E.; Itay, A.; Berger, R.; Halperin, S.; Jurkowicz, M.; Levin, E.G.; Olmer, L.; Regev-Yochay, G.; Lustig, Y.; et al. Seropositivity and Neutralising Antibodies at Six Months after BNT162b2 Vaccination in Patients with Solid Tumours. *Eur. J. Cancer* **2022**, *168*, 51–55. [CrossRef] [PubMed]
12. Massarweh, A.; Tschernichovsky, R.; Stemmer, A.; Benouaich-Amiel, A.; Siegal, T.; Eliakim-Raz, N.; Stemmer, S.M.; Yust-Katz, S. Immunogenicity of the BNT162b2 MRNA COVID-19 Vaccine in Patients with Primary Brain Tumors: A Prospective Cohort Study. *J. Neurooncol.* **2022**, *156*, 483–489. [CrossRef] [PubMed]
13. Fendler, A.; Shepherd, S.T.C.; Au, L.; Wilkinson, K.A.; Wu, M.; Byrne, F.; Cerrone, M.; Schmitt, A.M.; Joharatnam-Hogan, N.; Shum, B.; et al. Adaptive Immunity and Neutralizing Antibodies against SARS-CoV-2 Variants of Concern Following Vaccination in Patients with Cancer: The CAPTURE Study. *Nat. cancer* **2021**, *2*, 1305–1320. [CrossRef] [PubMed]
14. Singer, J.; Le, N.-S.; Mattes, D.; Klamminger, V.; Hackner, K.; Kolinsky, N.; Scherb, M.; Errhalt, P.; Kreye, G.; Pecherstorfer, M.; et al. Evaluation of Antibody Responses to COVID-19 Vaccines among Solid Tumor and Hematologic Patients. *Cancers* **2021**, *13*, 4312. [CrossRef] [PubMed]
15. Agha, M.; Blake, M.; Chilleo, C.; Wells, A.; Haidar, G. Suboptimal Response to COVID-19 MRNA Vaccines in Hematologic Malignancies Patients. *medRxiv* **2021**. [CrossRef]
16. Lim, S.H.; Stuart, B.; Joseph-Pietras, D.; Johnson, M.; Campbell, N.; Kelly, A.; Jeffrey, D.; Turaj, A.H.; Rolfvondenbaumen, K.; Galloway, C.; et al. Immune Responses against SARS-CoV-2 Variants after Two and Three Doses of Vaccine in B-Cell Malignancies: UK PROSECO Study. *Nat. Cancer* **2022**, *3*, 552–564. [CrossRef]
17. Tran, S.; Truong, T.H.; Narendran, A. Evaluation of COVID-19 Vaccine Response in Patients with Cancer: An Interim Analysis. *Eur. J. Cancer* **2021**, *159*, 259. [CrossRef]
18. Nelli, F.; Fabbri, A.; Onorato, A.; Giannarelli, D.; Silvestri, M.A.; Giron Berrios, J.R.; Virtuoso, A.; Marrucci, E.; Signorelli, C.; Chilelli, M.G.; et al. Effects of Active Cancer Treatment on Safety and Immunogenicity of COVID-19 MRNA-BNT162b2 Vaccine: Preliminary Results from the Prospective Observational Vax-On Study. *Ann. Oncol.* **2022**, *33*, 107–108. [CrossRef]
19. Cavanna, L.; Citterio, C.; Biasini, C.; Madaro, S.; Bacchetta, N.; Lis, A.; Cremona, G.; Muroni, M.; Bernuzzi, P.; Lo Cascio, G.; et al. COVID-19 Vaccines in Adult Cancer Patients with Solid Tumours Undergoing Active Treatment: Seropositivity and Safety. A Prospective Observational Study in Italy. *Eur. J. Cancer* **2021**, *157*, 441–449. [CrossRef]
20. Cavanna, L.; Proietto, M.; Citterio, C.; Anselmi, E.; Zaffignani, E.; Stroppa, E.M.; Borsotti, M.T.; Contini, A.; Di Girolamo, G.; Quitadamo, V.M.; et al. COVID-19 Vaccination in Cancer Patients Older than 70 Years Undergoing Active Treatment. Seroconversion Rate and Safety. *Vaccines* **2022**, *10*, 164. [CrossRef]
21. Corrie, P.G. Cytotoxic Chemotherapy: Clinical Aspects. *Medicine* **2008**, *36*, 24–28. [CrossRef]
22. Garcia, G.; Odaimi, M. Systemic Combination Chemotherapy in Elderly Pancreatic Cancer: A Review. *J. Gastrointest. Cancer* **2017**, *48*, 121–128. [CrossRef] [PubMed]
23. Mehta, S.R.; Suhag, V.; Semwal, M.; Sharma, N. Radiotherapy: Basic Concepts and Recent Advances. *Med. J. Armed Forces India* **2010**, *66*, 158. [CrossRef]
24. Figueiredo, J.C.; Merin, N.M.; Hamid, O.; Choi, S.Y.; Lemos, T.; Cozen, W.; Nguyen, N.; Finster, L.J.; Foley, J.; Darrah, J.; et al. Longitudinal SARS-CoV-2 MRNA Vaccine-Induced Humoral Immune Responses in Patients with Cancer. *Cancer Res.* **2021**, *81*, 6273–6280. [CrossRef] [PubMed]
25. Grinshpun, A.; Rottenberg, Y.; Ben-Dov, I.Z.; Djian, E.; Wolf, D.G.; Kadouri, L. Serologic Response to COVID-19 Infection and/or Vaccine in Cancer Patients on Active Treatment. *ESMO Open* **2021**, *6*, 100283. [CrossRef]
26. Ariamanesh, M.; Porouhan, P.; PeyroShabany, B.; Fazilat-Panah, D.; Dehghani, M.; Nabavifard, M.; Hatami, F.; Fereidouni, M.; Welsh, J.S.; Javadinia, S.A. Immunogenicity and Safety of the Inactivated SARS-CoV-2 Vaccine (BBIBP-CorV) in Patients with Malignancy. *Cancer Investig.* **2022**, *40*, 26–34. [CrossRef]
27. Agbarya, A.; Sarel, I.; Ziv-Baran, T.; Agranat, S.; Schwartz, O.; Shai, A.; Nordheimer, S.; Fenig, S.; Shechtman, Y.; Kozlener, E.; et al. Efficacy of the Mrna-Based Bnt162b2 COVID-19 Vaccine in Patients with Solid Malignancies Treated with Anti-Neoplastic Drugs. *Cancers* **2021**, *13*, 4191. [CrossRef]

28. Addeo, A.; Shah, P.K.; Bordry, N.; Hudson, R.D.; Albracht, B.; Di Marco, M.; Kaklamani, V.; Dietrich, P.Y.; Taylor, B.S.; Simand, P.F.; et al. Immunogenicity of SARS-CoV-2 Messenger RNA Vaccines in Patients with Cancer. *Cancer Cell* **2021**, *39*, 1091–1098.e2. [CrossRef]
29. Funakoshi, Y.; Yakushijin, K.; Ohji, G.; Hojo, W.; Sakai, H.; Takai, R.; Nose, T.; Ohata, S.; Nagatani, Y.; Koyama, T.; et al. Safety and Immunogenicity of the COVID-19 Vaccine BNT162b2 in Patients Undergoing Chemotherapy for Solid Cancer. *J. Infect. Chemother.* **2022**, *28*, 516–520. [CrossRef]
30. Ruggeri, E.M.; Nelli, F.; Fabbri, A.; Onorato, A.; Giannarelli, D.; Giron Berrios, J.R.; Virtuoso, A.; Marrucci, E.; Mazzotta, M.; Schirripa, M.; et al. Antineoplastic Treatment Class Modulates COVID-19 MRNA-BNT162b2 Vaccine Immunogenicity in Cancer Patients: A Secondary Analysis of the Prospective Vax-On Study. *ESMO Open* **2022**, *7*, 100350. [CrossRef]
31. Bowes, C.L.; Naranbhai, V.; St Denis, K.J.; Lam, E.C.; Bertaux, B.; Keane, F.K.; Khandekar, M.J.; Balazs, A.B.; Iafrate, J.A.; Gainor, J.F.; et al. Heterogeneous Immunogenicity of SARS-CoV-2 Vaccines in Cancer Patients Receiving Radiotherapy. *Radiother. Oncol.* **2022**, *166*, 88–91. [CrossRef] [PubMed]
32. Pardoll, D.M. The Blockade of Immune Checkpoints in Cancer Immunotherapy. *Nat. Rev. Cancer* **2012**, *12*, 252. [CrossRef] [PubMed]
33. Butte, M.J.; Keir, M.E.; Phamduy, T.B.; Sharpe, A.H.; Freeman, G.J. PD-L1 Interacts Specifically with B7-1 to Inhibit T Cell Proliferation. *Immunity* **2007**, *27*, 111. [CrossRef] [PubMed]
34. Karwacz, K.; Bricogne, C.; MacDonald, D.; Arce, F.; Bennett, C.L.; Collins, M.; Escors, D. PD-L1 Co-Stimulation Contributes to Ligand-Induced T Cell Receptor down-Modulation on $CD8^+$ T Cells. *EMBO Mol. Med.* **2011**, *3*, 581. [CrossRef] [PubMed]
35. Naranbhai, V.; Pernat, C.A.; Gavralidis, A.; St Denis, K.J.; Lam, E.C.; Spring, L.M.; Isakoff, S.J.; Farmer, J.R.; Zubiri, L.; Hobbs, G.S.; et al. Immunogenicity and Reactogenicity of SARS-CoV-2 Vaccines in Patients with Cancer: The CANVAX Cohort Study. *J. Clin. Oncol.* **2022**, *40*, 12–23. [CrossRef] [PubMed]
36. Ma, Y.; Liu, N.; Wang, Y.; Zeng, J.; Hu, Y.Y.; Hao, W.; Shi, H.; Zhu, P.; Lv, J.; Fan, W.; et al. Immune Checkpoint Blocking Impact and Nomogram Prediction of COVID-19 Inactivated Vaccine Seroconversion in Patients with Cancer: A Propensity-Score Matched Analysis. *J. Immunother. Cancer* **2021**, *9*, e003712. [CrossRef]
37. Lasagna, A.; Agustoni, F.; Percivalle, E.; Borgetto, S.; Paulet, A.; Comolli, G.; Sarasini, A.; Bergami, F.; Sammartino, J.C.; Ferrari, A.; et al. A Snapshot of the Immunogenicity, Efficacy and Safety of a Full Course of BNT162b2 Anti-SARS-CoV-2 Vaccine in Cancer Patients Treated with PD-1/PD-L1 Inhibitors: A Longitudinal Cohort Study. *ESMO Open* **2021**, *6*, 100272. [CrossRef]
38. Lasagna, A.; Lilleri, D.; Agustoni, F.; Percivalle, E.; Borgetto, S.; Alessio, N.; Comolli, G.; Sarasini, A.; Bergami, F.; Sammartino, J.C.; et al. Analysis of the Humoral and Cellular Immune Response after a Full Course of BNT162b2 Anti-SARS-CoV-2 Vaccine in Cancer Patients Treated with PD-1/PD-L1 Inhibitors with or without Chemotherapy: An Update after 6 Months of Follow-Up. *ESMO Open* **2022**, *7*, 100359. [CrossRef]
39. Wiseman, A.C. Immunosuppressive Medications. *Clin. J. Am. Soc. Nephrol.* **2016**, *11*, 332. [CrossRef]
40. Zitvogel, L.; Apetoh, L.; Ghiringhelli, F.; Kroemer, G. Immunological Aspects of Cancer Chemotherapy. *Nat. Rev. Immunol.* **2008**, *8*, 59–73. [CrossRef]
41. Ferrara, J.L.; Levine, J.E.; Reddy, P.; Holler, E. Graft-versus-Host Disease. *Lancet* **2009**, *373*, 1550. [CrossRef]
42. Sterner, R.C.; Sterner, R.M. CAR-T Cell Therapy: Current Limitations and Potential Strategies. *Blood Cancer J.* **2021**, *11*, 69. [CrossRef] [PubMed]
43. Srivastava, S.; Riddell, S.R. Engineering CAR-T Cells: Design Concepts. *Trends Immunol.* **2015**, *36*, 494–502. [CrossRef] [PubMed]
44. Thakkar, A.; Gonzalez-Lugo, J.D.; Goradia, N.; Gali, R.; Shapiro, L.C.; Pradhan, K.; Rahman, S.; Kim, S.Y.; Ko, B.; Sica, R.A.; et al. Seroconversion Rates Following COVID-19 Vaccination among Patients with Cancer. *Cancer Cell* **2021**, *39*, 1081–1090.e2. [CrossRef] [PubMed]
45. Shapiro, L.C.; Thakkar, A.; Campbell, S.T.; Forest, S.K.; Pradhan, K.; Gonzalez-Lugo, J.D.; Quinn, R.; Bhagat, T.D.; Choudhary, G.S.; McCort, M.; et al. Efficacy of Booster Doses in Augmenting Waning Immune Responses to COVID-19 Vaccine in Patients with Cancer. *Cancer Cell* **2022**, *40*, 3–5. [CrossRef] [PubMed]
46. Peeters, M.; Verbruggen, L.; Teuwen, L.; Vanhoutte, G.; Vande Kerckhove, S.; Peeters, B.; Raats, S.; Van der Massen, I.; De Keersmaecker, S.; Debie, Y.; et al. Reduced Humoral Immune Response after BNT162b2 Coronavirus Disease 2019 Messenger RNA Vaccination in Cancer Patients under Antineoplastic Treatment. *ESMO Open* **2021**, *6*, 100274. [CrossRef] [PubMed]
47. Nelli, F.; Fabbri, A.; Onorato, A.; Giannarelli, D.; Silvestri, M.A.; Pessina, G.; Giron Berrios, J.R.; Virtuoso, A.; Marrucci, E.; Schirripa, M.; et al. Six Month Immunogenicity of COVID-19 MRNA-BNT162b2 Vaccine in Actively Treated Cancer Patients: Updated Results of the Vax-On Study. *Ann. Oncol.* **2022**, *33*, 352–354. [CrossRef]
48. Pimpinelli, F.; Marchesi, F.; Piaggio, G.; Giannarelli, D.; Papa, E.; Falcucci, P.; Pontone, M.; Di Martino, S.; Laquintana, V.; La Malfa, A.; et al. Fifth-Week Immunogenicity and Safety of Anti-SARS-CoV-2 BNT162b2 Vaccine in Patients with Multiple Myeloma and Myeloproliferative Malignancies on Active Treatment: Preliminary Data from a Single Institution. *J. Hematol. Oncol.* **2021**, *14*, 81. [CrossRef]
49. Puhalla, S.; Bhattacharya, S.; Davidson, N.E. Hormonal Therapy in Breast Cancer: A Model Disease for the Personalization of Cancer Care. *Mol. Oncol.* **2012**, *6*, 222–236. [CrossRef]
50. Cortés, A.; Casado, J.L.; Longo, F.; Serrano, J.J.; Saavedra, C.; Velasco, H.; Martin, A.; Chamorro, J.; Rosero, D.; Fernández, M.; et al. Limited T Cell Response to SARS-CoV-2 MRNA Vaccine among Patients with Cancer Receiving Different Cancer Treatments. *Eur. J. Cancer* **2022**, *166*, 229–239. [CrossRef]

51. Khan, Q.J.; Bivona, C.R.; Martin, G.A.; Zhang, J.; Liu, B.; He, J.; Li, K.H.; Nelson, M.; Williamson, S.; Doolittle, G.C.; et al. Evaluation of the Durability of the Immune Humoral Response to COVID-19 Vaccines in Patients with Cancer Undergoing Treatment or Who Received a Stem Cell Transplant. *JAMA Oncol.* **2022**, *66210*, 1053–1058. [CrossRef] [PubMed]
52. Massarweh, A.; Eliakim-Raz, N.; Stemmer, A.; Levy-Barda, A.; Yust-Katz, S.; Zer, A.; Benouaich-Amiel, A.; Ben-Zvi, H.; Moskovits, N.; Brenner, B.; et al. Evaluation of Seropositivity Following BNT162b2 Messenger RNA Vaccination for SARS-CoV-2 in Patients Undergoing Treatment for Cancer. *JAMA Oncol.* **2021**, *7*, 1133–1140. [CrossRef] [PubMed]
53. Goshen-Lago, T.; Waldhorn, I.; Holland, R.; Szwarcwort-Cohen, M.; Reiner-Benaim, A.; Shachor-Meyouhas, Y.; Hussein, K.; Fahoum, L.; Baruch, M.; Peer, A.; et al. Serologic Status and Toxic Effects of the SARS-CoV-2 BNT162b2 Vaccine in Patients Undergoing Treatment for Cancer. *JAMA Oncol.* **2021**, *7*, 1507–1513. [CrossRef] [PubMed]
54. Joudi, M.; Moradi Binabaj, M.; Porouhan, P.; PeyroShabany, B.; Tabasi, M.; Fazilat-Panah, D.; Khajeh, M.; Mehrabian, A.; Dehghani, M.; Welsh, J.S.; et al. A Cohort Study on the Immunogenicity and Safety of the Inactivated SARS-CoV-2 Vaccine (BBIBP-CorV) in Patients with Breast Cancer; Does Trastuzumab Interfere with the Outcome? *Front. Endocrinol.* **2022**, *13*, 162. [CrossRef]
55. Trontzas, I.P.; Vathiotis, I.; Economidou, C.; Petridou, I.; Gomatou, G.; Grammoustianou, M.; Tsamis, I.; Syrigos, N.; Anagnostakis, M.; Fyta, E.; et al. Assessment of Seroconversion after SARS-CoV-2 Vaccination in Patients with Lung Cancer. *Vaccines* **2022**, *10*, 618. [CrossRef]
56. Di Noia, V.; Pimpinelli, F.; Renna, D.; Barberi, V.; Maccallini, M.T.; Gariazzo, L.; Pontone, M.; Monti, A.; Campo, F.; Taraborelli, E.; et al. Immunogenicity and Safety of COVID-19 Vaccine BNT162b2 for Patients with Solid Cancer: A Large Cohort Prospective Study from a Single Institution. *Clin. Cancer Res.* **2021**, *27*, 6815–6823. [CrossRef]
57. Shulman, R.M.; Weinberg, D.S.; Ross, E.A.; Ruth, K.; Rall, G.F.; Olszanski, A.J.; Helstrom, J.; Hall, M.J.; Judd, J.; Chen, D.Y.T.; et al. Adverse Events Reported by Patients with Cancer after Administration of a 2-Dose MRNA COVID-19 Vaccine. *J. Natl. Compr. Cancer Netw.* **2022**, *20*, 160–166. [CrossRef]
58. Kian, W.; Zemel, M.; Kestenbaum, E.H.; Rouvinov, K.; Alguayn, W.; Levitas, D.; Ievko, A.; Michlin, R.; Abod, M.A.; Massalha, I.; et al. Safety of the BNT162b2 MRNA COVID-19 Vaccine in Oncologic Patients Undergoing Numerous Cancer Treatment Options: A Retrospective Single-Center Study. *Medicine* **2022**, *101*, E28561. [CrossRef]
59. Kawaguchi, S.; Izumi, K.; Kadomoto, S.; Iwamoto, H.; Yaegashi, H.; Iijima, M.; Nohara, T.; Shigehara, K.; Kadono, Y.; Mizokami, A. Influence of the Coronavirus Disease 2019 Vaccine on Drug Therapy for Urological Cancer. *Anticancer Res.* **2022**, *42*, 2105–2111. [CrossRef]
60. So, A.C.P.; McGrath, H.; Ting, J.; Srikandarajah, K.; Germanou, S.; Moss, C.; Russell, B.; Monroy-Iglesias, M.; Dolly, S.; Irshad, S.; et al. COVID-19 Vaccine Safety in Cancer Patients: A Single Centre Experience. *Cancers* **2021**, *13*, 3573. [CrossRef]
61. Soyfer, V.; Gutfeld, O.; Shamai, S.; Schlocker, A.; Merimsky, O. COVID-19 Vaccine-Induced Radiation Recall Phenomenon. *Int. J. Radiat. Oncol. Biol. Phys.* **2021**, *110*, 957. [CrossRef] [PubMed]
62. Marples, R.; Douglas, C.; Xavier, J.; Collins, A.-J. Breast Radiation Recall Phenomenon after Astra-Zeneca COVID-19 Vaccine: A Case Series. *Cureus* **2022**, *14*, e21499. [CrossRef]
63. Scoccianti, S.; Delli Paoli, C.; Grilli Leonulli, B.; Paoletti, L.; Alpi, P.; Caini, S.; Barca, R.; Fondelli, S.; Russo, S.; Perna, M.; et al. Acute Tolerance of Moderna MRNA-1273 Vaccine against COVID-19 in Patients with Cancer Treated with Radiotherapy. *Lancet. Oncol.* **2021**, *22*, 1212. [CrossRef]
64. Waissengrin, B.; Agbarya, A.; Safadi, E.; Padova, H.; Wolf, I. Short-Term Safety of the BNT162b2 MRNA COVID-19 Vaccine in Patients with Cancer Treated with Immune Checkpoint Inhibitors. *Lancet Oncol.* **2021**, *22*, 581–583. [CrossRef]
65. Strobel, S.B.; Machiraju, D.; Kälber, K.A.; Hassel, J.C. Immune-Related Adverse Events of COVID-19 Vaccination in Skin Cancer Patients Receiving Immune-Checkpoint Inhibitor Treatment. *Cancer Immunol. Immunother.* **2021**, *71*, 2051–2056. [CrossRef] [PubMed]
66. Mei, Q.; Hu, G.; Yang, Y.; Liu, B.; Yin, J.; Li, M.; Huang, Q.; Tang, X.; Böhner, A.; Bryant, A.; et al. Impact of COVID-19 Vaccination on the Use of PD-1 Inhibitor in Treating Patients with Cancer: A Real-World Study. *J. Immunother. Cancer* **2022**, *10*, e004157. [CrossRef]
67. Au, L.; Fendler, A.; Shepherd, S.T.C.; Rzeniewicz, K.; Cerrone, M.; Byrne, F.; Carlyle, E.; Edmonds, K.; Del Rosario, L.; Shon, J.; et al. Cytokine Release Syndrome in a Patient with Colorectal Cancer after Vaccination with BNT162b2. *Nat. Med.* **2021**, *27*, 1362–1366. [CrossRef] [PubMed]
68. Bshesh, K.; Khan, W.; Vattoth, A.L.; Janjua, E.; Nauman, A.; Almasri, M.; Mohamed Ali, A.; Ramadorai, V.; Mushannen, B.; AlSubaie, M.; et al. Lymphadenopathy Post-COVID-19 Vaccination with Increased FDG Uptake May Be Falsely Attributed to Oncological Disorders: A Systematic Review. *J. Med. Virol.* **2022**, *94*, 1833. [CrossRef]
69. Avner, M.; Orevi, M.; Caplan, N.; Popovtzer, A.; Lotem, M.; Cohen, J.E. COVID-19 Vaccine as a Cause for Unilateral Lymphadenopathy Detected by 18F-FDG PET/CT in a Patient Affected by Melanoma. *Eur. J. Nucl. Med. Mol. Imaging* **2021**, *48*, 2659–2660. [CrossRef]
70. Hiller, N.; Goldberg, S.N.; Cohen-Cymberknoh, M.; Vainstein, V.; Simanovsky, N. Lymphadenopathy Associated with the COVID-19 Vaccine. *Cureus* **2021**, *13*, e13524. [CrossRef]
71. Bernstine, H.; Priss, M.; Anati, T.; Turko, O.; Gorenberg, M.; Steinmetz, A.P.; Groshar, D. Axillary Lymph Nodes Hypermetabolism after BNT162b2 MRNA COVID-19 Vaccination in Cancer Patients Undergoing ^{18}F-FDG PET/CT: A Cohort Study. *Clin. Nucl. Med.* **2021**, *46*, 396–401. [CrossRef] [PubMed]

72. Cohen, D.; Krauthammer, S.H.; Wolf, I.; Even-Sapir, E. Hypermetabolic Lymphadenopathy Following Administration of BNT162b2 MRNA COVID-19 Vaccine: Incidence Assessed by [^{18}F]FDG PET-CT and Relevance to Study Interpretation. *Eur. J. Nucl. Med. Mol. Imaging* **2021**, *48*, 1854. [CrossRef] [PubMed]
73. Eifer, M.; Tau, N.; Alhoubani, Y.; Kanana, N.; Domachevsky, L.; Shams, J.; Keret, N.; Gorfine, M.; Eshet, Y. COVID-19 MRNA Vaccination: Age and Immune Status and Its Association with Axillary Lymph Node PET/CT Uptake. *J. Nucl. Med.* **2022**, *63*, 134. [CrossRef] [PubMed]
74. Placke, J.M.; Reis, H.; Hadaschik, E.; Roesch, A.; Schadendorf, D.; Stoffels, I.; Klode, J. Coronavirus Disease 2019 Vaccine Mimics Lymph Node Metastases in Patients Undergoing Skin Cancer Follow-up: A Monocentre Study. *Eur. J. Cancer* **2021**, *154*, 167. [CrossRef] [PubMed]
75. Granata, V.; Fusco, R.; Setola, S.V.; Galdiero, R.; Picone, C.; Izzo, F.; D'aniello, R.; Miele, V.; Grassi, R.; Grassi, R.; et al. Lymphadenopathy after BNT162b2 COVID-19 Vaccine: Preliminary Ultrasound Findings. *Biology* **2021**, *10*, 214. [CrossRef]
76. Hagen, C.; Nowack, M.; Messerli, M.; Saro, F.; Mangold, F.; Bode, P.K. Fine Needle Aspiration in COVID-19 Vaccine-Associated Lymphadenopathy. *Swiss Med. Wkly.* **2021**, *151*, w20557. [CrossRef]
77. Ko, G.; Hota, S.; Cil, T.D. COVID-19 Vaccination and Breast Cancer Surgery Timing. *Breast Cancer Res. Treat.* **2021**, *188*, 825–826. [CrossRef]
78. Shirone, N.; Shinkai, T.; Yamane, T.; Uto, F.; Yoshimura, H.; Tamai, H.; Imai, T.; Inoue, M.; Kitano, S.; Kichikawa, K.; et al. Axillary Lymph Node Accumulation on FDG-PET/CT after Influenza Vaccination. *Ann. Nucl. Med.* **2012**, *26*, 248–252. [CrossRef]
79. Thomassen, A.; Lerberg Nielsen, A.; Gerke, O.; Johansen, A.; Petersen, H. Duration of 18F-FDG Avidity in Lymph Nodes after Pandemic H1N1v and Seasonal Influenza Vaccination. *Eur. J. Nucl. Med. Mol. Imaging* **2011**, *38*, 894–898. [CrossRef]
80. McIntosh, L.J.; Bankier, A.A.; Vijayaraghavan, G.R.; Licho, R.; Rosen, M.P. COVID-19 Vaccination-Related Uptake on FDG PET/CT: An Emerging Dilemma and Suggestions for Management. *Am. J. Roentgenol.* **2021**, *217*, 975–983. [CrossRef]
81. Becker, A.S.; Perez-Johnston, R.; Chikarmane, S.A.; Chen, M.M.; El Homsi, M.; Feigin, K.N.; Gallagher, K.M.; Hanna, E.Y.; Hicks, M.; Ilica, A.T.; et al. Multidisciplinary Recommendations Regarding Post-Vaccine Adenopathy and Radiologic Imaging: Radiology Scientific Expert Panel. *Radiology* **2021**, *300*, E323–E327. [CrossRef] [PubMed]
82. Lehman, C.D.; D'Alessandro, H.A.; Mendoza, D.P.; Succi, M.D.; Kambadakone, A.; Lamb, L.R. Unilateral Lymphadenopathy after COVID-19 Vaccination: A Practical Management Plan for Radiologists Across Specialties. *J. Am. Coll. Radiol.* **2021**, *18*, 843–852. [CrossRef] [PubMed]
83. Lane, D.L.; Neelapu, S.S.; Xu, G.; Weaver, O. COVID-19 Vaccine-Related Axillary and Cervical Lymphadenopathy in Patients with Current or Prior Breast Cancer and Other Malignancies: Cross-Sectional Imaging Findings on MRI, CT, and PET-CT. *Korean J. Radiol.* **2021**, *22*, 1938–1945. [CrossRef] [PubMed]
84. Locklin, J.N.; Woodard, G.A. Mammographic and Sonographic Findings in the Breast and Axillary Tail Following a COVID-19 Vaccine. *Clin. Imaging* **2021**, *80*, 202–204. [CrossRef] [PubMed]
85. Chung, H.; Whitman, G.; Leung, J.; Sun, J.; Middleton, L.; Le Petross, H. Ultrasound Features to Differentiate COVID-19 Vaccine-Induced Benign Adenopathy from Breast Cancer Related Malignant Adenopathy. *Acad. Radiol.* **2022**, *29*, 1004–1012. [CrossRef]
86. Adin, M.E.; Wu, J.; Isufi, E.; Tsui, E.; Pucar, D. Ipsilateral Malignant Axillary Lymphadenopathy and Contralateral Reactive Lymph Nodes in a COVID-19 Vaccine Recipient with Breast Cancer. *J. Breast Cancer* **2022**, *25*, 140. [CrossRef]
87. Granata, V.; Fusco, R.; Vallone, P.; Setola, S.V.; Picone, C.; Grassi, F.; Patrone, R.; Belli, A.; Izzo, F.; Petrillo, A. Not Only Lymphadenopathy: Case of Chest Lymphangitis Assessed with MRI after COVID 19 Vaccine. *Infect. Agent. Cancer* **2022**, *17*, 8. [CrossRef]
88. Moujaess, E.; Zeid, N.B.; Samaha, R.; Sawan, J.; Kourie, H.; Labaki, C.; Chebel, R.; Chahine, G.; Karak, F.E.; Nasr, F.; et al. Perceptions of the COVID-19 Vaccine among Patients with Cancer: A Single-Institution Survey. *Futur. Oncol.* **2021**, *17*, 4071–4079. [CrossRef]
89. Kufel-Grabowska, J.; Bartoszkiewicz, M.; Ramlau, R.; Litwiniuk, M. Cancer Patients and Internal Medicine Patients Attitude towards COVID-19 Vaccination in Poland. *Adv. Clin. Exp. Med.* **2021**, *30*, 805–811. [CrossRef]
90. Villarreal-Garza, C.; Vaca-Cartagena, B.F.; Becerril-Gaitan, A.; Ferrigno, A.S.; Mesa-Chavez, F.; Platas, A.; Platas, A. Attitudes and Factors Associated with COVID-19 Vaccine Hesitancy among Patients with Breast Cancer. *JAMA Oncol.* **2021**, *7*, 1242. [CrossRef]
91. Marijanović, I.; Kraljevic, M.; Buhovac, T.; Sokolovic, E. Acceptance of COVID-19 Vaccination and Its Associated Factors among Cancer Patients Attending the Oncology Clinic of University Clinical Hospital Mostar, Bosnia and Herzegovina: A Cross-Sectional Study. *Med. Sci. Monit.* **2021**, *27*, e932788-1. [CrossRef] [PubMed]
92. Chan, W.L.; Ho, Y.H.T.; Wong, C.K.H.; Choi, H.C.W.; Lam, K.O.; Yuen, K.K.; Kwong, D.; Hung, I. Acceptance of COVID-19 Vaccination in Cancer Patients in Hong Kong: Approaches to Improve the Vaccination Rate. *Vaccines* **2021**, *9*, 792. [CrossRef] [PubMed]
93. Forster, M.; Wuerstlein, R.; Koenig, A.; Amann, N.; Beyer, S.; Kaltofen, T.; Degenhardt, T.; Burges, A.; Trillsch, F.; Mahner, S.; et al. COVID-19 Vaccination in Patients with Breast Cancer and Gynecological Malignancies: A German Perspective. *Breast Off. J. Eur. Soc. Mastology* **2021**, *60*, 214. [CrossRef] [PubMed]
94. Tsai, R.; Hervey, J.; Hoffman, K.; Wood, J.; Johnson, J.; Deighton, D.; Clermont, D.; Loew, B.; Goldberg, S.L. COVID-19 Vaccine Hesitancy and Acceptance among Individuals with Cancer, Autoimmune Diseases, or Other Serious Comorbid Conditions: Cross-Sectional, Internet-Based Survey. *JMIR Public Health Surveill.* **2022**, *8*, e29872. [CrossRef]

95. Khiari, H.; Cherif, I.; M'ghirbi, F.; Mezlini, A.; Hsairi, M. COVID-19 Vaccination Acceptance and Its Associated Factors among Cancer Patients in Tunisia. *Asian Pac. J. Cancer Prev.* **2021**, *22*, 3499. [CrossRef]
96. Mejri, N.; Berrazega, Y.; Ouertani, E.; Rachdi, H.; Bohli, M.; Kochbati, L.; Boussen, H. Understanding COVID-19 Vaccine Hesitancy and Resistance: Another Challenge in Cancer Patients. *Support. Care Cancer* **2022**, *30*, 289. [CrossRef]
97. Peng, X.; Gao, P.; Wang, Q.; Wu, H.G.; Yan, Y.L.; Xia, Y.; Wang, J.Y.; Lu, F.; Pan, H.; Yang, Y.; et al. Prevalence and Impact Factors of COVID-19 Vaccination Hesitancy among Breast Cancer Survivors: A Multicenter Cross-Sectional Study in China. *Front. Med.* **2021**, *8*, 741204. [CrossRef]
98. Heyne, S.; Esser, P.; Werner, A.; Lehmann-Laue, A.; Mehnert-Theuerkauf, A. Attitudes toward a COVID-19 Vaccine and Vaccination Status in Cancer Patients: A Cross-Sectional Survey. *J. Cancer Res. Clin. Oncol.* **2022**, *148*, 1363. [CrossRef]
99. Chun, J.Y.; Kim, S.I.; Park, E.Y.; Park, S.Y.; Koh, S.J.; Cha, Y.; Yoo, H.J.; Joung, J.Y.; Yoon, H.M.; Eom, B.W.; et al. Cancer Patients' Willingness to Take COVID-19 Vaccination: A Nationwide Multicenter Survey in Korea. *Cancers* **2021**, *13*, 3883. [CrossRef]
100. Erdem, D.; Karaman, I. Impact of Corona-Phobia on Attitudes and Acceptance towards COVID-19 Vaccine among Cancer Patients: A Single-Center Study. *Futur. Oncol.* **2021**, *18*, 457–469. [CrossRef]
101. Home—ClinicalTrials.gov. Available online: https://clinicaltrials.gov/ct2/home (accessed on 18 October 2022).
102. Shroff, R.T.; Chalasani, P.; Wei, R.; Pennington, D.; Quirk, G.; Schoenle, M.V.; Peyton, K.L.; Uhrlaub, J.L.; Ripperger, T.J.; Jergović, M.; et al. Immune Responses to Two and Three Doses of the BNT162b2 MRNA Vaccine in Adults with Solid Tumors. *Nat. Med.* **2021**, *27*, 2002–2011. [CrossRef] [PubMed]
103. Herishanu, Y.; Avivi, I.; Aharon, A.; Shefer, G.; Levi, S.; Bronstein, Y.; Morales, M.; Ziv, T.; Shorer Arbel, Y.; Scarfò, L.; et al. Efficacy of the BNT162b2 MRNA COVID-19 Vaccine in Patients with Chronic Lymphocytic Leukemia. *Blood* **2021**, *137*, 3165. [CrossRef] [PubMed]
104. Polack, F.P.; Thomas, S.J.; Kitchin, N.; Absalon, J.; Gurtman, A.; Lockhart, S.; Perez, J.L.; Marc, G.P.; Moreira, E.D.; Zerbini, C.; et al. Safety and Efficacy of the BNT162b2 MRNA COVID-19 Vaccine. *N. Engl. J. Med.* **2020**, *383*, 2603–2615. [CrossRef] [PubMed]
105. Seneviratne, S.L.; Yasawardene, P.; Wijerathne, W.; Somawardana, B. COVID-19 Vaccination in Cancer Patients: A Narrative Review. *J. Int. Med. Res.* **2022**, *50*, 3000605221086155. [CrossRef]
106. He, Y.; Ding, Y.; Cao, B.; Huang, Y.; Wang, X. COVID-19 Vaccine Development from the Perspective of Cancer Patients. *Hum. Vaccin. Immunother.* **2021**, *17*, 3281–3287. [CrossRef]
107. Hwang, J.K.; Zhang, T.; Wang, A.Z.; Li, Z. COVID-19 Vaccines for Patients with Cancer: Benefits Likely Outweigh Risks. *J. Hematol. Oncol.* **2021**, *14*, 38. [CrossRef]
108. Yekedüz, E.; Ayasun, R.; Köksoy, E.B.; Utkan, G.; Ürün, Y.; Akbulut, H. MRNA-Based COVID-19 Vaccines Appear Not to Increase Immune Events in Cancer Patients Receiving Immune Checkpoint Inhibitors. *Future Virol.* **2021**, *16*, 583–585. [CrossRef]
109. Malek, A.E.; Cornejo, P.P.; Daoud, N.; Alam, M. The MRNA COVID-19 Vaccine in Patients with Cancer Receiving Checkpoint Inhibitor Therapy: What We Know and What We Don't. *Immunotherapy* **2021**, *14*, 91–94. [CrossRef]
110. Esechie, A.; Fang, X.; Banerjee, P.; Rai, P.; Thottempudi, N. A Case Report of Longitudinal Extensive Transverse Myelitis: Immunotherapy Related Adverse Effect vs. COVID-19 Related Immunization Complications. *Int. J. Neurosci.* **2022**; *online ahead of print*. [CrossRef]

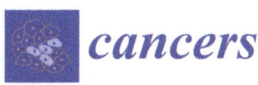

Review

The Impact of the COVID-19 Pandemic on Oncology Care and Clinical Trials

Jennyfa K. Ali and John C. Riches *

Centre for Haemato-Oncology, Barts Cancer Institute, Queen Mary University of London, 3rd Floor John Vane Science Centre, Charterhouse Square, London EC1M 6BQ, UK; jennyfa.ali@rmh.nhs.uk
* Correspondence: j.riches@qmul.ac.uk

Simple Summary: The coronavirus pandemic has had a considerable impact on all parts of society. Unsurprisingly, healthcare has been particularly affected, including cancer care and trials of new drugs. This article will summarize the impact the pandemic has had on cancer healthcare taking into consideration how the pandemic affected potential cancer patients and stopped them seeking medical advice for new symptoms. The pandemic also affected the ability of people to access healthcare services and undergo the tests necessary to diagnose cancer. This article will also discuss the impact of the pandemic on existing treatments and the trials of new drugs. In light of the unprecedented speed of development of new treatments and vaccines for the virus itself, it will also review whether some of these adaptations could be used to accelerate the development of novel cancer therapies.

Abstract: The coronavirus disease 2019 (COVID-19) pandemic has caused considerable global disruption to clinical practice. This article will review the impact that the pandemic has had on oncology clinical trials. It will assess the effect of the COVID-19 situation on the initial presentation and investigation of patients with suspected cancer. It will also review the impact of the pandemic on the subsequent management of cancer patients, and how clinical trial approval, recruitment, and conduct were affected during the pandemic. An intriguing aspect of the pandemic is that clinical trials investigating treatments for COVID-19 and vaccinations against the causative virus, SARS-CoV-2, have been approved and conducted at an unprecedented speed. In light of this, this review will also discuss the potential that this enhanced regulatory environment could have on the running of oncology clinical trials in the future.

Keywords: SARS-Cov-2; COVID-19; oncology; cancer screening; clinical trials

1. Introduction

The emergence of the novel coronavirus severe acute respiratory syndrome coronavirus 2 (SARS-CoV-2) caused a global healthcare crisis that reshaped both standard cancer care practices and oncology research [1]. The reasons for this were multifactorial. Firstly, efforts to contain transmission led to the withdrawal of face-to-face consultations, the suspension of normal diagnostic services, and the rapid expansion of telemedicine, all with the aim of reducing viral spread from healthcare worker to the patient and vice versa [2]. Secondly, the impact of severe coronavirus disease 2019 (COVID-19) on healthcare systems led to a redeployment of healthcare workers to deal with the pandemic, which inevitably had an impact on cancer pathways. These factors also affected clinical trials, which were often initially suspended, before being restarted with substantial amendments to facilitate their conduct in the pandemic-era world. Furthermore, it was clear from initial reports that patients with significant co-morbidities, including cancer, were at increased risk of having severe disease and death [3,4]. Mortality rates for patients with cancer and symptomatic COVID-19 have been reported at 24–28% [5,6]. Consequently, cancer patients and healthcare professionals often faced difficult decisions regarding treatment, with the benefit of therapy having to be factored against the increased risk of acquiring SARS-CoV-2 from hospitalization/increased frequency of visits to hospital and developing more severe COVID-19 due to modulation of the immune system by therapy. This article will review the many impacts of COVID-19 on cancer care, from the initial point of entry into cancer care pathways through to the longer-term implications (Figure 1). In addition, it will focus on the impact on oncology clinical trials. Interestingly, implementing a more patient-centric approach in clinical trials somewhat inadvertently improved working efficiency, patient experience, and trial running costs. In addition, given the unprecedented speed with which COVID-19 clinical trials were approved and conducted, it will also review whether there are lessons that could be learnt to benefit the oncology community.

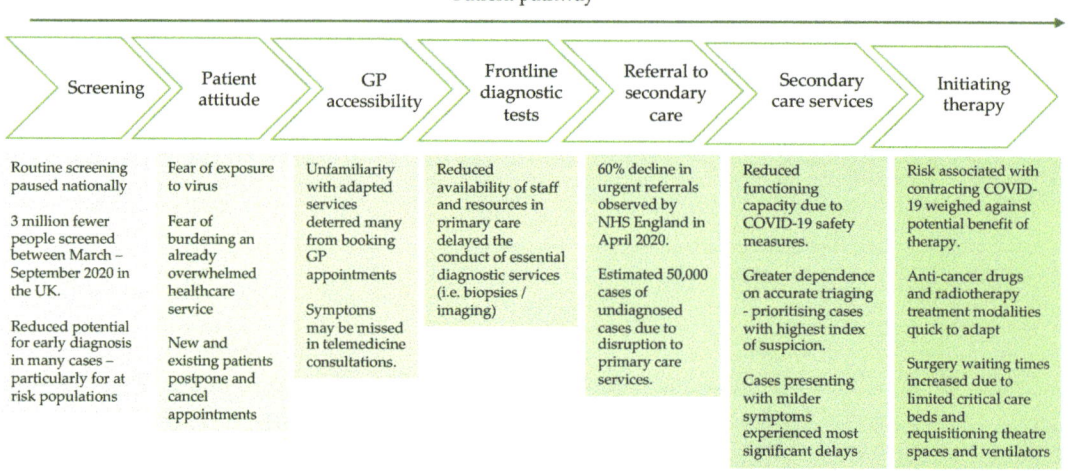

Figure 1. Impact of COVID-19 on the oncology care pathway.

2. Impact on the Initial Presentation of Patients with Potential Cancer

The COVID-19 pandemic affected how patients were first suspected of having cancer in several different ways. Routine screening services were typically paused in the early stages of the pandemic over concerns over viral transmission and as staff were redirected toward COVID-19-directed care. Disruption to screening services decreases the potential for early cancer detection in many cases, particularly in routine screening of at-risk populations such as breast screening of women with high familial risk and colorectal cancer (CRC) screening for individuals with inflammatory bowel disease (IBD) or Familial Adenomatous Polyposis (FAP) [7–10]. In the United Kingdom (UK), it has been estimated that 3 million fewer people were screened between the months of March to September 2020. This resulted in a 42% reduction in the number of patients initiating treatment following diagnosis via screening in the year April 2020–March 2021 [11]. This raises the rather alarming question of what happened to all those missing cases: were they diagnosed in good time through alternative pathways or do they still remain undiagnosed? Therefore, a long-term consequence of the pandemic may well be that these missed diagnoses will be picked up later, indirectly adding to the morbidity and mortality from SARS-CoV-2 [12].

A further impact is reflected in the behavior of the common populace themselves. A common feature of many governmental responses to the pandemic was to enforce a widespread "lockdown", essentially confining people to their homes. In the UK, a National Health Service (NHS) survey conducted in April 2020 to gain insight into public attitudes towards seeking medical advice for suspected cancer found that over 50% of the public had concerns and were hesitant about seeking help due to the pandemic. While shopping for essentials and seeking medical care were typically allowed, the overall impact of lockdown measures combined with the degree and nature of media coverage effectively discouraged people from seeking medical advice. Symptoms that may have normally provoked a visit to a primary care physician were not acted on, as people sought to adhere to the regulations in an attempt to avoid the virus or out of fear of burdening an already overwhelmed healthcare service [11]. In addition, there has also been concern that individuals were not reporting potential symptoms of cancer due to mis-attributing them to COVID-19. The prime example of this is lung cancer, where the development of respiratory symptoms such as a cough could be easily attributed to SARS-CoV-2 [13,14]. This is particularly worrying given the association of lung cancer mortality with more advanced stage presentation with metastatic disease [15]. Currently, there are little data to confirm an excess of lung cancer deaths due to this phenomenon, although this may change over the coming months and years.

A further consideration is the impact of the pandemic on primary care services. Many general practitioners ceased face-to-face services altogether, which also included a significant reduction in basic frontline diagnostics such as blood tests and X-rays. Primary care services were also forced to adapt to prevent the spread of SARS-CoV-2, particularly to the elderly and vulnerable at greater risk of fatal COVID-19. Social contact was avoided wherever possible, resulting in a switch to the widespread usage of telemedicine platforms to replace in-person consultations [16]. It can be argued that deviation from the normal process is enough to deter people from seeking advice regarding their health concerns, particularly those with limited access/familiarity with online portals. It is also noteworthy that symptoms that would have been observed in a physical appointment may not have been noticed by the primary care physicians or may be subjectively downplayed by the patient during a telephone/video call appointment.

All of these factors would have contributed to early cancer symptoms being missed, which was reflected in the reduction in referrals to secondary care. It has been widely noted that there was a significant decrease in the number of urgent referrals after the first lockdown was imposed in March 2020. The largest declines were observed specifically during the peaks of each wave of the pandemic. In England, NHS statistics recorded the largest fall in April 2020 when a 60% decrease in urgent referrals was recorded compared with April 2019 [17]. Overall, it was estimated that there have potentially been ~50,000 cases of undiagnosed cancer because of the disruption caused to normal primary care services and routine screening—equating to approximately 1 in 1000 of the UK population. However, the negative effects of COVID-19 on oncology care are not exclusively a consequence of the impact on primary care services and screening, but also have been significantly impacted by public healthcare seeking attitudes due to fear of exposure to the virus [11].

3. Impact on the Investigation of Patients with Suspected Cancer

In addition to the impacts on primary care, the COVID-19 pandemic has also had a massive impact on secondary care. Hospitals and health centers reduced their functioning capacity to maintain social distancing measures in accordance with government guidelines, which consequently delayed cancer diagnosis. Furthermore, any staff who displayed symptoms/tested positive for COVID-19 (or were exposed to someone who has tested positive) were also required to self-isolate as part of government guidelines, which further disrupted staffing levels and limited functioning capacity [18]. The UK NHS operational standard for the 2 week-wait urgent referral system states that 93% of patients with suspected cancer should be seen by a specialist within 14 days from primary care referral. This standard was not met in 2020/2021, when 88.7% of all urgent cancer referrals were seen within 14 days, representing a 2.8% decrease from the previous year (90.8%). Impact varied based on cancer type, therefore case burden should also be considered when considering the impact on diagnostic services. For example, suspected breast cancer referrals displayed the poorest performance with only 80.8% of urgent referrals meeting the 2-week timeframe. It is likely the larger case burden of breast cancer overwhelmed breast cancer services operating at reduced capacity due to the pandemic [19]. The reduced functioning capacity introduced a greater dependence on triaging patients in order of urgency, with resources being prioritized to cases with a high index of suspicion of cancer [20]. Subsequently, patients displaying experiencing milder symptoms who did not meet the criteria for urgent referral experienced the most significant delay in referral to secondary care [21]. The delays were not just confined to the initial assessment in secondary care, but were found throughout the pathway. For example, there was a significant reduction in surgical procedures such as biopsies, as surgeons, theatre staff, anesthesiologists, and ventilators were redeployed to assist with the pandemic [22]. A recent study conducted using data from Irish hospitals observed a 21.5% reduction in the number of biopsy procedures carried out between January–June of 2020 in comparison with the same time in 2019. When examined more closely, it is noted that the largest decline (−48%) was recorded between the period of April to June, which was soon after lockdown restrictions went into place in mid-March 2020 [23]. While diagnostic delays will clearly have an impact on the likelihood of successfully treating a particular tumor, a later diagnosis also causes significant mental and emotional stress [9]. This likely to have been particularly magnified due to the nature of the pandemic, with physical distancing contributing to the distress caused by removal from personal support systems such as family and friends [24].

4. Impact of the Management of Patients with Cancer

It was observed early in the pandemic that patients with cancer were at higher risk of developing severe and fatal COVID-19 [3,4]. This was due to cancers generally occurring more commonly in a higher risk population (e.g., the elderly), the immunosuppressive, and/or deconditioning effect of many malignancies, as well as the immune-modulatory effects of some treatments [25]. Somewhat surprisingly, large meta-analyses and registry studies have shown that systemic anticancer therapy per se does not increase the risk of dying from COVID-19. Instead, factors such as having cancer, older age, and the presence of other significant co-morbidities have been repeatedly demonstrated to be the major risk factors [25,26]. Several different strategies were adopted to try and deal with these problems. Risk–benefit analyses were typically conducted on a patient-by-patient basis, with treatments being postponed or withdrawn where the benefit offered by therapy was marginal [27–29]. Where possible, chemotherapy regimens were switched to the oral route to reduce the need for patients to attend hospital where they would run the risk of acquiring SARS-CoV-2 [30]. There were also recommendations made to supportive care, for example for the widespread use of granulocyte colony stimulating factor injections to reduce the risk of hospitalization from febrile neutropenia [31]. Consequently, more stringent measures were taken to shelter this population from contracting the virus and many scheduled treatments (i.e., chemotherapy, radiotherapy, and surgery) during the beginning of the pandemic were postponed while adaptive approaches of delivering therapy were established [32,33]. Cancer services rapidly developed strategies to overcome this setback and continue cancer care while minimizing the risk of COVID-19 transmission. COVID free hubs were set-up, distinct from hospitals, where cancer patients could receive their treatment with a reduced risk of virus transmission [34]. This included the use of "chemo buses" that could be parked on site of hospitals or moved to a more convenient location for patients. This effectively minimized the exposure to SARS-CoV-2 transmission in clinical settings while receiving therapy.

In the UK, NHS operational standards for new primary cancers state that treatment should commence within 31 days for 98% of patients receiving chemotherapy or other anti-cancer drugs, and for 94% of patients for radiotherapy and surgery. The overall performance for anti-cancer drugs and radiotherapy in 2020/2021 was above operational standards, which shows that services were able to adapt and continue with these treatments. However, despite efforts to maintain service levels, surgery was more significantly impacted during the pandemic and failed to meet operational standards, with only 88% of patients receiving surgery within 31 days [19]. Despite measures enforced to prevent SARS-CoV-2 infection, patients themselves also chose to delay their treatment in fear of contracting the virus by leaving self-isolation to receive treatment. One retrospective study of 165 lung cancer patients found that 9.1% of patients experienced a delay in receiving their treatment, although 80% of this population chose to delay their treatment themselves [35]. This is another instance where fear of exposure to the virus influenced decisions made by patients for medical intervention.

A further evolving area is the use of COVID-19 vaccinations in patients with cancer. Given the higher mortality rates from SARS-CoV-2 infection seen in these patients, the establishment of a safe and effective vaccine is crucial. Recent reports have suggested that COVID-19 vaccination for cancer patients is safe, immunogenic, and effective in protecting against symptomatic disease. However, the rates of seroconversion and protection offered by vaccination are generally lower in patients with cancer compared with the general population. Patients with hematological malignancies appear to be at particular risk, especially those who have received B-cell-depleting agents in the past 12 months [36]. Therefore, despite the relatively high coverage of COVID-19 vaccination programs in some countries, patients with cancer continue to remain at risk. Measures to address this include testing for antibody responses in cancer patients, and, in those found to have a deficient SARS-CoV-2 immune response, continuing to recommend adherence to infection-risk reduction measures and/or consideration of prophylactic treatment with COVID-19-neutralising monoclonal antibodies [37].

5. Impact on Clinical Trials

The effects of the pandemic on clinical trials were felt throughout administrative and clinical practices. Clinical trial initiation and recruitment were typically halted at the beginning of the pandemic as infection control measures were implemented [38]. Furthermore, trials of investigational medical products (IMPs) known to be immune-suppressive, or cause pneumonitis, were ceased due to concerns about the potential to exacerbate the severity of SARS-CoV-2 infection [39]. In a March 2021 report, a 60% decrease in new oncology clinical trials during the pandemic was noted, fueling concerns regarding slowing the development of new cancer therapies [40]. A major UK-based cancer research charity, Cancer Research UK, halted recruitment in 95% of their clinical trials, both to protect cancer patients, and to cope with the redeployment of clinical research staff to support frontline COVID-19-facing healthcare services. However, it is noteworthy that trials for pediatric and adolescent patients were affected to a lesser extent, following observations that young adults, children, and infants were less likely to develop severe SARS-CoV-2 infection and transmit it to others [41]. By halting start up and further trial recruitment, resources were prioritized to patients already enrolled in existing trials, who were benefiting from treatment and continued where possible. A further consideration was that the extensive monitoring and face-to-face physical assessments characteristic of normal clinical trial practice were no longer considered appropriate given the risks of exposure to the virus, either in hospital or during travel to and from the healthcare institution. This called for dramatic changes in routine practices and trial protocols to prevent the spread of COVID-19 while preserving trial integrity and patient welfare [42].

In the UK, the Medicines and Healthcare Products Regulatory Agency (MHRA) released guidelines in accordance with government restrictions to guide clinical trial management [43]. The shift in clinical trial protocol began with the scrutinization of every in-person appointment, with the aim of determining whether face-to-face assessment was necessary, or whether alternative strategies could be implemented to achieve the same objectives [44]. For example, standard physical examinations of marginal benefit such as weight, height, and blood pressure measurements, were typically excluded to reduce the need for hospital visits. Furthermore, screening tests such as echocardiograms and multi-gated acquisition (MUGA) scans were dispensed with in patients without risk factors or a history of cardio-vascular disease, as the risk of exposure to patients and healthcare workers could not be justified [45]. Other measures included the posting of informed consent (IC) forms and other documentation to patient's homes instead of them being signed during in-person consultations; the option to e-sign documents was also incorporated and recognized as an accepted form of consent by regulatory organizations [44]. These bodies also typically encouraged the switch to IMPs in oral form where appropriate, as the IMP could be delivered directly to the patient's home and be self-administered at the agreed schedule, reducing the need for them to travel to the trial site [43].

Telemedicine was also widely embraced as the best mode of communication to deliver the essential information to patients in remote video consultations, reducing the need for an in-person visit [44,46]. Notably, a systematic review has also provided evidence that supportive care and counselling delivered by telephone can be more convenient and noninferior to standard care for all outcomes, including knowledge, decision conflict, cancer distress, and perceived stress [47]. However, varying levels of computer literacy among trial participants must be taken into consideration. Pre-pandemic, one of the major obstacles faced by telemedicine was termed the "digital divide", as there was a substantial disparity in IT literacy between elder and younger demographics [48]. Unsurprisingly, the most recent report highlighted this disparity, as data showed that 54% of adults aged 75 and over did not use the internet compared to 99% of individuals aged 16–44 years [49]. Despite this, the pandemic has resulted in a wider uptake of digital technology by older people, as meeting in person has not been feasible [46]. Study visits that could be conducted remotely were identified and adapted, such as the reporting of adverse events or suspected adverse events by video consultation or questionnaires/patient diary cards. Furthermore, some protocols also allowed for physical assessments and tests that would normally occur at the trial site to be carried out locally by primary care physicians and other health professionals [50]. Where these assessments could not be performed locally due to the nature of the assessment, the interval between assessments was increased to reduce the total number of patient visits to hospital. In addition, in-person tests such as imaging scans and follow-up sample collections were planned to occur within one visit to further minimize risk of exposure to the virus, which also inadvertently improved the patient experience [51]. Remote monitoring systems were also implemented, allowing patients to be followed-up from their homes. For example, the use of wearable devices that provide a stream of real time data (e.g., blood pressure/heart rate monitors) was also expanded. This is a welcome innovation, as these approaches have the advantage that the data can be collected over extended periods of time and in a more natural and relaxed environment, mitigating issues such as "whitecoat hypertension" [52,53].

A further demonstration of clinical trial modification during the COVID-19 pandemic, albeit outside of cancer research, was the Randomised Evaluation of Covid-19 Therapy (RECOVERY) trial. The RECOVERY trial took on an unorthodox approach to set up a large-scale randomized clinical trial using a digital portal. DigiTrials is a data platform that consolidates patient data across the UK health system, which made the patient population in critical care units across the UK more accessible for recruitment into the trial. The DigiTrial system also provided a universal platform for data collection and processing, which allowed for quicker analysis and reporting of results [54]. The RECOVERY trial took a flexible approach with its protocol, which allowed for trial arms to be added as new research unveiled potential COVID-19 treatment modalities, while also allowing for arms to be halted as soon as data (which was being analyzed on an ongoing basis) determined that the therapy was ineffective (e.g., the anti-malarial drug Hydroxychloroquine) [55]. This also made clinical trial management less arduous for healthcare workers who were already under extreme pressure. This was reflected in the speed of the results: the trial established that dexamethasone reduced the number of deaths by one-third in ventilated critical care patients in just 98 days [56].

6. Lessons Learnt for the Future of Oncology Clinical Trials

The RECOVERY trial and other trials have served as an example demonstrating how a flexible protocol, the use of a data platform, and integration with standard care can considerably improve trial efficiency and turnaround time. With a simplified consent form and a carefully thought-out "trial by design" approach, the RECOVERY trial astoundingly received regulatory approval within 9 days, which is drastic compared to the average

30–60-day time frame. Many health research authorities are still currently fast-tracking ethical approval for COVID-19 research and have managed to bring the normal 60-day cycle down to just 10 days. Another paradigm shifting example has been the development of SARS-CoV-2 vaccines. Prior to the pandemic, the timeline from basic science and target identification through the phases of clinical development and licensing typically took 10–20 years, a time not inconsistent with the time it takes to develop a new anti-cancer drug. However, effective vaccines for COVID-19 were developed, tested, and licensed within a year of the virus first being discovered [57–59]. Undoubtedly, there were several factors that contributed to this, with the global nature of the pandemic meaning that pharmaceutical companies, research institutions, and governments made/had access to massive resources available for this purpose. However, this period established the proof of principal that effective treatments can be safely developed in a fraction of the time that it has historically taken.

The acceleration of drug development aside, there are many other examples of innovative practice that have emerged during the pandemic, that can be further adapted and taken forward. As discussed above, the intensity and frequency of monitoring assessments for patients on study was streamlined during the pandemic, with the aim of avoiding exposure to the virus [44]. As it now seems that many of these visits are unnecessary, future protocols should be designed with reduced numbers of visits to improve efficiency and patient experience, if retrospective analyses show no impact upon trial integrity [60]. This includes repeat biopsies and venepunctures, as it has been observed that the reduction in sample collection during the pandemic inadvertently contributed to an improved patient experience. Reducing the intensity of monitoring also reduces the inconvenience of traveling, which in turn helps address existing issues with patient retention in clinical trials. Patient drop-out and insufficient recruitment are often the cause of trials failing to complete accrual within the study period [61]. This is frustrating from a clinical perspective, as it prolongs the approval of beneficial therapies to reach a wider patient population. However, from a pharmaceutical and clinical research organization (CRO) perspective, failing to complete trials within aliquoted time frames can have financial implications and tarnish the reputation of the investigators. The cost to complete clinical trial research is then reflected in the costing of the therapy, driving up prices of new therapies. Ethical and regulatory standards in clinical trials have effectively managed risk and protected against litigation, at the expense of increased bureaucracy. Paradoxically, these stringent measures enforced to maximize patient safety and prevent malpractice have a wider negative impact on patients in standard care, as the elongation of trials/trial initiation ultimately delays the accessibility of more efficacious therapies.

Many healthcare systems are permanently under a degree of stress, which was experienced even before the COVID-19 pandemic, both financially and due to a shortage of appropriately trained staff. Efforts should be made to integrate trial design more closely with standard hospital workflow to lessen the burden on health services, promote an increase in clinical trial activity, and to develop resilience so that clinical trials can continue, should there be future waves of COVID-19 or another novel infectious agent [50]. One advantage of this is that if the clinical trial experience mimics the normal standard of care, then this should improve the quality of clinical trial data. A common problem is that the results of major clinical trials are not always recapitulated in the "real-world" setting, in part due to patient selection, but also due the increased monitoring and physical and psychological support given to the participants. If clinical trials resemble standard care more closely, then disparities between clinical trial and "real-world" data are less likely to be as apparent. The pandemic also offered significant training opportunities as staff were redeployed. For example, in some centers, oncology research nurses were redeployed to assist with COVID-19 vaccination trials, due to their experienced research nurses in trialing IMPs with significant side effect profiles [62]. Standardized "cross-training" of clinical research staff would allow for interchangeability of research staff between different studies. This would reduce staffing burden and potential burn-out in the event of unforeseen circumstances that result in clinical staffing shortages when running trials [60].

There have been many examples for how the administrative and regulatory burden imposed on research sites can be improved. New policies were implemented by CROs, sponsors, and regulatory authorities during the pandemic that facilitated a magnitude of administrative duties surrounding recruitment, site selection, and study monitoring by leveraging technology and simplifying reporting processes. This included implementing virtual online meeting platforms (i.e., Zoom/Microsoft Teams) and protected e-DocuSign (via AdobeSign) to support remote work for many administrative employees for a reduced dependence on physical paperwork. Standard practice in clinical trials requires all protocol violations to be thoroughly documented within the details of the trial to allow for accurate analysis of the data. The deviation reporting process during the pandemic was scaled back to combat the surge of administrative work because of the several protocol violations put in place to adapt trials. Only major deviations were reported in stand-alone deviation reports and all minor protocol deviations were reported on a weekly basis collectively, opposed to raising a report per deviation, whether it be major or minor [63]. Furthermore, there is considerable variability in the methods of how protocol deviations and trial amendments are documented across different CROs, which makes comparative analysis between studies much more complex. Standardizing how deviations are recorded, potentially using an inter-operator technology platform, would reduce administrative paperwork, allowing protocol violations to be reported in a more accessible and consistent manner. Accessibility of patient records and medical notes remotely was a significant issue faced by clinical trial monitors during the pandemic. Patient information is strictly confidential, which limits the modes it can be shared as this raises several issues with general data protection regulation (GDPR). The digitalization of data collection during the pandemic played a huge role in delivering rapid trial results. A similar approach should be adopted for the recording and processing of trial data on a secure and regulatory-approved digital platform, which anonymizes patient information and facilitates the remote access of trial data. As modern trials have become progressively complex with increases in the sophistication of therapy, it seems reasonable that the nature of regulation and administration should evolve as well.

7. Conclusions

The impacts of the COVID-19 pandemic on oncology care and clinical trials have been immense, and there is no doubt that the pandemic will leave a permanent impression on healthcare services. As devastating as the disruption has been, the response to the pandemic has seen many innovations and adaptations that will continue to be of great value in the future [64] (Figure 2). The pandemic has provided an opportunity to address some of the inefficiencies in the conduct of clinical trials, such as excessive bureaucracy and patient monitoring, and has driven improvements that offer the potential for future trials to be carried out more quickly and safely. Major successes include the rapid set up of COVID free cancer hubs that facilitated the provision of anti-cancer drug, radiotherapy, and surgery could continue where possible, with a reduced risk of virus transmission In addition, the swift implementation of telehealth platforms as a form of virtual meetings between patients and health professionals, as well as meetings between colleagues and professionals from other organizations within healthcare, has been a substantial leap in the maturation of digitalizing healthcare services [65]. However, the notion of solely relying on telehealth platforms post pandemic is far from reality. It is most likely that telehealth will become an integrated part of patient—doctor communication as a means to improve working efficiency and patient convenience. However, it is probable that the option for face-to-face consultations will still be available in consideration of the issue of digital exclusion, particularly among the elderly population where low computer literacy is most prominent [66].

In clinical trials, the COVID-19 pandemic caused a momentary pause that necessitated a step back to begin initiating change on very complicated and established practices. In a matter of months, the clinical trial industry has made a huge leap in leveraging technology that may have taken years to implement into normal practices without these drivers. The successful digitalization of many administrative processes has opened the door for the application of innovative technologies and methodologies to improve working efficiency. In the longer term, this offers the potential to reduce the burden of clinical documentation and increase the speed of data acquisition and interpretation, which should also result in a faster translation to the clinic. The experience from the pandemic should also inform the development of new measures to make healthcare systems and clinical trial networks more resilient to future healthcare crises, such as further waves of COVID-19, novel infectious agents, or other challenges.

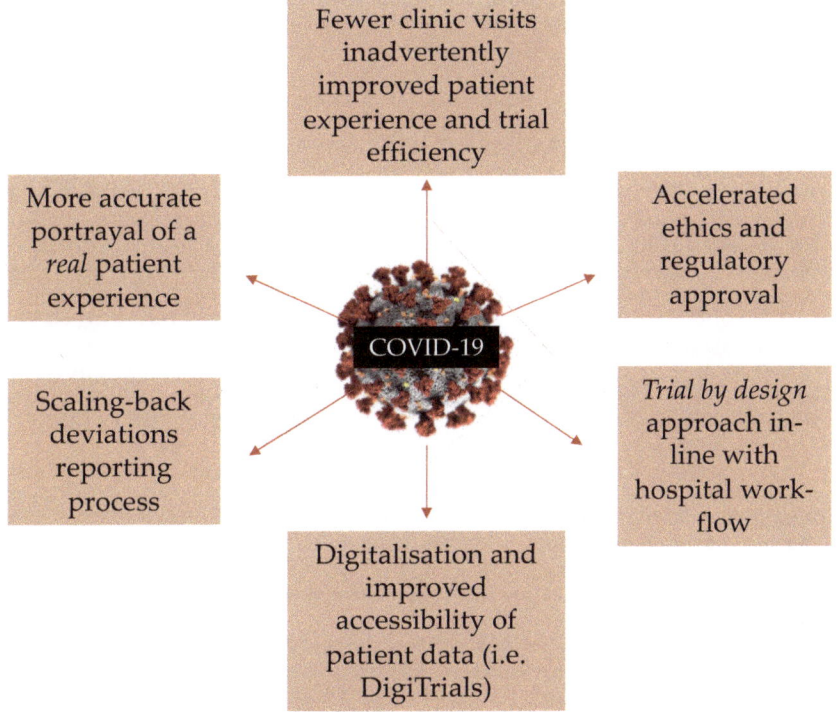

Figure 2. Potential positive impacts on oncology clinical trials due to COVID-19.

Author Contributions: J.K.A. and J.C.R. prepared the original draft and wrote and edited the manuscript. All authors have read and agreed to the published version of the manuscript.

Funding: This work was supported by Wellcome Trust grant 110020/Z/15/Z and Kay Kendall Leukaemia Fund grant KKL1248 to JCR.

Conflicts of Interest: The authors declare no conflict of interest.

References

1. Zhu, N.; Zhang, D.; Wang, W.; Li, X.; Yang, B.; Song, J.; Zhao, X.; Huang, B.; Shi, W.; Lu, R.; et al. A Novel Coronavirus from Patients with Pneumonia in China, 2019. *N. Engl. J. Med.* **2020**, *382*, 727–733. [CrossRef] [PubMed]
2. Wijesooriya, N.R.; Mishra, V.; Brand, P.L.; Rubin, B.K. COVID-19 and telehealth, education, and research adaptations. *Paediatr. Respir. Rev.* **2020**, *35*, 38–42. [CrossRef] [PubMed]
3. Liang, W.; Guan, W.; Chen, R.; Wang, W.; Li, J.; Xu, K.; Li, C.; Ai, Q.; Lu, W.; Liang, H.; et al. Cancer patients in SARS-CoV-2 infection: A nationwide analysis in China. *Lancet Oncol.* **2020**, *21*, 335–337. [CrossRef]
4. Guan, W.-J.; Ni, Z.-Y.; Hu, Y.; Liang, W.-H.; Ou, C.-Q.; He, J.-X.; Liu, L.; Shan, H.; Lei, C.-L.; Hui, D.S.C.; et al. Clinical Characteristics of Coronavirus Disease 2019 in China. *N. Engl. J. Med.* **2020**, *382*, 1708–1720. [CrossRef] [PubMed]

5. Erdal, G.S.; Polat, O.; Erdem, G.U.; Korkusuz, R.; Hindilerden, F.; Yilmaz, M.; Yasar, K.K.; Isiksacan, N.; Tural, D. The mortality rate of COVID-19 was high in cancer patients: A retrospective single-center study. *Int. J. Clin. Oncol.* **2021**, *26*, 826–834. [CrossRef] [PubMed]
6. Lee, L.Y.W.; Cazier, J.-B.; Angelis, V.; Arnold, R.; Bisht, V.; Campton, A.N.; Chackathayil, J.; Cheng, V.W.; Curley, H.M.; Fittall, M.W.T.; et al. COVID-19 mortality in patients with cancer on chemotherapy or other anticancer treatments: A prospective cohort study. *Lancet* **2020**, *395*, 1919–1926. [CrossRef]
7. Cancino, R.S.; Su, Z.; Mesa, R.; Tomlinson, G.E.; Wang, J. The Impact of COVID-19 on Cancer Screening: Challenges and Opportunities. *JMIR Cancer* **2020**, *6*, e21697. [CrossRef]
8. Dekker, E.; Chiu, H.M.; Lansdorp-Vogelaar, I.; WEO Colorectal Cancer Screening Committee. Colorectal Cancer Screening in the Novel Coronavirus Disease-2019 Era. *Gastroenterology* **2020**, *159*, 1998–2003. [CrossRef]
9. Hesary, F.B.; Salehiniya, H. The Impact of the COVID-19 Epidemic on Diagnosis, Treatment, Concerns, Problems, and Mental Health in Patients with Gastric Cancer. *J. Gastrointest. Cancer* **2021**, 1–8. [CrossRef]
10. Mazidimoradi, A.; Tiznobaik, A.; Salehiniya, H. Impact of the COVID-19 Pandemic on Colorectal Cancer Screening: A Systematic Review. *J. Gastrointest. Cancer* **2021**, 1–15. [CrossRef]
11. Macmillan Cancer Support. *The Forgotten 'C'? The Impact of Covid-19 on Cancer*; Macmillan Cancer Support: London, UK, 2020.
12. Fagundes, T.P.; Albuquerque, R.M.; Miranda, D.L.P.; Landeiro, L.C.G.; Ayres, G.S.F.; Correia, C.C.E.; Nogueira-Rodrigues, A. Dealing with cancer screening in the COVID-19 era. *Rev. Assoc. Med. Bras. (1992)* **2021**, *67*, 86–90. [CrossRef]
13. Birt, L.; Hall, N.; Emery, J.; Banks, J.; Mills, K.; Johnson, M.; Hamilton, W.; Walter, F.M. Responding to symptoms suggestive of lung cancer: A qualitative interview study. *BMJ Open Respir. Res.* **2014**, *1*, e000067. [CrossRef]
14. Hannaford, P.C.; Thornton, A.J.; Murchie, P.; Whitaker, K.L.; Adam, R.; Elliott, A.M. Patterns of symptoms possibly indicative of cancer and associated help-seeking behaviour in a large sample of United Kingdom residents—The USEFUL study. *PLOS ONE* **2020**, *15*, e0228033. [CrossRef]
15. Buccheri, G. Lung cancer: Clinical presentation and specialist referral time. *Eur. Respir. J.* **2004**, *24*, 898–904. [CrossRef]
16. Al-Shamsi, H.O.; Alhazzani, W.; Alhuraiji, A.; Coomes, E.A.; Chemaly, R.F.; Almuhanna, M.; Wolff, R.A.; Ibrahim, N.K.; Chua, M.L.; Hotte, S.J.; et al. A Practical Approach to the Management of Cancer Patients During the Novel Coronavirus Disease 2019 (COVID-19) Pandemic: An International Collaborative Group. *Oncologist* **2020**, *25*, e936–e945. [CrossRef]
17. NHS England. NHS Warning to Seek Help for Cancer Symptoms, as Half of Public Report Concerns with Getting Checked. Available online: https://www.england.nhs.uk/2020/04/nhs-warning-seek-help-cancer-symptoms/ (accessed on 1 October 2021).
18. Sideris, G.A.; Nikolakea, M.; Karanikola, A.-E.; Konstantinopoulou, S.; Giannis, D.; Modahl, L. Imaging in the COVID-19 era: Lessons learned during a pandemic. *World J. Radiol.* **2021**, *13*, 192–222. [CrossRef]
19. Coward, A.; Moon, K.; McDonnell, P. *Waiting Times for Suspected and Diagnosed Cancer Patients: 2020–21 Annual Report*; NHS: Leeds, UK, 2021.
20. Bakouny, Z.; Hawley, J.E.; Choueiri, T.K.; Peters, S.; Rini, B.I.; Warner, J.L.; Painter, C.A. COVID-19 and Cancer: Current Challenges and Perspectives. *Cancer Cell* **2020**, *38*, 629–646. [CrossRef]
21. Round, T.; L'Esperance, V.; Bayly, J.; Brain, K.; Dallas, L.; Edwards, J.G.; Haswell, T.; Hiley, C.; Lovell, N.; McAdam, J.; et al. COVID-19 and the multidisciplinary care of patients with lung cancer: An evidence-based review and commentary. *Br. J. Cancer* **2021**, *125*, 629–640. [CrossRef]
22. Rashid, S.; Tsao, H. Effect of the COVID-19 Pandemic on Delayed Skin Cancer Services. *Dermatol. Clin.* **2021**, *39*, 627–637. [CrossRef]
23. Phelan, N.; Behan, L.A.; Owens, L. The Impact of the COVID-19 Pandemic on Women's Reproductive Health. *Front. Endocrinol.* **2021**, *12*, 642755. [CrossRef]
24. Bandinelli, L.; Ornell, F.; von Diemen, L.; Kessler, F.H.P. The Sum of Fears in Cancer Patients Inside the Context of the COVID-19. *Front. Psychiatry* **2021**, *12*, 557834. [CrossRef]
25. Vijenthira, A.; Gong, I.Y.; Fox, T.A.; Booth, S.; Cook, G.; Fattizzo, B.; Martín-Moro, F.; Razanamahery, J.; Riches, J.C.; Zwicker, I.J.; et al. Outcomes of patients with hematologic malignancies and COVID-19: A systematic review and meta-analysis of 3377 patients. *Blood* **2020**, *136*, 2881–2892. [CrossRef]
26. Lee, A.J.X.; Purshouse, K. COVID-19 and cancer registries: Learning from the first peak of the SARS-CoV-2 pandemic. *Br. J. Cancer* **2021**, *124*, 1777–1784. [CrossRef]
27. Travassos, T.C.; De Oliveira, J.M.I.; Selegatto, I.B.; Reis, L.O. COVID-19 impact on bladder cancer-orientations for diagnosing, decision making, and treatment. *Am. J. Clin. Exp. Urol.* **2021**, *9*, 132–139.
28. Moslim, M.A.; Hall, M.J.; Meyer, J.E.; Reddy, S.S. Pancreatic cancer in the era of COVID-19 pandemic: Which one is the lesser of two evils? *World J. Clin. Oncol.* **2021**, *12*, 54–60. [CrossRef]
29. Jacome, L.S.; Deshmukh, S.K.; Thulasiraman, P.; Holliday, N.P.; Singh, S. Impact of COVID-19 Pandemic on Ovarian Cancer Management: Adjusting to the New Normal. *Cancer Manag. Res.* **2021**, *13*, 359–366. [CrossRef]
30. Ray, U.; Aziz, F.; Shankar, A.; Biswas, A.S.; Chakraborty, A. COVID-19: The Impact in Oncology Care. *SN Compr. Clin. Med.* **2020**, *2*, 2621–2630. [CrossRef]
31. Aapro, M.; Lyman, G.; Bokemeyer, C.; Rapoport, B.; Mathieson, N.; Koptelova, N.; Cornes, P.; Anderson, R.; Gascón, P.; Kuderer, N. Supportive care in patients with cancer during the COVID-19 pandemic. *ESMO Open* **2021**, *6*, 100038. [CrossRef]

32. Wang, A.; Chang, S.H.; Kim, E.J.; Bessich, J.L.; Sabari, J.K.; Cooper, B.; Geraci, T.C.; Cerfolio, R.J. Dynamic Management of Lung Cancer Care During Surging COVID-19. *Front. Surg.* **2021**, *8*, 663364. [CrossRef]
33. Gundavda, M.K.; Gundavda, K.K. Cancer or COVID-19? A Review of Guidelines for Safe Cancer Care in the Wake of the Pandemic. *SN Compr. Clin. Med.* **2020**, *2*, 2691–2701. [CrossRef]
34. Academy of Medical Royal Colleges; NHS England. *Clinical Guide for the Management of Essential Cancer Surgery for Adults during the Coronavirus Pandemic*; NHS England: Leeds, UK, 2020.
35. Fujita, K.; Ito, T.; Saito, Z.; Kanai, O.; Nakatani, K.; Mio, T. Impact of COVID-19 pandemic on lung cancer treatment scheduling. *Thorac. Cancer* **2020**, *11*, 2983–2986. [CrossRef] [PubMed]
36. Corti, C.; Antonarelli, G.; Scotté, F.; Spano, J.; Barrière, J.; Michot, J.; André, F.; Curigliano, G. Seroconversion rate after vaccination against COVID-19 in cancer patients—a systematic review. *Ann. Oncol.* **2021**. [CrossRef] [PubMed]
37. Ludwig, H.; Sonneveld, P.; Facon, T.; San-Miguel, J.; Avet-Loiseau, H.; Mohty, M.; Mateos, M.-V.; Moreau, P.; Cavo, M.; Pawlyn, C.; et al. COVID-19 vaccination in patients with multiple myeloma: A consensus of the European Myeloma Network. *Lancet Haematol.* **2021**. [CrossRef]
38. Li, Y.; Wang, X.; Wang, W. The Impact of COVID-19 on Cancer. *Infect. Drug Resist.* **2021**, *14*, 3809–3816. [CrossRef] [PubMed]
39. Gulati, S.; Muddasani, R.; Bergerot, P.G.; Pal, S.K. Systemic therapy and COVID19: Immunotherapy and chemotherapy. *Urol. Oncol. Semin. Orig. Investig.* **2021**, *39*, 213–220. [CrossRef]
40. Wilkinson, E. Dramatic drop in new cancer drug trials during the COVID-19 pandemic. *Lancet Oncol.* **2021**, *22*, 305. [CrossRef]
41. Crowe, T. *Viewpoint: How We're Keeping Children's Cancer Trials Going*; The Royal Marsden: London, UK, 2020.
42. Gongora, A.L.; Jardim, D.; Bastos, D.A. Oncology Clinical Trials During the COVID-19 Pandemic. *Oncology* **2020**, *34*, 265–269. [CrossRef]
43. Medicines and Healthcare products Regulatory Agency. *Managing Clinical Trials During Coronavirus (COVID-19)*; Medicines and Healthcare products Regulatory Agency: London, UK, 2021.
44. Upadhaya, S.; Yu, J.X.; Oliva, C.; Hooton, M.; Hodge, J.; Hubbard-Lucey, V.M. Impact of COVID-19 on oncology clinical trials. *Nat. Rev. Drug Discov.* **2020**, *19*, 376–377. [CrossRef]
45. Doherty, G.J.; Goksu, M.; De Paula, B.H.R. Rethinking cancer clinical trials for COVID-19 and beyond. *Nat. Rev. Cancer* **2020**, *1*, 568–572. [CrossRef]
46. Mann, D.M.; Chen, J.; Chunara, R.; Testa, P.; Nov, O. COVID-19 transforms health care through telemedicine: Evidence from the field. *J. Am. Med Inform. Assoc.* **2020**, *27*, 1132–1135. [CrossRef]
47. Singh, S.; Fletcher, G.G.; Yao, X.; Sussman, J. Virtual Care in Patients with Cancer: A Systematic Review. *Curr. Oncol.* **2021**, *28*, 3488–3506. [CrossRef]
48. Kulkarni, R.; Malouin, A.R. State of Telehealth. *N. Engl. J. Med.* **2016**, *375*, 1399–1400. [CrossRef]
49. Prescott, C. *Internet Users, UK: 2020*; Office for National Statistics: Newport, UK, 2021.
50. Shiely, F.; Foley, J.; Stone, A.; Cobbe, E.; Browne, S.; Murphy, E.; Kelsey, M.; Walsh-Crowley, J.; Eustace, J.A. Managing clinical trials during COVID-19: Experience from a clinical research facility. *Trials* **2021**, *22*, 1–7. [CrossRef]
51. NHS Health Research Authority. Making Changes to a Research Study to Manage the Impact of COVID-19. Available online: https://www.hra.nhs.uk/covid-19-research/covid-19-guidance-sponsors-sites-and-researchers/ (accessed on 1 October 2021).
52. Celis, H.; Fagard, R.H. White-coat hypertension: A clinical review. *Eur. J. Intern. Med.* **2004**, *15*, 348–357. [CrossRef]
53. Izmailova, E.S.; Ellis, R.; Benko, C. Remote Monitoring in Clinical Trials During the COVID-19 Pandemic. *Clin. Transl. Sci.* **2020**, *13*, 838–841. [CrossRef]
54. NHS Digital. NHS DigiTrials. Available online: https://digital.nhs.uk/services/nhs-digitrials (accessed on 1 October 2021).
55. Mather, N. How we accelerated clinical trials in the age of coronavirus. *Nat. Cell Biol.* **2020**, *584*, 326. [CrossRef]
56. The RECOVERY Collaborative Group. Dexamethasone in Hospitalized Patients with Covid-19. *N. Engl. J. Med.* **2021**, *384*, 693–704. [CrossRef]
57. Jackson, L.A.; Anderson, E.J.; Rouphael, N.G.; Roberts, P.C.; Makhene, M.; Coler, R.N.; McCullough, M.P.; Chappell, J.D.; Denison, M.R.; Stevens, L.J.; et al. An mRNA Vaccine against SARS-CoV-2—Preliminary Report. *N. Engl. J. Med.* **2020**, *383*, 1920–1931. [CrossRef]
58. Polack, F.P.; Thomas, S.J.; Kitchin, N.; Absalon, J.; Gurtman, A.; Lockhart, S.; Perez, J.L.; Pérez Marc, G.; Moreira, E.D.; Zerbini, C.; et al. Safety and efficacy of the BNT162b2 mRNA COVID-19 vaccine. *N. Engl. J. Med.* **2020**, *383*, 2603–2615. [CrossRef]
59. Walsh, E.E.; Frenck, R.W., Jr.; Falsey, A.R.; Kitchin, N.; Absalon, J.; Gurtman, A.; Lockhart, S.; Neuzil, K.; Mulligan, M.J.; Bailey, R.; et al. Safety and Immunogenicity of Two RNA-Based COVID-19 Vaccine Candidates. *N. Engl. J. Med.* **2020**, *383*, 2439–2450. [CrossRef]
60. Pennell, N.A.; Dillmon, M.; Levit, L.A.; Moushey, E.A.; Alva, A.S.; Blau, S.; Cannon, T.L.; Dickson, N.R.; Diehn, M.; Gonen, M.; et al. American Society of Clinical Oncology Road to Recovery Report: Learning From the COVID-19 Experience to Improve Clinical Research and Cancer Care. *J. Clin. Oncol.* **2021**, *39*, 155–169. [CrossRef]
61. Gogtay, N.J.; Chaudhari, N.; Ravi, R.; Thatte, U.M. Recruitment and retention of the participants in clinical trials: Challenges and solutions. *Perspect. Clin. Res.* **2020**, *11*, 64–69. [CrossRef]
62. Cancer Research UK. Getting cancer services back on track during the coronavirus pandemic. Available online: https://news.cancerresearchuk.org/2020/06/22/getting-cancer-services-back-on-track-during-the-covid-19-pandemic/ (accessed on 1 October 2021).

63. Croudass, A. *Applying Lessons from COVID-19: Shaping the Delivery of Cancer Clinical Trials*; Cancer Research UK: London, UK, 2020.
64. Ashbury, F.D. COVID-19 and supportive cancer care: Key issues and opportunities. *Curr. Opin. Oncol.* **2021**, *33*, 295–300. [CrossRef]
65. Shirke, M.M.; Shaikh, S.A.; Harky, A. Implications of Telemedicine in Oncology during the COVID-19 Pandemic. *Acta Bio Med.* **2020**, *91*, e2020022.
66. Richards, M.; Anderson, M.; Carter, P.; Ebert, B.L.; Mossialos, E. The impact of the COVID-19 pandemic on cancer care. *Nat. Rev. Cancer* **2020**, *1*, 565–567. [CrossRef]

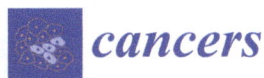

Article

Effect of Obesity among Hospitalized Cancer Patients with or without COVID-19 on a National Level

Jonathan Cottenet [1,2], Solène Tapia [1,2], Patrick Arveux [3], Alain Bernard [4], Tienhan Sandrine Dabakuyo-Yonli [5,6] and Catherine Quantin [1,2,7,8,9,*]

1. Biostatistics and Bioinformatics (DIM), University Hospital, BP 77908, 21079 Dijon, France
2. University of Bourgogne Franche-Comté, 21000 Dijon, France
3. Center for Primary Care and Public Health, Unisanté, University of Lausanne, 1015 Lausanne, Switzerland
4. Department of Thoracic and Cardiovascular Surgery, Dijon-Bourgogne University Hospital, 14 Rue Gaffarel, BP 77908, 21079 Dijon, France
5. Breast and Gynaecologic Cancer Registry of Côte d'Or/Epidemiology and Quality of Life Research Unit, Georges François Leclerc Centre-UNICANCER, 1 Rue Professeur Marion, 21000 Dijon, France
6. Lipids, Nutrition, Cancer Research Center, INSERM U1231, 21000 Dijon, France
7. Inserm, CIC 1432, 21000 Dijon, France
8. Clinical Epidemiology/Clinical Trials Unit, Dijon-Bourgogne University Hospital, Clinical Investigation Center, 21000 Dijon, France
9. Inserm, High-Dimensional Biostatistics for Drug Safety and Genomics, Le Centre de Recherche en Epidémiologie et Santé des Populations (CESP), Université Paris-Saclay (UVSQ), 94800 Villejuif, France
* Correspondence: catherine.quantin@chu-dijon.fr; Tel.: +33-3-80-29-34-65

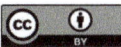

Citation: Cottenet, J.; Tapia, S.; Arveux, P.; Bernard, A.; Dabakuyo-Yonli, T.S.; Quantin, C. Effect of Obesity among Hospitalized Cancer Patients with or without COVID-19 on a National Level. *Cancers* 2022, *14*, 5660. https://doi.org/10.3390/cancers14225660

Academic Editors: Maria Dalamaga, Narjes Nasiri-Ansari and Nikolaos Spyrou

Received: 3 October 2022
Accepted: 14 November 2022
Published: 17 November 2022

Publisher's Note: MDPI stays neutral with regard to jurisdictional claims in published maps and institutional affiliations.

Copyright: © 2022 by the authors. Licensee MDPI, Basel, Switzerland. This article is an open access article distributed under the terms and conditions of the Creative Commons Attribution (CC BY) license (https://creativecommons.org/licenses/by/4.0/).

Simple Summary: Few papers have looked for an association between obesity and mortality risk in cancer patients with COVID-19 but, to our knowledge, none have studied this association in relation to the severity of obesity. We performed a study using data from the French national hospital database to study the effect of obesity (and its severity) on the risk of intensive care unit (ICU) admission, severe complications, and in-hospital mortality in cancer patients hospitalized for COVID-19 or not. The risk of ICU admission or severe complications was higher in cancer patients with obesity compared to cancer patients without obesity, regardless of cancer type and obesity severity. We did not find an excess obesity-related risk for in-hospital mortality, except for massive obesity in COVID-19 patients with hematological cancer and in non-COVID-19 patients with solid cancer. Further studies are warranted to better understand the relationship between obesity, and especially massive obesity, the prognosis of SARS-CoV-2 infection in cancer patients.

Abstract: Cancer and obesity are well-known prognostic factors in COVID-19. Our objective was to study the effect of obesity (and its severity) on the risk of intensive care unit (ICU) admission, severe complications, and in-hospital mortality, in a population of cancer patients hospitalized with or without COVID-19. All patients hospitalized in France for cancer from 1 March 2020 to 28 February 2022 were included from the French national administrative database. The effect of obesity was estimated in COVID-19 and in non-COVID-19 cancer patients using logistic and survival regressions, taking into account age, sex, comorbidities, and different types of cancer. Among the 992,899 cancer patients, we identified 53,090 patients with COVID-19 (5.35%), of which 3260 were obese (6.1%). After adjustment, for patients with or without COVID-19, there is an increased risk of ICU admission or severe complications in obese patients, regardless of the type of obesity. Regarding in-hospital mortality, there is no excess risk associated with overall obesity. However, massive obesity appears to be associated with an increased risk of in-hospital mortality, with a significantly stronger effect in solid cancer patients without COVID-19 and a significantly stronger effect in hematological cancer patients with COVID-19. This study showed that in France, among hospitalized patients with cancer and with or without COVID-19, increased vigilance is needed for obese patients, both in epidemic and non-epidemic periods. This vigilance should be further strengthened in patients with massive obesity for whom the risk of in-hospital mortality is higher, particularly in epidemic periods for patients with hematological cancers.

Keywords: obesity; COVID-19; cancer; tumor subtype; mortality; intensive care unit; medico-administrative data; SARS-CoV-2; France

---

1. Introduction

The World Health Organization declared a global pandemic in March 2020 [1] as a result of the severe acute respiratory syndrome coronavirus 2 (SARS-CoV2) outbreak. The 2019 coronavirus disease (COVID-19), caused by SARS-CoV-2, is still present and continues to cause significant mortality and morbidity worldwide. Indeed, COVID-19, as an extremely communicable virus, displays a range of conditions from no symptoms at all to severe illness and death [2–5], which has led to a shift in the focus of healthcare systems. As a result of health recommendations and changes in patient behavior, the pandemic also had indirect effects on morbidity and mortality

As of 28 January 2021, the COVID-19 epidemic was responsible for 99,727,853 confirmed cases worldwide, including 32,218,360 in Europe, and 2,137,670 deaths worldwide, 166,613 of which were in Europe [6]. In France, there were 3,053,617 confirmed cases and 73,049 deaths [7]. Based on expert opinion and data from the literature [8–12], the Haut Conseil de la Santé Publique (HCSP) considers that several factors can lead to severe SARS-Cov-2 infection. These include cardiovascular disease, diabetes (including unbalanced insulin-dependent diabetes or diabetes with secondary complications), chronic respiratory disease, and patients with congenital or acquired immunosuppression. In particular, patients treated for cancer (e.g., cancer chemotherapy, immunosuppressive therapy, biotherapy) are at increased risk of developing a severe form. People with morbid obesity are also cited as being at higher risk [13–16].

Cancer patients, due to the disease and specific treatments such as chemotherapy or surgery, are considered immunocompromised and therefore have a higher risk of infection [17–20]. Several publications have shown that cancer patients are three times more likely to develop serious complications from COVID-19 [9–11,15,21]. More specifically, in a study focused on lung cancer [22], we showed that, in this population, SARS-CoV-2 was associated with a 7-fold increased risk of in-hospital mortality and an almost 5-fold increased risk of serious complications.

Obesity is also a well-known prognostic factor in COVID-19. In numerous studies, obesity is associated with increased morbidity and mortality in patients with COVID-19 [23–27]. However, in some populations, there seems to be an obesity paradox, especially in severely ill populations such as respiratory failure or cancer patients [23,28–33]. Indeed, it appears that in these studies, obesity was not significantly associated with increased morbidity and mortality in cancer patients with COVID-19. Some studies even found that the risk of mortality was lower in cancer patients with metabolic comorbidities. However, the controversy persists as most of these studies were small and may have lacked power. Moreover, they did not take into account the different waves of the epidemic and more specifically 2021 and/or 2022.

There are very few data describing the natural history of cancer patients with COVID-19. Some papers have looked for an association between obesity and mortality risk but, to our knowledge, none have studied this association in relation to the severity of obesity. We hypothesized that there may be an intercorrelated relationship between obesity and cancer and that their mutual pathogenetic attributes may predispose individuals to a different prognosis when they develop a SARS-CoV-2 infection.

Using data from the French national hospital database, which includes more than 1,000,000 patients hospitalized for cancer between March 2020 and March 2022, our aim was, therefore, to investigate the effect of obesity (and its severity) on the risk of intensive care unit (ICU) admission, severe complications and in-hospital mortality in cancer patients hospitalized with or without COVID-19.

2. Materials and Methods

2.1. Database

We conducted a retrospective cohort study using the national hospital Programme de Médicalisation des Systèmes d'Information (PMSI) database, which is designed to include discharge abstracts for all inpatient admissions to public and private hospitals in France. Inspired by the American DRG (diagnosis-related groups) model, the information in these abstracts is anonymous and covers both medical and administrative data. Diagnoses identified during the hospital stay are coded according to the 10th edition of the International Classification of Diseases (ICD-10), and procedures performed during hospitalization are coded according to the French Common Classification of Medical Procedures. The fact that these national data are used for the allocation of hospital budgets encourages improvement in data quality in terms of coherence, accuracy, and exhaustiveness. Therefore, these hospital data have been used in medical research for many years [34–44], and their quality has been confirmed in recent studies on COVID-19 [5,45–50].

2.2. Population

We included all patients hospitalized for or with cancer from 1 March 2020 to 28 February 2022. Hospital stays of more than one day (i.e., excluding a day of hospitalization, such as a chemotherapy session) for cancer were identified using the International Classification of Diseases, 10th Revision (ICD-10) codes, via principal diagnoses (PD), related diagnoses (RD) or associated diagnoses (AD). It should be noted that only the 1st stay identified during the inclusion period has been retained so that a patient is counted only once. We considered all cancers corresponding to malignant tumors (all those beginning with 'C', Table S1), with and without metastases, and separated them into different tumor subtypes (solid cancers with metastases, solid cancers with localized tumor, and hematological cancers).

Among these patients, we separated a group of patients with mention of COVID-19 at the time of oncology stay, and another group of patients without mention of COVID-19 either at the time of inclusion or during the whole study period. COVID-19 patients were identified using ICD-10 codes (U0710, U0711, U0712, U0714 or U0715). We also identified obese patients at the time of oncology stay using ICD-10 codes E66 (except overweight) in PD, RD, or AD. The diagnosis of obesity was based on a body mass index (BMI) of ≥ 30 kg/m^2. Obesity was also classified according to its severity: massive obesity (BMI ≥ 50 kg/m^2), morbid obesity (BMI 40 to 49 kg/m^2), and standard obesity (BMI 30 to 39 kg/m^2). The classification of the ICD-10 codes used is given in Table S2.

2.3. Outcomes

Our primary outcome was transferring to the intensive care unit (ICU), which was determined by the presence of an ICU stay indicator in the filed claims during the cancer stay. Our second outcome was severe complications (including acute respiratory and kidney diseases, stroke, myocardial infarction, atrial fibrillation, and venous thrombosis including pulmonary embolism) during the cancer stay and 90 days after discharge. Finally, our third outcome was in-hospital mortality, defined as any patient who died in hospital during the cancer stay and within 90 days after discharge.

2.4. Variables

Patient characteristics such as age (seven age classes were defined: ≤ 40, 41–50, 51–60, 61–70, 71–80, 81–90, and >90) and gender were also retrieved. We also extracted all diagnoses from the discharge abstracts to retrieve patients' comorbidities: hypertension, diabetes, dementia, HIV, heart failure, chronic respiratory and renal diseases, cirrhosis, peripheral vascular disease, dyslipidemia, deficiency anemia, and pulmonary bacterial infection. Finally, we identified chemotherapy in the previous 2 years and in the month following the inclusion stay, via ICD-10 code Z511.

2.5. Statistical Analysis

Qualitative variables are provided as frequencies (percentages) and were compared using the Chi-2 test or Fisher's exact test. Quantitative variables are provided as means ± standard deviation (SD) and medians [interquartile range (Q1–Q3)], and were compared using the Student's *t* test or Mann-Whitney test.

Our outcomes were compared for all patients and then according to the type of tumor (solid cancers with metastasis, with localized tumors, hematological cancers) and the type of obesity (massive, morbid, standard).

To estimate the effect of obesity in cancer patients hospitalized depending on the COVID-19 infection, all the following models were performed in both COVID-19 and non-COVID-19 patients, after adjustment on age, sex, chemotherapy, and other comorbidities:

- Logistic regression models to estimate the effect of obesity on the risk of transfer to ICU, severe complications, and in-hospital mortality at inclusion.
- Fine and Gray models to estimate the effect of obesity on the risk of severe complications within 90 days after discharge. This model takes into account the competing risk between severe complications and in-hospital mortality, as, death may prevent the observation of severe complications.
- Cox models to estimate the effect of obesity on the risk of in-hospital mortality within 90 days after discharge.

We also performed sensitivity analyses by separating the analyses into two different periods of the epidemic corresponding to two different viral periods: March–December 2020 (the original virus) and January 2021–February 2022 (the emergence of the alpha variant in France in late 2020).

The statistical significance threshold was set at < 0.05. All analyses were performed using SAS (SAS Institute Inc, Version 9.4, Cary, NC, USA).

3. Results

3.1. Patient Characteristics

We included 922,899 patients diagnosed with cancer, among whom we identified 53,090 patients with COVID-19 (5.35%). Among these patients, 3260 were classified as obese (6.14%) (Table 1).

Table 1. Characteristics of COVID-19 cancer patients by obesity.

	No Obesity (1)	Obesity (2)	*p*-Value (1 vs. 2)	Standard Obesity (3)	Morbid Obesity (4)	Massive Obesity (5)	*p*-Value (1 vs. 3)	*p*-Value (1 vs. 4)	*p*-Value (1 vs. 5)
N	49,830	3260		2704	497	59			
Men, *n*(%)	29,939 (60.08)	1695 (51.99)	<0.01	1494 (55.25)	182 (36.62)	19 (32.20)	<0.01	<0.01	<0.01
Age, mean (std)	72.58 (14.32)	68.99 (11.61)	<0.01	69.43 (11.55)	67.32 (11.64)	62.88 (11.13)	<0.01	<0.01	<0.01
Age group (years)			<0.01				<0.01	<0.01	<0.01
≤40	1379 (2.77)	55 (1.69)		40 (1.48)	12 (2.41)	3 (5.08)			
41–50	1817 (3.65)	158 (4.85)		124 (4.59)	28 (5.63)	6 (10.17)			
51–80	30,644 (61.50)	2550 (78.22)		2105 (77.85)	396 (79.68)	49 (83.05)			
81–90	12,846 (25.78)	443 (13.59)		386 (14.28)	56 (11.27)	1 (1.69)			
>90	3144 (6.31)	54 (1.66)		49 (1.81)	5 (1.01)	0			
Chemotherapy, n(%)	22,967 (46.09)	1207 (37.02)	<0.01	1009 (37.32)	174 (35.01)	24 (40.68)	<0.01	<0.01	0.40
Comorbidities, n(%)									
Hypertension	16,747 (33.61)	1869 (57.33)	<0.01	1536 (56.80)	296 (59.56)	37 (62.71)	<0.01	<0.01	<0.01
Dementia	2612 (5.24)	81 (2.48)	<0.01	68 (2.51)	13 (2.62)	0	<0.01	<0.01	0.08
HIV	191 (0.38)	7 (0.21)	0.13	6 (0.22)	1 (0.20)	0	0.18	1	1
Heart failure	4467 (8.96)	416 (12.76)	<0.01	316 (11.69)	91 (18.31)	9 (15.25)	<0.01	<0.01	0.09

Table 1. Cont.

	No Obesity (1)	Obesity (2)	p-Value (1 vs. 2)	Standard Obesity (3)	Morbid Obesity (4)	Massive Obesity (5)	p-Value (1 vs. 3)	p-Value (1 vs. 4)	p-Value (1 vs. 5)
Chronic respiratory disease	924 (1.85)	154 (4.72)	<0.01	112 (4.14)	38 (7.65)	4 (6.78)	<0.01	<0.01	0.02
Chronic kidney disease	4767 (9.57)	438 (13.44)	<0.01	363 (13.42)	74 (14.89)	1 (1.69)	<0.01	<0.01	0.04
Cirrhosis	1114 (2.24)	133 (4.08)	<0.01	112 (4.14)	17 (3.42)	4 (6.78)	<0.01	0.08	0.04
Diabetes	9275 (18.61)	1320 (40.49)	<0.01	1064 (39.35)	234 (47.08)	22 (37.29)	<0.01	<0.01	<0.01
Peripheral vascular disease	2315 (4.65)	196 (6.01)	<0.01	166 (6.14)	29 (5.84)	1 (1.69)	<0.01	0.21	0.53
Dyslipidemia	2533 (5.08)	379 (11.63)	<0.01	315 (11.65)	59 (11.87)	5 (8.47)	<0.01	<0.01	0.23
Deficiency Anemia	2881 (5.78)	223 (6.84)	0.01	186 (6.88)	33 (6.64)	4 (6.78)	0.02	0.42	0.78
COPD	3674 (7.37)	362 (11.10)	<0.01	300 (11.09)	56 (11.27)	6 (10.17)	<0.01	0.001	0.45
Pulmonary bacterial infection	3149 (6.32)	379 (11.63)	<0.01	331 (12.24)	41 (8.25)	7 (11.86)	<0.01	0.08	0.10
Outcomes, n(%)									
Admission to ICU	6753 (13.55)	992 (30.43)	<0.01	825 (30.51)	146 (29.38)	21 (35.59)	<0.01	<0.01	<0.01
Severe complication during the inclusion stay	33,599 (67.43)	2589 (79.42)	<0.01	2154 (79.66)	385 (77.46)	50 (84.75)	<0.01	<0.01	<0.01
In-hospital mortality during the inclusion stay	15,313 (30.73)	805 (24.69)	<0.01	653 (24.15)	132 (26.56)	20 (33.90)	<0.01	0.04	0.60
Severe complication within 90 days	36,583 (73.42)	2724 (83.56)	<0.01	2262 (83.65)	409 (82.29)	53 (89.83)	<0.01	<0.01	<0.01
In-hospital mortality within 90 days	19,377 (38.89)	981 (30.09)	<0.01	801 (29.62)	156 (31.39)	24 (40.68)	<0.01	<0.01	0.78

In cancer patients with COVID-19 (Table 1), the rate of men was lower in obese than in non-obese patients (51.99% vs. 60.08%, $p < 0.01$), and obese patients were younger than non-obese patients.

In addition, the rates of the majority of comorbidities studied were higher in obese patients than in non-obese patients, except for dementia and HIV (Table 1). Finally, regarding outcomes (Table 1), the rate of ICU admission was two times higher in obese than in non-obese patients (30.4% vs. 13.6%, $p < 0.01$). The rate of severe complications was also higher whether at inclusion (79.4% vs. 67.4, $p < 0.01$) or within 90 days (83.6% vs. 73.4%, $p < 0.01$). In contrast, the in-hospital mortality rate was lower in obese patients than in non-obese patients whether at inclusion (24.7% vs. 30.7%, $p < 0.01$) or within 90 days (30.1% vs. 38.9%, $p < 0.01$).

Among obese patients (N = 3260), 83% were classified as standard obesity (N = 2704), 15% as morbid obesity (N = 497), and 2% as massive obesity (N = 59). Regardless of the type of obesity, patients were younger than non-obese patients and less often male (Table 1). It should be noted that men represent only 30% of the patients with morbid or massive obesity. Concerning comorbidities, the majority of comorbidities studied were significantly higher in standard obese patients than in non-obese patients, except for dementia and HIV (Table 1). We found the same results for morbidly obese patients even if the discrepancy was not significant for cirrhosis, peripheral vascular disease, deficiency anemia, and pulmonary bacterial infection. For the comparison between non-obese patients and those with massive obesity, we found that the rates of hypertension, chronic respiratory and kidney disease, cirrhosis, and diabetes were significantly higher in massively obese patients.

Whatever the type of obesity, the rate of ICU admission or severe complications was higher in obese patients than in non-obese patients (Table 1). Regarding in-hospital mortality, rates were significantly lower in patients with standard or morbid obesity than in non-obese patients, either at inclusion (respectively 24.2%, 26.6%, and 30.7%) or at 90 days (29.6%, 31.4%, and 38.9%). In contrast, the rates were higher in massively obese patients, although this difference was not significant, either at inclusion (33.9% vs. 30.7%, $p = 0.60$) or at 90 days (40.7% vs. 38.9%, $p = 0.78$).

For non-COVID-19 patients, we found similar results regarding patient characteristics to those for COVID-19 patients (Table S1).

3.2. Outcomes Depending on the Type of Tumor

When we look at the type of tumor (Table 2), the rate of hematological cancer was similar between obese and non-obese patients (26.29% vs. 25.45%, $p = 0.29$). However, the rate of solid cancer with metastasis was higher in non-obese patients (39.67% vs. 31.07%, $p < 0.01$), while the rate of solid cancer with localized tumor was higher in obese patients (42.64% vs. 34.88%, $p < 0.01$). The same results were found whatever the type of obesity, although the differences were not significant for patients with massive obesity (Table 2).

Table 2. Type of cancer by obesity among COVID-19 cancer patients.

	No Obesity (1)	Obesity (2)	p-Value (1 vs. 2)	Standard Obesity (3)	Morbid Obesity (4)	Massive Obesity (5)	p-Value (1 vs. 3)	p-Value (1 vs. 4)	p-Value (1 vs. 5)
N	49,830	3260		2704	497	59			
Hematological cancer, n(%)	12,682 (25.45)	857 (26.29)	0.29	731 (27.03)	110 (22.13)	16 (27.12)	0.07	0.09	0.77
Solid Cancer with metastasis, n(%)	19,767 (39.67)	1013 (31.07)	<0.01	840 (31.07)	156 (31.39)	17 (28.81)	<0.01	<0.01	0.09
Solid Cancer with localized tumor, n(%)	17,381 (34.88)	1390 (42.64)	<0.01	1133 (41.90)	231 (46.48)	26 (44.07)	<0.01	<0.01	0.14

Regarding the description of the type of cancer, among non-COVID-19 patients (Table S2), the rate of patients with hematological cancer or solid cancer with metastasis was lower in obese patients than in non-obese patients (8.49% vs. 10.45% for hematological cancer and 24.62% vs. 29.69% for solid cancer with metastasis). Furthermore, it should be noted that among non-COVID-19 patients with massive obesity, the rate of patients with hematological cancer was similar to that in patients without obesity (11% vs. 10.45 %, $p = 0.58$). Conversely, and as observed in the population of patients with cancer and COVID-19, the rate of solid cancer with localized tumors was higher in obese patients (whatever the type of obesity).

Concerning our outcomes, for COVID-19 patients, whatever the type of tumor and the type of obesity, the rate of ICU admission or severe complications was higher in obese patients than in non-obese patients (Table 3).

However, the in-hospital mortality rate appears to differ according to the type of tumor and the type of obesity (Table 3). In hematological cancer, the more severe the obesity, the higher the mortality rate. Compared to non-obese patients, the mortality rate is lower for standard obese patients, similar for morbidly obese patients, and higher for massive obese patients. In solid cancer with metastasis, compared to non-obese patients, the mortality rate is lower for standard obese patients and massively obese patients, while it is equivalent for morbidly obese patients. In solid cancer with localized tumors, compared to non-obese patients, the mortality rate is lower for standard obese patients and morbidly obese patients, while it is equivalent massively obese patients.

Compared to the COVID-19 population, the results are similar for ICU admissions or complications in the non-COVID-19 population but are not the same for in-hospital mortality, especially in the population with massive obesity (Table S3). Thus, for patients with hematological cancer, the mortality rate for massive obesity is similar to that of patients without obesity. For patients with solid cancers (with metastases or with localized tumors), the in-hospital mortality rate is higher in patients with massive obesity than in patients without obesity.

Table 3. Admission to ICU, severe complication and in-hospital mortality of COVID-19 cancer patients by type of cancer and obesity.

Hematological Cancer	No Obesity (1) 12,682	Obesity (2) 857	p-Value (1 vs. 2)	Standard Obesity (3) 731	Morbid Obesity (4) 110	Massive Obesity (5) 16	p-Value (1 vs. 3)	p-Value (1 vs. 4)	p-Value (1 vs. 5)
Admission to ICU	2770 (21.84)	349 (40.72)	<0.01	295 (40.36)	48 (43.64)	6 (37.50)	<0.01	<0.01	0.14
Severe complication during the inclusion stay	8975 (70.77)	703 (82.03)	<0.01	593 (81.12)	94 (85.45)	16 (100)	<0.01	<0.01	0.01
In-hospital mortality during the inclusion stay	3798 (29.95)	238 (27.77)	0.18	196 (26.81)	34 (30.91)	8 (50)	0.07	0.83	0.10
Severe complication within 90 days	9735 (76.76)	730 (85.18)	<0.01	618 (84.54)	96 (87.27)	16 (100)	<0.01	0.01	0.03
In-hospital mortality within 90 days	4528 (35.70)	270 (31.51)	0.01	222 (30.37)	38 (34.55)	10 (62.50)	<0.01	0.80	0.03
Solid Cancer with metastasis	19,767	1013		840	156	17			
Admission to ICU	1727 (8.74)	218 (21.52)	<0.01	181 (21.55)	32 (20.51)	5 (29.41)	<0.01	<0.01	0.01
Severe complication during the inclusion stay	12,788 (64.69)	798 (78.78)	<0.01	671 (79.88)	113 (72.44)	14 (82.35)	<0.01	0.04	0.13
In-hospital mortality during the inclusion stay	7281 (36.83)	296 (29.22)	<0.01	236 (28.10)	55 (35.26)	5 (29.41)	<0.01	0.68	0.53
Severe complication within 90 days	14,015 (70.90)	851 (84.01)	<0.01	714 (85)	123 (78.85)	14 (82.35)	<0.01	0.03	0.43
In-hospital mortality within 90 days	9570 (48.41)	378 (37.31)	<0.01	305 (36.31)	67 (42.95)	6 (35.29)	<0.01	0.17	0.28
Solid Cancer with localized tumor	17,381	1390		1133	231	26			
Admission to ICU	2256 (12.98)	425 (30.58)	<0.01	349 (30.80)	66 (28.57)	10 (38.46)	<0.01	<0.01	<0.01
Severe complication during the inclusion stay	11,836 (68.10)	1088 (78.27)	<0.01	890 (78.55)	178 (77.06)	20 (76.92)	<0.01	<0.01	0.33
In-hospital mortality during the inclusion stay	4234 (24.36)	271 (19.5)	<0.01	221 (19.51)	43 (18.61)	7 (26.92)	<0.01	0.04	0.76
Severe complication within 90 days	12,833 (73.83)	1143 (82.23)	<0.01	930 (82.08)	190 (82.25)	23 (88.46)	<0.01	<0.01	0.09
In-hospital mortality within 90 days	5279 (30.37)	333 (23.96)	<0.01	274 (24.18)	51 (22.08)	8 (30.77)	<0.01	0.01	0.96

3.3. Multivariate Analyses

Regarding the effect of obesity on COVID-19 cancer patients, after adjusting for age, sex, chemotherapy, and comorbidities, we found that those with obesity have twice the risk of admission to ICU compared to those without obesity, regardless of cancer type (Table 4). We found the same results concerning the risk of severe complications, especially for severe complications during the admission stay (Table 4). With regard to hospital mortality, there was no excess risk linked to obesity, in cancer patients with COVID-19 (Table 4), regardless of cancer type.

In the multivariate analyses for the non-COVID-19 patients (Table S4), we found the same results by type of cancer and in COVID-19 patients, i.e., obesity was associated with an increased risk of ICU admission and severe complications, but not with an increased risk of hospital mortality.

For COVID-19 patients, if we focus on the effect according to the severity of the obesity, we found that the risk of admission to ICU was two times higher whatever the severity and whatever the type of cancer (Table 5), even if this risk was not significant for massive obese patients in hematological cancer and solid cancer with metastasis. The risk of severe complications within 90 days was also higher, although not significant, for patients with solid cancer with metastasis and morbid or massive obesity (Table 5).

Table 4. Effect of obesity by type of cancer on the different outcomes, among COVID-19 cancer patients.

	In-Hospital Mortality during the Stay *	Severe Complications during the Stay *	Intensive Care Support during the Stay *	In-Hospital Mortality within 90 Days **	Severe Complications within 90 Days ***
	OR [95% CI]	OR [95% CI]	OR [95% CI]	HR [95% CI]	HR [95% CI]
All cancer	0.783 [0.719–0.852]	1.682 [1.531–1.847]	2.130 [1.952–2.323]	0.791 [0.741–0.844]	1.117 [1.094–1.139]
Hematological cancer	0.977 [0.831–1.148]	1.728 [1.424–2.096]	1.909 [1.631–2.233]	0.929 [0.820–1.053]	1.093 [1.053–1.134]
Solid Cancer with metastasis	0.733 [0.636–0.844]	1.791 [1.521–2.108]	2.225 [1.877–2.639]	0.762 [0.687–0.846]	1.153 [1.113–1.195]
Solid cancer with localized tumor	0.814 [0.705–0.939]	1.592 [1.378–1.840]	2.053 [1.791–2.354]	0.827 [0.738–0.925]	1.101 [1.067–1.137]

OR = Odds ratio; HR = Hazard ratio; CI = confidence interval * Logistic model adjusted on age class, sex, chemotherapy, dementia, heart failure, chronic respiratory disease, cirrhosis, diabetes, deficiency anemia and pulmonary bacterial infection; ** Cox model adjusted on age class, sex, dementia, heart failure, chronic respiratory disease, cirrhosis, diabetes, deficiency anemia and pulmonary bacterial infection; *** Fine & Gray model adjusted on age class, sex, dementia, heart failure, chronic respiratory disease, cirrhosis, diabetes, deficiency anemia and pulmonary bacterial infection.

Table 5. Effect of obesity according to its severity and by type of cancer on the different outcomes, among COVID-19 cancer patients.

	In-Hospital Mortality during the Stay *	Severe Complications during the Stay *	Intensive Care Support during the Stay *	In-Hospital Mortality within 90 Days **	Severe Complications within 90 Days ***
	OR [95% CI]	OR [95% CI]	OR [95% CI]	HR [95% CI]	HR [95% CI]
All cancer					
Standard obesity	0.750 [0.684–0.823]	1.714 [1.547–1.899]	2.136 [1.944–2.347]	0.772 [0.719–0.829]	1.118 [1.095–1.143]
Morbid obesity	0.914 [0.745–1.121]	1.433 [1.138–1.804]	2.063 [1.674–2.543]	0.860 [0.734–1.008]	1.091 [1.039–1.146]
Massive obesity	1.401 [0.806–2.434]	2.796 [1.320–5.922]	2.378 [1.353–4.179]	1.178 [0.789–1.759]	1.251 [1.113–1.406]
Hematological cancer					
Standard obesity	0.915 [0.768–1.090]	1.599 [1.302–1.963]	1.880 [1.587–2.226]	0.887 [0.774–1.016]	1.082 [1.040–1.127]
Morbid obesity	1.247 [0.819–1.899]	2.462 [1.406–4.312]	2.247 [1.505–3.353]	1.073 [0.778–1.480]	1.137 [1.040–1.243]
Massive obesity	3.094 [1.117–8.570]		1.197 [0.409–3.503]	2.202 [1.182–4.100]	1.303 [1.135–1.497]
Solid Cancer with metastasis					
Standard obesity	0.690 [0.590–0.807]	1.954 [1.632–2.341]	2.260 [1.880–2.717]	0.734 [0.654–0.824]	1.175 [1.132–1.221]
Morbid obesity	0.991 [0.709–1.385]	1.086 [0.735–1.607]	1.982 [1.301–3.019]	0.926 [0.727–1.179]	1.035 [0.941–1.139]
Massive obesity	0.808 [0.283–2.311]	2.482 [0.668–9.218]	2.742 [0.912–8.246]	0.757 [0.340–1.687]	1.162 [0.89–1.517]
Solid Cancer with localized tumor					
Standard obesity	0.793 [0.678–0.928]	1.617 [1.380–1.895]	2.067 [1.781–2.400]	0.821 [0.725–0.928]	1.096 [1.058–1.134]
Morbid obesity	0.863 [0.613–1.215]	1.446 [1.028–2.035]	1.881 [1.377–2.570]	0.820 [0.622–1.083]	1.112 [1.034–1.197]
Massive obesity	1.531 [0.618–3.794]	1.847 [0.690–4.948]	3.132 [1.366–7.181]	1.183 [0.591–2.370]	1.283 [1.065–1.546]

OR = Odds ratio; HR = Hazard ratio; CI = confidence interval; * Logistic model adjusted on age class, sex, chemotherapy, dementia, heart failure, chronic respiratory disease, cirrhosis, diabetes, deficiency anemia and pulmonary bacterial infection; ** Cox model adjusted on age class, sex, dementia, heart failure, chronic respiratory disease, cirrhosis, diabetes, deficiency anemia and pulmonary bacterial infection; *** Fine & Gray model adjusted on age class, sex, dementia, heart failure, chronic respiratory disease, cirrhosis, diabetes, deficiency anemia and pulmonary bacterial infection.

Finally, concerning in-hospital mortality (Table 5), massive obesity seems to be a risk factor, particularly in patients with hematological cancer, where this risk is significant (OR = 3.09 [1.12–8.57] during the inclusion stay and HR = 2.20 [1.18–4.10] within 90 days).

For the other types of obesity (standard or morbid), there was no excess risk due to obesity in patients with solid cancer (with metastasis or with localized tumor).

In the non-COVID-19 population, after looking at the type of obesity, we still found that the risk of admission to intensive care was higher for all types of obesity and all types of cancer (Table S5). We found the same results for the excess risk of severe complications. Regarding in-hospital mortality, massive obesity again seems to be a risk factor, and even more so in patients with solid cancer (with metastasis or with localized tumor).

In the sensitivity analyses, separating the analyses according to the health conditions of the pandemic in France, we found the same trends as in the results above, whatever the period considered (2020 or 2021–2022).

4. Discussion

Our results showed that in France, for patients with or without COVID-19, there is an increased risk of ICU admission or severe complications in obese patients, regardless of the type of obesity. Regarding in-hospital mortality, there is no excess risk associated with overall obesity. However, massive obesity appears to be associated with an increased risk of in-hospital mortality, with a significantly stronger effect in solid cancer patients without COVID-19 and a significantly stronger effect in hematological cancer patients with COVID-19. We also found an increased risk of in-hospital mortality in solid cancer patients with localized tumors among COVID-19 patients, but this result was not significant. However, we can hypothesize a lack of power in this subgroup with few patients with massive obesity. Focusing on COVID-19, cancer patients with obesity are twice as likely to be admitted to ICU compared to cancer patients without obesity, regardless of cancer type and obesity severity. We found the same results for the risk of severe complications. However, surprisingly, we did not find a significant excess obesity-related risk for in-hospital mortality among cancer patients hospitalized for COVID-19, except for massive obesity in patients with hematological cancer.

The fact that an increased risk of complications and ICU admissions were shown in obese cancer patients was to be expected. Indeed, many studies have shown similar results in the general population and cancer patients.

However, we did not find that obesity had a negative effect on in-hospital mortality in cancer patients hospitalized for COVID-19. While this result may seem surprising since obesity is classically considered as contributing to a worse prognosis in the COVID-19 population [23–27], it is consistent with other studies [23,28–33,51] in cancer patients which did not find that mortality was increased (most ORs were close to 1 even after adjustment). This is the case, for example, for the cancer consortium cohort study, which found that obesity was not significantly associated with the risk of 30-day mortality, either in univariate analysis or after adjustment for age, sex, and smoking (OR = 0.99 [0.58–1.71]). This result is also consistent with a meta-analysis including 2117 mixed ambulatory and hospitalized cancer patients (OR = 0.92 [0.66–1.28]. Secondly, it is well known that obese patients may paradoxically have lower mortality than non-obese patients [23].

This "obesity paradox" is observed in several epidemiological studies of chronic diseases, acute illnesses, and cancer, where mortality in non-obese patients is higher than in obese patients [52–55]. This phenomenon was also observed during the COVID-19 pandemic and has been supported in the US, using a mathematical model [56]. The lean mass found in obese people could be a possible explanation for the obesity paradox. Indeed, even if the increase in BMI is mainly due to fat mass, obese people have an increase in lean mass, including muscle mass, in particular cardiac muscle mass. The obesity paradox could therefore be linked to a protective effect of increased lean mass. [52]. According to Park et al., "the leading hypothesis for this phenomenon points to the greater metabolic reserve represented by the abundant adipose tissue, which enables the patient to withstand the course of severe acute or chronic illness".

Of course, the obesity paradox cannot be the only reason associated with these results. Indeed, in the most advanced stages, a characteristic feature of cancer is cachexia. Cancer cachexia is a multifactorial syndrome that leads to substantial weight loss, primarily due to skeletal muscle loss, and can have a substantially negative impact on the response to immune checkpoint inhibitors therapy, particularly inpatients with advanced non-small cell lung cancer [57]. Furthermore, cachexia is frequently obscured by obesity, leading to underdiagnosis and excess mortality [58]. In particular, Martin et al. showed that skeletal muscle depletion is a powerful prognostic factor of mortality, independent of body mass index [59]. However, we cannot reliably identify cachexia in our database. This is not necessarily surprising since cachexia is usually not recorded in hospital cohorts. Moreover, there still exists a gap in the clinical management of cachexia due to the complex nature of the condition, which may affect the ability to identify cachectic patients and appropriate treatment, for which there is no globally recognized 'gold standard' [60]. Therefore, cachexia remains a largely underestimated condition.

Considering the severity of obesity, compared to patients without obesity, we did not find an excess mortality risk for patients with standard or with morbid obesity. This result is consistent with other studies looking at this impact on COVID-19 patients and chronic illnesses [18,61,62]. Again, this may be related to the obesity paradox. Indeed, studies confirming the "obesity paradox" showed that patients with standard or morbid BMI had severe symptoms that led to admission to intensive care, but not to increased mortality. However, other papers have shown that the risk is increased for both the general and COVID-19 populations [63–65]. To our knowledge, this is the first study to show the effect of massive obesity in cancer patients with COVID-19, as we did not find any study that took into account a BMI of more than 50 kg/m2. We found an excess risk for all types of cancer, but this excess risk is in fact significant in patients with hematological cancer (this type of cancer is particularly associated with a severe form of COVID-19) [63,66,67], even if our number of patients is small. Further studies are thus needed to investigate the relationship between massive obesity and mortality in patients with cancer and COVID-19 infection.

Not all cancer patients have the same risk of developing severe COVID-19. Indeed, the mechanisms underlying the progression of COVID-19 to a severe form include host factors such as age or cachexia, hypercoagulable states caused by cancer or drugs, and possible hyperexpression of entry factors such as angiotensin-2 converting enzyme or neurophilin-1 [68]. Other factors affecting viral immunity include myeloid cell dysfunction and cancer-related T-cell depletion [69]. The immune system is also involved in the virus-induced cytokine storm [70], which may be tempered or delayed by cancer- or drug-related immune depression [71]. For example, in a previous study [19], we found that among COVID cancer patients, those with hematological cancer had a slight risk of developing more complications during their stay than those with solid tumors. This could be explained by the treatment of these patients and the resulting immunosuppression during and after treatment, and probably throughout their lives. [68–71]. However, our data show that the effects of obesity on severe complications, admission to ICU, or mortality are nearly the same whatever the type of cancer and notably those with the worst prognosis such as hematological cancers and metastatic solid tumors. These results suggest that the influence of obesity on the prognosis of SARS-CoV-2 infection may be independent of the type of cancer, which may also seem surprising. Further studies are needed to further investigate the association between obesity and the prognosis of COVID-19 infection, regardless of cancer type.

4.1. Strengths

In France, the national hospital database includes information from all French private and public hospitals, including data on COVID-19 patients and cancer patients. The fact that these national data are used for hospital budget allocation encourages high levels of data consistency, accuracy, and completeness. As a result, this study includes national data for more than 40,000 cancer patients and COVID-19, making it one of the largest studies in terms of the number of patients included and the completeness of the data. This study is also one of the few to provide data with full hospital follow-up, including all in-hospital mortality, regardless of the length of stay, and 90 days of follow-up. In addition, we were able to obtain information on the metastatic status of all solid tumors as well as on the patients' comorbidities. We were also able to separate the different severities of obesity in our analyses by considering three categories (standard, morbid, and massive) and to our knowledge, none have studied this association in relation to the severity of obesity in cancer patients with COVID-19. We also considered two different periods of the epidemic corresponding to two different viral periods: the original virus and the emergence of the alpha variant in France in late 2020.

4.2. Limitations

We recognize that there are several limitations. First, we included only hospitalized patients and we only measured hospital mortality, even if mortality in France mainly occurs in hospitals. Thus we cannot discount that a number of patients infected with COVID-19 were not hospitalized. Our study thus included only severe cases of COVID-19. Secondly, the data used to identify obesity are based on ICD-10 codes identified in the PMSI hospital database, and these data are collected for medico-economic purposes. However, we can assume that the completeness is satisfactory because hospitals have a strong financial incentive to collect these data. Indeed, the information is sometimes not filled in the discharge abstract when there is no impact on the patient's care, which is often the case for ambulatory care, but this was not the case for the hospitalizations considered. We cannot ignore a misclassification between our different obesity groups. We may also have a lack of power in the massive obesity group, although we do have significant results for hematological cancers.

Given the reliance on ICD-10 codes for the selection of patients and the ascertainment of outcomes, there was a potential for misclassification-related or under-detection-related bias, especially for comorbidities [72,73]. Coding practices may vary among institutions as the people who perform the coding of diagnoses can be clinicians or information system technicians. Nevertheless, the quality of coding is checked in a standardized way by medical information professionals in each hospital in order to correct diagnoses (internal quality assessment), and the level of recording of co-morbidities has increased significantly in recent years, following its impact on the tariff of hospital stays. Because of the impact on hospital budget allocation, it has been shown that hospital claims data are becoming more accurate. In addition, a national external quality assessment program has been implemented to verify the quality of discharge abstracts in each hospital. Moreover, the use of hospital data to identify all hospitalized cancer cases may be questionable. It seems unlikely that cancer was not recorded in the PMSI data, as cancer is a serious condition that is difficult to ignore when summarizing a patient's history as the coding of cancer has an impact on the hospital's budget allocation.

In addition, we had no information on the stage of cancer or on the treatments, whether anti-cancer treatments (which would have allowed us to evaluate the potentially induced immuno-suppression) such as hormonal therapy, or other treatments used in other pathologies, which may influence (for good or bad) the severity of COVID-19 in hospitalized patients, such as different inhibitors (tyrosine kinase, IL6, ARA2). Finally, we do not have access to vaccination data, but cancer patients were a priority in the French regulations and the rate of completion of the initial vaccination schedule was over 90% for these patients in 2022.

5. Conclusions

This study showed that in France, among hospitalized patients with cancer and with or without COVID-19, increased vigilance is needed for obese patients, both in epidemic and non-epidemic periods. This vigilance should be further strengthened in patients with massive obesity for whom the risk of in-hospital mortality is higher, particularly in epidemic periods for patients with hematological cancers.

Focusing on COVID-19, obese patients have an increased risk of admission to the ICU (a two-fold increase) and severe complications compared to non-obese patients. Surprisingly, we did not find any excess risk related to obesity regarding in-hospital mortality, suggesting that the paradigm of the "obesity paradox" may also apply to this population. Considering the severity of obesity, compared to patients without obesity, we did not find an excess mortality risk for patients with standard or morbid obesity. However, to our knowledge, this is the first study to show an effect the massive obesity, especially in hematological cancer patients.

This study also provides information about the role of obesity according to the different types of cancer for which the prognosis is worse such as hematological cancers and all metastatic cancers. We found nearly the same results as described above, whatever the type of cancer. These results suggest that the influence of obesity on the prognosis of SARS-CoV-2 infection may be independent of the type of cancer. Further studies are warranted to better understand the relationship between obesity, especially massive obesity, and the prognosis of SARS-CoV-2 infection in cancer patients.

Supplementary Materials: The following supporting information can be downloaded at: https://www.mdpi.com/article/10.3390/cancers14225660/s1, Table S1: ICD-10 codes used for identification of tumor subtypes; Table S2: ICD-10 codes used for obesity; Table S3: Admission to ICU, severe complication and in-hospital mortality of non COVID-19 cancer patients by type of cancer and obesity; Table S4: Effect of obesity by type of cancer on the different outcomes, among non COVID-19 cancer patients; Table S5: Effect of obesity according to its severity and by type of cancer on the different outcomes, among non COVID-19 cancer patients.

Author Contributions: J.C. and C.Q. were involved in the conception and design of the study. C.Q. was the coordinator of the study. J.C. and C.Q. were responsible for the data collection. J.C. and T.S.D.-Y. wrote the first draft. S.T. was in charge of the analysis. J.C., S.T. and C.Q. accessed and verified the data. J.C., S.T., P.A., A.B., T.S.D.-Y. and C.Q. were involved in the interpretation, critically reviewed the first draft, and approved the final version. All authors have read and agreed to the published version of the manuscript.

Funding: This research received no external funding.

Institutional Review Board Statement: The study was conducted according to the guidelines of the Declaration of Helsinki, and approved by the National Committee for data protection: declaration of conformity to the methodology of reference 05 obtained on 7 August 2018 under the number 2204633 v0.

Informed Consent Statement: Patient consent was not needed for this study as it was a retrospective study and that the national data used were anonymous.

Data Availability Statement: The PMSI database was transmitted by the national agency for the management of hospitalization data. The use of these data by our department was approved by the National Committee for data protection. We are not allowed to transmit these data. PMSI data are available for researchers who meet the criteria for access to these French confidential data (this access is submitted to the approval of the National Committee for data protection) from the national agency for the management of hospitalization (ATIH—Agence technique de l'information sur l'hospitalisation, 117 boulevard Marius Vivier Merle, 69329 Lyon Cedex 03, France).

Acknowledgments: The authors thank Suzanne Rankin for reviewing the English and Gwenaëlle Periard for her help with the layout and management of this article.

Conflicts of Interest: The authors declare no conflict of interest.

References

1. World Health Organization. World Health Organization Coronavirus disease (COVID-19): Herd immunity, lockdowns and COVID-19. 2020. Available online: https://www.who.int/news-room/questions-and-answers/item/herd-immunity-lockdowns-and-covid-19 (accessed on 10 April 2021).
2. Bénézit, F.; Loubet, P.; Galtier, F.; Pronier, C.; Lenzi, N.; Lesieur, Z.; Jouneau, S.; Lagathu, G.; L'Honneur, A.-S.; Foulongne, V.; et al. Non-influenza respiratory viruses in adult patients admitted with influenza-like illness: A 3-year prospective multicenter study. *Infection* 2020, *48*, 489–495. [CrossRef]
3. Bernard Stoecklin, S.; Rolland, P.; Silue, Y.; Mailles, A.; Campese, C.; Simondon, A.; Mechain, M.; Meurice, L.; Nguyen, M.; Bassi, C.; et al. First cases of coronavirus disease 2019 (COVID-19) in France: Surveillance, investigations and control measures, January 2020. Euro Surveill. Bull. Eur. Sur Mal. Transm. *Eur. Commun. Dis. Bull.* 2020, *25*, 2000094. [CrossRef]
4. Bouadma, L.; Lescure, F.-X.; Lucet, J.-C.; Yazdanpanah, Y.; Timsit, J.-F. Severe SARS-CoV-2 infections: Practical considerations and management strategy for intensivists. *Intensive Care Med.* 2020, *46*, 579–582. [CrossRef] [PubMed]
5. Piroth, L.; Cottenet, J.; Mariet, A.-S.; Bonniaud, P.; Blot, M.; Tubert-Bitter, P.; Quantin, C. Comparison of the characteristics, morbidity, and mortality of COVID-19 and seasonal influenza: A nationwide, population-based retrospective cohort study. *Lancet Respir. Med.* 2021, *9*, 251–259. [CrossRef]
6. Sources Sources—Worldwide Data on COVID-19. Available online: https://www.ecdc.europa.eu/en/publications-data/sources-worldwide-data-covid-19 (accessed on 10 November 2022).
7. Santé Publique France. L'épidémie de COVID-19 en Chiffres. Available online: https://www.santepubliquefrance.fr/maladies-et-traumatismes/maladies-et-infections-respiratoires/infection-a-coronavirus/articles/infection-au-nouveau-coronavirus-sars-cov-2-covid-19-france-et-monde#block-242818 (accessed on 4 October 2020).
8. Chen, G.; Wu, D.; Guo, W.; Cao, Y.; Huang, D.; Wang, H.; Wang, T.; Zhang, X.; Chen, H.; Yu, H.; et al. Clinical and immunological features of severe and moderate coronavirus disease 2019. *J. Clin. Investig.* 2020, *130*, 2620–2629. [CrossRef] [PubMed]
9. Zhang, L.; Zhu, F.; Xie, L.; Wang, C.; Wang, J.; Chen, R.; Jia, P.; Guan, H.Q.; Peng, L.; Chen, Y.; et al. Clinical characteristics of COVID-19-infected cancer patients: A retrospective case study in three hospitals within Wuhan, China. *Ann. Oncol. Off. J. Eur. Soc. Med. Oncol.* 2020, *31*, 894–901. [CrossRef]
10. Liu, W.; Tao, Z.-W.; Wang, L.; Yuan, M.-L.; Liu, K.; Zhou, L.; Wei, S.; Deng, Y.; Liu, J.; Liu, H.-G.; et al. Analysis of factors associated with disease outcomes in hospitalized patients with 2019 novel coronavirus disease. *Chin. Med. J.* 2020, *133*, 1032–1038. [CrossRef]
11. Simonnet, A.; Chetboun, M.; Poissy, J.; Raverdy, V.; Noulette, J.; Duhamel, A.; Labreuche, J.; Mathieu, D.; Pattou, F.; Jourdain, M.; et al. High Prevalence of Obesity in Severe Acute Respiratory Syndrome Coronavirus-2 (SARS-CoV-2) Requiring Invasive Mechanical Ventilation. *Obes. Silver Spring Md* 2020, *28*, 1195–1199. [CrossRef]
12. Chen, N.; Zhou, M.; Dong, X.; Qu, J.; Gong, F.; Han, Y.; Qiu, Y.; Wang, J.; Liu, Y.; Wei, Y.; et al. Epidemiological and clinical characteristics of 99 cases of 2019 novel coronavirus pneumonia in Wuhan, China: A descriptive study. *Lancet Lond. Engl.* 2020, *395*, 507–513. [CrossRef]
13. Du, R.-H.; Liang, L.-R.; Yang, C.-Q.; Wang, W.; Cao, T.-Z.; Li, M.; Guo, G.-Y.; Du, J.; Zheng, C.-L.; Zhu, Q.; et al. Predictors of mortality for patients with COVID-19 pneumonia caused by SARS-CoV-2: A prospective cohort study. *Eur. Respir. J.* 2020, *55*, 2000524. [CrossRef]
14. Verity, R.; Okell, L.C.; Dorigatti, I.; Winskill, P.; Whittaker, C.; Imai, N.; Cuomo-Dannenburg, G.; Thompson, H.; Walker, P.G.T.; Fu, H.; et al. Estimates of the severity of coronavirus disease 2019: A model-based analysis. *Lancet Infect. Dis.* 2020, *20*, 669–677. [CrossRef]
15. Wang, B.; Li, R.; Lu, Z.; Huang, Y. Does comorbidity increase the risk of patients with COVID-19: Evidence from meta-analysis. *Aging* 2020, *12*, 6049–6057. [CrossRef] [PubMed]
16. Zhou, F.; Yu, T.; Du, R.; Fan, G.; Liu, Y.; Liu, Z.; Xiang, J.; Wang, Y.; Song, B.; Gu, X.; et al. Clinical course and risk factors for mortality of adult inpatients with COVID-19 in Wuhan, China: A retrospective cohort study. *Lancet Lond. Engl.* 2020, *395*, 1054–1062. [CrossRef]
17. Arayici, M.E.; Kipcak, N.; Kayacik, U.; Kelbat, C.; Keskin, D.; Kilicarslan, M.E.; Kilinc, A.V.; Kirgoz, S.; Kirilmaz, A.; Kizilkaya, M.A.; et al. Effects of SARS-CoV-2 infections in patients with cancer on mortality, ICU admission and incidence: A systematic review with meta-analysis involving 709,908 participants and 31,732 cancer patients. *J. Cancer Res. Clin. Oncol.* 2022. Online ahead of print. [CrossRef]
18. Sezer, H.; Bulut Canbaz, H.; Yurdakul, F.; Özserezli, B.; Yazıcı, D. Is obesity paradox valid for critically-ill COVID-19 patients with respiratory failure? *Turk. Thorac. J.* 2022, *23*, 268–276. [CrossRef] [PubMed]
19. Bernard, A.; Cottenet, J.; Bonniaud, P.; Piroth, L.; Arveux, P.; Tubert-Bitter, P.; Quantin, C. Comparison of Cancer Patients to Non-Cancer Patients among COVID-19 Inpatients at a National Level. *Cancers* 2021, *13*, 1436. [CrossRef] [PubMed]
20. Lee, M.; Quinn, R.; Pradhan, K.; Fedorov, K.; Levitz, D.; Fromowitz, A.; Thakkar, A.; Shapiro, L.C.; Kabarriti, R.; Ruiz, R.E.; et al. Impact of COVID-19 on case fatality rate of patients with cancer during the Omicron wave. *Cancer Cell* 2022, *40*, 343–345. [CrossRef]
21. Liang, W.; Guan, W.; Chen, R.; Wang, W.; Li, J.; Xu, K.; Li, C.; Ai, Q.; Lu, W.; Liang, H.; et al. Cancer patients in SARS-CoV-2 infection: A nationwide analysis in China. *Lancet Oncol.* 2020, *21*, 335–337. [CrossRef]
22. Pagès, P.-B.; Cottenet, J.; Mariet, A.-S.; Bernard, A.; Quantin, C. In-hospital mortality following lung cancer resection: Nationwide administrative database. *Eur. Respir. J.* 2016, *47*, 1809–1817. [CrossRef]

23. Park, R.; Wulff-Burchfield, E.; Sun, W.; Kasi, A. Is obesity a risk factor in cancer patients with COVID-19? *Future Oncol. Lond. Engl.* **2021**, *17*, 3541–3544. [CrossRef]
24. Aboueshia, M.; Hussein, M.H.; Attia, A.S.; Swinford, A.; Miller, P.; Omar, M.; Toraih, E.A.; Saba, N.; Safah, H.; Duchesne, J.; et al. Cancer and COVID-19: Analysis of patient outcomes. *Future Oncol. Lond. Engl.* **2021**, *17*, 3499–3510. [CrossRef] [PubMed]
25. Rossi, A.P.; Gottin, L.; Donadello, K.; Schweiger, V.; Nocini, R.; Taiana, M.; Zamboni, M.; Polati, E. Obesity as a risk factor for unfavourable outcomes in critically ill patients affected by Covid 19. *Nutr. Metab. Cardiovasc. Dis. NMCD* **2021**, *31*, 762–768. [CrossRef] [PubMed]
26. Gao, M.; Piernas, C.; Astbury, N.M.; Hippisley-Cox, J.; O'Rahilly, S.; Aveyard, P.; Jebb, S.A. Associations between body-mass index and COVID-19 severity in 6·9 million people in England: A prospective, community-based, cohort study. *Lancet Diabetes Endocrinol.* **2021**, *9*, 350–359. [CrossRef]
27. Robinson, K.N.; Saber, D.A. Obesity: Policy and Practice Recommendations for High-Risk Populations Influenced by the COVID-19 Pandemic. *mSystems* **2022**, *7*, e0008922. [CrossRef] [PubMed]
28. Benderra, M.-A.; Aparicio, A.; Leblanc, J.; Wassermann, D.; Kempf, E.; Galula, G.; Bernaux, M.; Canellas, A.; Moreau, T.; Bellamine, A.; et al. Clinical Characteristics, Care Trajectories and Mortality Rate of SARS-CoV-2 Infected Cancer Patients: A Multicenter Cohort Study. *Cancers* **2021**, *13*, 4749. [CrossRef]
29. Jee, J.; Foote, M.B.; Lumish, M.; Stonestrom, A.J.; Wills, B.; Narendra, V.; Avutu, V.; Murciano-Goroff, Y.R.; Chan, J.E.; Derkach, A.; et al. Chemotherapy and COVID-19 Outcomes in Patients With Cancer. *J. Clin. Oncol. Off. J. Am. Soc. Clin. Oncol.* **2020**, *38*, 3538–3546. [CrossRef] [PubMed]
30. Kuderer, N.M.; Choueiri, T.K.; Shah, D.P.; Shyr, Y.; Rubinstein, S.M.; Rivera, D.R.; Shete, S.; Hsu, C.-Y.; Desai, A.; de Lima Lopes, G.; et al. Clinical impact of COVID-19 on patients with cancer (CCC19): A cohort study. *Lancet Lond. Engl.* **2020**, *395*, 1907–1918. [CrossRef]
31. Park, R.; Wulff-Burchfield, E.M.; Mehta, K.; Sun, W.; Kasi, A. Prognostic impact of obesity in cancer patients with COVID-19 infection: A systematic review and meta-analysis. *J. Clin. Oncol.* **2021**, *39*, e18578. [CrossRef]
32. Sanchez-Pina, J.M.; Rodríguez Rodriguez, M.; Castro Quismondo, N.; Gil Manso, R.; Colmenares, R.; Gil Alos, D.; Paciello, M.L.; Zafra, D.; Garcia-Sanchez, C.; Villegas, C.; et al. Clinical course and risk factors for mortality from COVID-19 in patients with haematological malignancies. *Eur. J. Haematol.* **2020**, *105*, 597–607. [CrossRef]
33. Fox, T.A.; Troy-Barnes, E.; Kirkwood, A.A.; Chan, W.Y.; Day, J.W.; Chavda, S.J.; Kumar, E.A.; David, K.; Tomkins, O.; Sanchez, E.; et al. Clinical outcomes and risk factors for severe COVID-19 in patients with haematological disorders receiving chemo- or immunotherapy. *Br. J. Haematol.* **2020**, *191*, 194–206. [CrossRef]
34. Vuagnat, A.; Jollant, F.; Abbar, M.; Hawton, K.; Quantin, C. Recurrence and mortality 1 year after hospital admission for non-fatal self-harm: A nationwide population-based study. *Epidemiol. Psychiatr. Sci.* **2019**, *29*, e20. [CrossRef]
35. Jollant, F.; Goueslard, K.; Hawton, K.; Quantin, C. Self-harm, somatic disorders and mortality in the 3 years following a hospitalisation in psychiatry in adolescents and young adults. *Evid. Based Ment. Health* **2022**. *Online ahead of print.* [CrossRef]
36. Goueslard, K.; Jollant, F.; Petit, J.M.; Quantin, C. Self-harm hospitalization following bariatric surgery in adolescents and young adults. *Clin. Nutr. Edinb. Scotl.* **2022**, *41*, 238–245. [CrossRef] [PubMed]
37. Quantin, C.; Yamdjieu Ngadeu, C.; Cottenet, J.; Escolano, S.; Bechraoui-Quantin, S.; Rożenberg, P.; Tubert-Bitter, P.; Gouyon, J.-B. Early exposure of pregnant women to non-steroidal anti-inflammatory drugs delivered outside hospitals and preterm birth risk: Nationwide cohort study. *BJOG Int. J. Obstet. Gynaecol.* **2021**, *128*, 1575–1584. [CrossRef]
38. Goueslard, K.; Petit, J.-M.; Cottenet, J.; Chauvet-Gelinier, J.-C.; Jollant, F.; Quantin, C. Increased Risk of Rehospitalization for Acute Diabetes Complications and Suicide Attempts in Patients With Type 1 Diabetes and Comorbid Schizophrenia. *Diabetes Care* **2018**, *41*, 2316–2321. [CrossRef]
39. Maitre, T.; Cottenet, J.; Beltramo, G.; Georges, M.; Blot, M.; Piroth, L.; Bonniaud, P.; Quantin, C. Increasing burden of noninfectious lung disease in persons living with HIV: A 7-year study using the French nationwide hospital administrative database. *Eur. Respir. J.* **2018**, *52*, 1800359. [CrossRef]
40. Creuzot-Garcher, C.; Benzenine, E.; Mariet, A.-S.; de Lazzer, A.; Chiquet, C.; Bron, A.M.; Quantin, C. Incidence of Acute Postoperative Endophthalmitis after Cataract Surgery: A Nationwide Study in France from 2005 to 2014. *Ophthalmology* **2016**, *123*, 1414–1420. [CrossRef] [PubMed]
41. Abdulmalak, C.; Cottenet, J.; Beltramo, G.; Georges, M.; Camus, P.; Bonniaud, P.; Quantin, C. Haemoptysis in adults: A 5-year study using the French nationwide hospital administrative database. *Eur. Respir. J.* **2015**, *46*, 503–511. [CrossRef] [PubMed]
42. Le Teuff, G.; Abrahamowicz, M.; Wynant, W.; Binquet, C.; Moreau, T.; Quantin, C. Flexible modeling of disease activity measures improved prognosis of disability progression in relapsing-remitting multiple sclerosis. *J. Clin. Epidemiol.* **2015**, *68*, 307–316. [CrossRef]
43. Quantin, C.; Benzenine, E.; Velten, M.; Huet, F.; Farrington, C.P.; Tubert-Bitter, P. Self-controlled case series and misclassification bias induced by case selection from administrative hospital databases: Application to febrile convulsions in pediatric vaccine pharmacoepidemiology. *Am. J. Epidemiol.* **2013**, *178*, 1731–1739. [CrossRef]
44. Lorgis, L.; Cottenet, J.; Molins, G.; Benzenine, E.; Zeller, M.; Aube, H.; Touzery, C.; Hamblin, J.; Gudjoncik, A.; Cottin, Y.; et al. Outcomes after acute myocardial infarction in HIV-infected patients: Analysis of data from a French nationwide hospital medical information database. *Circulation* **2013**, *127*, 1767–1774. [CrossRef] [PubMed]

45. Jollant, F.; Roussot, A.; Corruble, E.; Chauvet-Gelinier, J.C.; Falissard, B.; Mikaeloff, Y.; Quantin, C. Prolonged impact of the COVID-19 pandemic on self-harm hospitalizations in France: A nationwide retrospective observational study. *Eur. Psychiatry J. Assoc. Eur. Psychiatr.* **2022**, *65*, e35. [CrossRef]
46. Mariet, A.S.; Giroud, M.; Benzenine, E.; Cottenet, J.; Roussot, A.; Aho-Glélé, L.S.; Tubert-Bitter, P.; Béjot, Y.; Quantin, C. Hospitalizations for stroke in France during the COVID-19 pandemic before, during and after the national lockdown. *Stroke* **2020**, *52*, 1362–1369. [CrossRef] [PubMed]
47. Beltramo, G.; Cottenet, J.; Mariet, A.-S.; Georges, M.; Piroth, L.; Tubert-Bitter, P.; Bonniaud, P.; Quantin, C. Chronic respiratory diseases are predictors of severe outcome in COVID-19 hospitalised patients: A nationwide study. *Eur. Respir. J.* **2021**, *58*, 2004474. [CrossRef] [PubMed]
48. Simon, E.; Cottenet, J.; Mariet, A.-S.; Bechraoui-Quantin, S.; Rozenberg, P.; Gouyon, J.-B.; Quantin, C. Impact of the COVID-19 pandemic on preterm birth and stillbirth: A nationwide, population-based retrospective cohort study. *Am. J. Obstet. Gynecol.* **2021**, *225*, 347–348. [CrossRef] [PubMed]
49. Quantin, C.; Tubert-Bitter, P. COVID-19 and social inequalities: A complex and dynamic interaction. *Lancet Public Health* **2022**, *7*, e204–e205. [CrossRef]
50. Karila, L.; Roussot, A.; Mariet, A.-S.; Benyamina, A.; Falissard, B.; Mikaeloff, Y.; Quantin, C. Effects of the 2020 health crisis on acute alcohol intoxication: A nationwide retrospective observational study. *Drug Alcohol Depend.* **2021**, *228*, 109062. [CrossRef]
51. Castelo-Branco, L.; Tsourti, Z.; Gennatas, S.; Rogado, J.; Sekacheva, M.; Viñal, D.; Lee, R.; Croitoru, A.; Vitorino, M.; Khallaf, S.; et al. COVID-19 in patients with cancer: First report of the ESMO international, registry-based, cohort study (ESMO-CoCARE). *ESMO Open* **2022**, *7*, 100499. [CrossRef]
52. Abdoul Carime, N.; Cottenet, J.; Clerfond, G.; Eschalier, R.; Quilliot, D.; Eicher, J.-C.; Joly, B.; Quantin, C. Impact of nutritional status on heart failure mortality: A retrospective cohort study. *Nutr. J.* **2022**, *21*, 1–9. [CrossRef] [PubMed]
53. Bryere, J.; Dejardin, O.; Launay, L.; Colonna, M.; Grosclaude, P.; Launoy, G. French Network of Cancer Registries (FRANCIM) Socioeconomic status and site-specific cancer incidence, a Bayesian approach in a French Cancer Registries Network study. *Eur. J. Cancer Prev. Off. J. Eur. Cancer Prev. Organ. ECP* **2018**, *27*, 391–398. [CrossRef]
54. Gupta, S.; Hayek, S.S.; Wang, W.; Chan, L.; Mathews, K.S.; Melamed, M.L.; Brenner, S.K.; Leonberg-Yoo, A.; Schenck, E.J.; Radbel, J.; et al. Factors Associated With Death in Critically Ill Patients With Coronavirus Disease 2019 in the US. *JAMA Intern. Med.* **2020**, *180*, 1436–1447. [CrossRef] [PubMed]
55. Lee, L.Y.W.; Cazier, J.-B.; Starkey, T.; Briggs, S.E.W.; Arnold, R.; Bisht, V.; Booth, S.; Campton, N.A.; Cheng, V.W.T.; Collins, G.; et al. COVID-19 prevalence and mortality in patients with cancer and the effect of primary tumour subtype and patient demographics: A prospective cohort study. *Lancet Oncol.* **2020**, *21*, 1309–1316. [CrossRef]
56. Arbel, Y.; Fialkoff, C.; Kerner, A.; Kerner, M. Can reduction in infection and mortality rates from coronavirus be explained by an obesity survival paradox? An analysis at the US statewide level. *Int. J. Obes. 2005* **2020**, *44*, 2339–2342. [CrossRef]
57. Hakozaki, T.; Nolin-Lapalme, A.; Kogawa, M.; Okuma, Y.; Nakamura, S.; Moreau-Amaru, D.; Tamura, T.; Hosomi, Y.; Takeyama, H.; Richard, C.; et al. Cancer Cachexia among Patients with Advanced Non-Small-Cell Lung Cancer on Immunotherapy: An Observational Study with Exploratory Gut Microbiota Analysis. *Cancers* **2022**, *14*, 5405. [CrossRef]
58. Fearon, K.; Arends, J.; Baracos, V. Understanding the mechanisms and treatment options in cancer cachexia. *Nat. Rev. Clin. Oncol.* **2013**, *10*, 90–99. [CrossRef]
59. Martin, L.; Birdsell, L.; Macdonald, N.; Reiman, T.; Clandinin, M.T.; McCargar, L.J.; Murphy, R.; Ghosh, S.; Sawyer, M.B.; Baracos, V.E. Cancer cachexia in the age of obesity: Skeletal muscle depletion is a powerful prognostic factor, independent of body mass index. *J. Clin. Oncol. Off. J. Am. Soc. Clin. Oncol.* **2013**, *31*, 1539–1547. [CrossRef] [PubMed]
60. Vaughan, V.C.; Martin, P.; Lewandowski, P.A. Cancer cachexia: Impact, mechanisms and emerging treatments. *J. Cachexia Sarcopenia Muscle* **2013**, *4*, 95–109. [CrossRef]
61. Singh, R.; Rathore, S.S.; Khan, H.; Karale, S.; Chawla, Y.; Iqbal, K.; Bhurwal, A.; Tekin, A.; Jain, N.; Mehra, I.; et al. Association of Obesity With COVID-19 Severity and Mortality: An Updated Systemic Review, Meta-Analysis, and Meta-Regression. *Front. Endocrinol.* **2022**, *13*, 780872. [CrossRef]
62. Lavie, C.J.; Coursin, D.B.; Long, M.T. The Obesity Paradox in Infections and Implications for COVID-19. *Mayo Clin. Proc.* **2021**, *96*, 518–520. [CrossRef]
63. Williamson, E.J.; Walker, A.J.; Bhaskaran, K.; Bacon, S.; Bates, C.; Morton, C.E.; Curtis, H.J.; Mehrkar, A.; Evans, D.; Inglesby, P.; et al. OpenSAFELY: Factors associated with COVID-19 death in 17 million patients. *Nature* **2020**, *584*, 430–436. [CrossRef]
64. Booth, A.; Reed, A.B.; Ponzo, S.; Yassaee, A.; Aral, M.; Plans, D.; Labrique, A.; Mohan, D. Population risk factors for severe disease and mortality in COVID-19: A global systematic review and meta-analysis. *PLoS ONE* **2021**, *16*, e0247461. [CrossRef]
65. Vulturar, D.-M.; Crivii, C.-B.; Orăsan, O.H.; Palade, E.; Buzoianu, A.-D.; Zehan, I.G.; Todea, D.A. Obesity Impact on SARS-CoV-2 Infection: Pros and Cons "Obesity Paradox"-A Systematic Review. *J. Clin. Med.* **2022**, *11*, 3844. [CrossRef] [PubMed]
66. Albiges, L.; Foulon, S.; Bayle, A.; Gachot, B.; Pommeret, F.; Willekens, C.; Stoclin, A.; Merad, M.; Griscelli, F.; Lacroix, L.; et al. Determinants of the outcomes of patients with cancer infected with SARS-CoV-2: Results from the Gustave Roussy cohort. *Nat. Cancer* **2020**, *1*, 965–975. [CrossRef] [PubMed]
67. Mehta, V.; Goel, S.; Kabarriti, R.; Cole, D.; Goldfinger, M.; Acuna-Villaorduna, A.; Pradhan, K.; Thota, R.; Reissman, S.; Sparano, J.A.; et al. Case Fatality Rate of Cancer Patients with COVID-19 in a New York Hospital System. *Cancer Discov.* **2020**, *10*, 935–941. [CrossRef]

68. Cantuti-Castelvetri, L.; Ojha, R.; Pedro, L.D.; Djannatian, M.; Franz, J.; Kuivanen, S.; van der Meer, F.; Kallio, K.; Kaya, T.; Anastasina, M.; et al. Neuropilin-1 facilitates SARS-CoV-2 cell entry and infectivity. *Science* **2020**, *370*, 856–860. [CrossRef]
69. McKinney, E.F.; Smith, K.G.C. Metabolic exhaustion in infection, cancer and autoimmunity. *Nat. Immunol.* **2018**, *19*, 213–221. [CrossRef]
70. Roncati, L.; Ligabue, G.; Fabbiani, L.; Malagoli, C.; Gallo, G.; Lusenti, B.; Nasillo, V.; Manenti, A.; Maiorana, A. Type 3 hypersensitivity in COVID-19 vasculitis. *Clin. Immunol. Orlando Fla* **2020**, *217*, 108487. [CrossRef] [PubMed]
71. Moore, D.; Aveyard, P.; Connock, M.; Wang, D.; Fry-Smith, A.; Barton, P. Effectiveness and safety of nicotine replacement therapy assisted reduction to stop smoking: Systematic review and meta-analysis. *BMJ* **2009**, *338*, b1024. [CrossRef]
72. Goldberg, M.; Jougla, E.; Fassa, M.; Padieu, R.; Quantin, C. The French public health information system. *J. Int. Assoc. Stat.* **2012**, *28*, 31–41.
73. Setoguchi, S.; Solomon, D.H.; Glynn, R.J.; Cook, E.F.; Levin, R.; Schneeweiss, S. Agreement of diagnosis and its date for hematologic malignancies and solid tumors between medicare claims and cancer registry data. *Cancer Causes Control* **2007**, *18*, 561–569. [CrossRef]

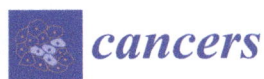

Article

A Multicenter Analysis of the Outcome of Cancer Patients with Neutropenia and COVID-19 Optionally Treated with Granulocyte-Colony Stimulating Factor (G-CSF): A Comparative Analysis

María Sereno [1,2,*,†], Ana María Jimenez-Gordo [1,2,†], Javier Baena-Espinar [3], Carlos Aguado [4], Xabier Mielgo [5], Ana Pertejo [6], Rosa Álvarez-Álvarez [7], Ana Sánchez [8], Jose Luis López [9], Raquel Molina [9], Ana López-Alfonso [10], Berta Hernández [11], Luis Enrique Chiara [12], Ana Manuela Martín [13], Ana López-Martín [14], Miriam Dorta [15], Ana Collazo-Lorduy [16], Enrique Casado [1,2], Ana Ramirez de Molina [2] and Gonzalo Colmenarejo [2]

1. Infanta Sofía University Hospital, 28702 Madrid, Spain; ajgordo@salud.madrid.org (A.M.J.-G.); enriquecasado@salud.madrid.org (E.C.)
2. IMDEA-Food Institute, CEI UAM+CSIC, 28702 Madrid, Spain; aramirez@iib.uam.es (A.R.d.M.); gonzalo.colmenarejo@imdea.org (G.C.)
3. Doce de Octubre University Hospital, 28702 Madrid, Spain; javier.baena@salud.madrid.org
4. San Carlos University Hospital, 28040 Madrid, Spain; carlos.aguado@salud.madrid.org
5. Fundación-University Alcorcón Hospital, 28922 Madrid, Spain; xmielgo@salud.madrid.org
6. La Paz University Hospital, 28046 Madrid, Spain; pertejo.ana@salud.madrid.org
7. Gregorio Marañón University Hospital, 28009 Madrid, Spain; rosa.alvarez.al@salud.madrid.org
8. Getafe University Hospital, 28905 Madrid, Spain; anasanpen@salud.madrid.org
9. Príncipe de Asturias University Hospital, 28805 Madrid, Spain; jllopez@salud.madrid.org (J.L.L.); raquel.molina@salud.madrid.org (R.M.)
10. Infanta Leonor University Hospital, 28031 Madrid, Spain; ana.lopez2@salud.madrid.org
11. La Princesa University Hospital, 28006 Madrid, Spain; bertahernandezmarin@salud.madrid.org
12. Guadalajara University Hospital, 19001 Castilla La Mancha, Spain; lucho_chara@salud.castillaylamancha.com
13. Fuenlabrada University Hospital, 28942 Madrid, Spain; anamanuela.martin@salud.madrid.org
14. Leganés-Severo Ochoa University Hospital, 28914 Madrid, Spain; ana5lomar@salud.madrid.org
15. Clara Campall CIOCC, 28050 Madrid, Spain; mdorta@hmhospitales.com
16. Puerta de Hierro University Hospital, 28220 Madrid, Spain; anaclorduy@salud.madrid.org
* Correspondence: maria.sereno@salud.madrid.org
† Both authors are co-first authors because we have contributed as a first author for the design, redaction, review and providing patients for this study.

Simple Summary: Infections with COVID-19 in neutropenic cancer patients are related to poor outcomes. A G-CSF treatment used in neutropenic cancer with SARS-CoV-2 infections is related to a higher rate of respiratory failure according to progressive and growing evidence. In this small retrospective non-randomized study, we found an association between G-CSF treatment and the parameters predisposing for worse infections with COVID-19 and neutropenia compared with patients not treated with G-CSF. We also found that the number of days on G-CSF treatment was related to a higher risk of mortality in a multivariable analysis among patients treated with G-CSF.

Abstract: Background: Approximately 15% of patients infected by SARS-CoV-2 develop a distress syndrome secondary to a host hyperinflammatory response induced by a cytokine storm. Myelosuppression is associated with a higher risk of infections and mortality. There are data to support methods of management for neutropenia and COVID-19. We present a multicenter experience during the first COVID-19 outbreak in neutropenic cancer patients infected by SARS-CoV-2. Methods: Clinical retrospective data were collected from neutropenic cancer patients with COVID-19. Comorbidities, tumor type, stage, treatment, neutropenia severity, G-CSF, COVID-19 parameters, and mortality were analyzed. A bivariate analysis of the impact on mortality was carried out. Additionally, we performed a multivariable logistic regression to predict respiratory failure and death. Results: Among the 943 cancer patients screened, 83 patients (11.3%) simultaneously had neutropenia and an infection with COVID-19. The lungs (26%) and breasts (22%) were the primary locations affected, and most

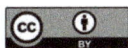

patients had advanced disease (67%). In the logistic model, as adjusted covariates, sex, age, treatment (palliative vs. curative), tumor type, and the lowest level of neutrophils were used. A significant effect was obtained for the number of days of G-CSF treatment (OR = 1.4, 95% CI [1,1,03,92], p-value = 0.01). Conclusions: Our findings suggest that a prolonged G-CSF treatment could be disadvantageous for these cancer patients with infections by COVID-19, with a higher probability of worse outcome.

Keywords: COVID-19; neutropenia; G-CSF treatment; respiratory failure

1. Introduction

Coronavirus disease 2019 (COVID-19), caused by severe acute respiratory syndrome coronavirus 2 (SARS-CoV-2), has become a global pandemic. Infections by SARS-CoV-2 can turn into acute respiratory proliferation, which is cleared in most cases by the immune system after 7 to 14 days [1]. However, approximately 15% of patients infected by COVID-19 develop severe lung disease and multiorgan failure, which are major causes of mortality [2]. Two different but overlapping phases can be distinguished in COVID-19: an initial mild response to the virus infection, followed by a severe phase with a host hyperinflammatory response induced by a cytokine storm [3,4]. The development of novel therapies are critical to overcome this pandemic [5]. It is well known that cancer patients are more vulnerable to infections [6]. Jung et al. described a rate of 0.79% SARS-CoV-2 infections in 1,524 cancer patients compared with a rate of 0.37% in the general population of Wuhan [7]. Kim et al. described a much higher mortality in patients with hematologic malignancies and infection with COVID-19 compared with others without this condition (40 vs. 3.6%, $p < 0.001$) [8]. Furthermore, most of the patients with comorbidities such as hypertension, diabetes, obesity, chronic obstructive pulmonary disease (COPD), tobacco consumption, vascular disease, advanced age, and other chronic diseases require frequent visits to the hospital, which is correlated with a higher risk of severe complications in the case of infection with SARS-CoV-2 [9,10].

Chemotherapy is one of the most common treatments in cancer patients. Myelosuppression, more specifically the development of febrile neutropenia, is an undesirable secondary effect in these patients [11]. Soon after the onset of the pandemic, several panels of experts in Spanish, European, and American oncology associations recommended the modification of oncological treatments to induce less neutropenia and to consider expanding the indications of Filgrastim (G-CSF) use to patients with intermediate (10–20%) and higher neutropenia risk. Scarce data have been reported about the effect of G-CSF in patients with cancer and infections by COVID-19. Lymphocyte T-mediated immunity has been implicated in SARS-CoV-2 infections [12]. G-CSF has been associated with a reduction in hospitalization days and a quicker recovery of neutrophil counts, including in older febrile neutropenia patients [13]. The mechanism of action of G-CSF includes the stimulation of both cytokines and neutrophils. This has been associated with lung injury, including adult respiratory distress syndrome (SDRA) [14]. Moreover, neutrophilia and a high neutrophil/lymphocyte ratio (NLR) have been described as bad prognostic factors in patients infected with COVID-19 [15]. Thus, there is uncertainty about the use of G-CSF and its impact in the clinical outcome of cancer patients treated with it [16].

To shed some light on this convoluted issue, in this work, we present a multi-center experience in several hospitals in Spain during the first COVID-19 outbreak with a cohort of patients with neutropenia cancer and infected with COVID-19.

2. Materials and Methods

This is a retrospective and observational analysis (without randomized design) and includes patients with neutropenic cancer and simultaneously infected with SARS-CoV-2. We collected cases from 14 hospitals from Madrid and Guadalajara in Spain (H. 12 de Octubre, H. Clínico San Carlos, HF. Alcorcón, H. Infanta Sofía, H. Infanta Leonor, H.

Guadalajara, H. Puerta de Hierro, H. Severo Ochoa, H. Alcalá de Henares, H. Getafe, H. La Paz, H. Princesa, H. Gregorio Marañón, and H. Fuenlabrada) that appeared during the first epidemic wave between March and June 2020. The patients included had to be receiving active cancer treatment, have a neutrophile count <1500/mL, have a fever (38 °C or more), and be infected with SARS-CoV-2 confirmed through a positive oropharingeal PCR. The anonymized data were collected in Excel 16.38. We included data on the variables related to demographics (age, sex, and hospital) as well as general clinical features: ECOG, performance status, smoking, body mass index, cardiovascular disease, or diabetes mellitus. We also collected information about the neoplastic disease (tumor location and stage), the anti-tumoral treatment (chemotherapy immunotherapy, targeted or endocrine treatments; time from last cycle; and COVID-19 diagnostic treatment intention), and multiple analytical parameters (neutrophil and lymphocyte counts, D-dimer, lactate dehydrogenase (LDH), pro-calcitonin, and C-reactive protein). Filgrastim® administration (30–48 MU/0.5 mL subcutaneous per day) and treatment duration were also noted. Data related to SARS-CoV-2 infections were also included: severity and duration, as well as presence of pneumonia and/or thrombosis. Different COVID-19 treatments such as antibiotics, chloroquine, remdesivir, corticoids, anti-IL6 or anti-IL1, anticoagulants, and colchicine were collected, when applicable. Data about admission to the intensive care unit and the final outcome after SARS-CoV-2 infection were gathered: complete recovery, sequels, death, as well as cancer treatment modifications. This study was approved by the Ethical Committee for Clinical Research in La Paz University Hospital, code (PI-4194), on 4 May 2020.

All of the statistical analyses were performed with the R 3.6.1 software [17]. Distributions of the quantitative variables were described through their mean, median, standard deviation, interquartile range, maximum, and minimum, and their normality was tested through the Shapiro–Wilk test. Distributions of qualitative variables were described though the corresponding absolute and relative frequencies. Bivariate analyses were performed for the categorical variables (e.g., related to basal factors, COVID-19 severity, etc.) vs. categorical (death, respiratory distress, etc.) or continuous-variables (e.g., lowest neutrophil levels, highest CRP, etc.). The significance of associations with the former was tested through Fisher's exact test, while that with the latter was tested through one-way ANOVA or the Kruskal–Wallis test, depending on the normality of the quantitative variables. Multivariable models were derived in the form of logistic regressions to test the significance of the number of G-CSF treatment days in COVID19-related outcomes such as death or respiratory distress after adjusting for appropriate covariables unbalanced in the sample. All of the statistical tests were bilateral, and a significance level of 0.05 was used throughout. Statistical inferences in the logistic models used 95% profile confidence intervals.

3. Results

Among the 943 patients with cancer and COVID-19, only 83 patients (11.3%) presented concomitant neutropenia during the first SARS-CoV-2 outbreak.

3.1. Descriptive Analysis of Baseline Clinical Characteristics

Eighty-three patients were selected from 14 hospitals in Spain. The baseline characteristics and different parameters related to cancer are presented in Table 1, both as totals and split by G-CSF treatment. The median age was 67 years, and the majority of patients presented ECOG 0-2 (79/95%). Cardiovascular disease was present in 35 (42.68%) patients, and 13 (15.8%) of total patients had diabetes. Weight data were also collected, observing 37/83 (54%) of patients with BMI > 25 (overweight), and the majority of patients were current smokers (17/83, 20.7%) or former smokers (31/83, 37.8%). On the other hand, the most frequent tumors, in decreasing order, were lung cancer (26%), breast cancer (22%), colon cancer (13%), and non-colon digestive cancers (17%), while the rest of the tumors included prostate cancer, ovarian cancer, gynecological cancer, sarcoma, and others. Advanced (IV) stage was the most common stage (67%), followed by stage III

(19.5%) and stage II (13.4%). The most frequent cancer treatment was chemotherapy in 87.7% of the patients, followed by chemoimmunotherapy and other types in the rest of the participants. Finally, palliation was the main intention of the treatment (67.9%). Three patients who received a chemo-immunotherapy combination had a severe outcome and died. Table 1 also includes the p-value of the test for association of these variables with G-CSF treatment (Filgrastim®), from which we can see that the patients displayed similar clinical baseline features irrespective of receiving G-CSF treatment. The only exception was type of treatment, which is expected given that G-CSF treatment is more frequently administered in chemotherapy settings, even in a preventive way prior to cancer treatment (8 in our dataset).

Table 1. Baseline characteristics of all patients included: total and split by G-CSF treatment. No attempt was made to impute missing values present in some variables. The p-value of association with G-CSF is also shown.

Baseline Characteristics	Total	Without G-CSF	With G-CSF	p-Value
Age				
<70	36 (43.4%)	19 (44.2%)	17 (42.5%)	0.8
>70	47 (56.6%)	24 (55.8%)	23 (57.5%)	
Sex				
Male	41 (49.4%)	21 (48.8%)	20 (50%)	1
Female	42 (50.6%)	22 (51.2%)	20 (50%)	
ECOG				
0	24 (30%)	14 (34%)	10 (25.6%)	
1	46 (37.5%)	25 (61%)	21 (53.8%)	0.15
2	9 (11.25%)	2 (4.9%)	7 (18%)	
3	1 (1.25%)	0	1 (2.6%)	
Cardiovascular disease *				
No	47 (57.3%)	24 (57.14%)	23 (57.5%)	1
Yes	35 (42.7%)	18 (42.9%)	17 (42.5%)	
Diabetes mellitus				
No	69 (84.1%)	37 (88.1%)	32 (80%)	0.37
Yes	13 (15.9%)	5 (11.9%)	8 (20%)	
Body Mass Index				
<20	7 (10.1%)	5 (16.13%)	2 (5.26%)	
20–25	25 (36.2%)	9 (29%)	16 (42.11%)	0.44
25–30	23 (33.3%)	11 (35.5%)	12 (31.6%)	
>30	14 (20.3%)	6 (19.3%)	8 (21%)	
Smoking				
No	34 (41.5%)	17 (40.5%)	17 (42.5%)	
Smoker	17 (20.7%)	7 (16.7%)	10 (25%)	0.57
Previous smoker	31 (37.8%)	18 (19.3%)	13 (32.5%)	
Primary tumor				
Lung	22 (26.8%)	11 (26.2%)	11 (27.5%)	
Colorectal	11 (13.4%)	8 (19%)	3 (7.5%)	
Other digestive	14 (17.1%)	5 (11.9%)	9 (22.5%)	
Breast	18 (22%)	9 (21.4%)	9 (22.5%)	0.66
Gynecological	6 (7.3%)	4 (9.5%)	2 (5%)	
Urothelial	3 (3.7%)	1 (2.4%)	2 (5%)	
Sarcoma	2 (2.4%)	0	2 (5%)	
Head and neck	5 (6.1%)	3 (7.1%)	2 (5%)	
Others	1 (1.22%)	1 (2.4%)	0	

Table 1. Cont.

Baseline Characteristics	Total	Without G-CSF	With G-CSF	p-Value
Stage				
II	11 (13.4%)	5 (11.9%)	6 (15%)	
III	16 (19.5%)	9 (21.4%)	7 (17.5%)	0.88
IV	55 (67.1%)	28 (66.7%)	27 (67.5%)	
Type of treatment				
Chemotherapy	63 (75.6%)	25 (59.5%)	38 (95%)	
Immunotherapy	1 (1.2%)	1 (2.4%)	0	0.001
Chemoimmunotherapy	15 (12.2%)	13 (31%)	2 (5%)	
Other	3 (3.7%)	3 (7.1%)	0	
Treatment intention				
Curative	27 (32.9%)	14 (33.3%)	13 (32.5%)	1
Palliative	55 (67.1%)	28 (66.7%)	27 (67.5%)	

* Ischemic cardiac disease; history of high blood pressure; peripheral ischemic disease; other miocardiopathies.

3.2. Descriptive Analysis of COVID-19 Disease and Treatments

The SARS-CoV-2 infection variables as well as treatments are presented in Table 2. Respiratory failure was detected in 63.4% of cases, and only 25,61% of patients did not require any oxygen supplementation. Nevertheless, 31 patients (37.8%) needed FiO_2 supplementation of higher than 35%, whereas the rest of the patients required 24% oxygen flow or no extra oxygen flow. Fever or low-grade fever was referred to in 86.6% of the patients, while clinical and radiological pneumonia were confirmed in 63 patients (77%), being bilateral or multi-lobar in a considerable number of cases (45/83, 54.9%). The majority of the patients received antibiotics (77/83, 92.7%), mainly ceftriaxone and carbapenems. In addition to antibiotics, around 88% of the patients were treated with chloroquine, and antiviral therapy was used in 38 (46%) patients, predominantly lopinavir/ritonavir as first options (35%) followed by a combination of lopinavir/ritonavir and remdesivir (11%). Corticoids were administered in around 38% of the cases, 23% as high doses of methylprednisolone and 14% as standard doses. Other treatments were reported: anti-IL6 and colchicine, although with a very small amount of cases (14 and 1, respectively). The majority of patients (82%) received some kind of anti-thrombotic therapy, mainly prophylactic low-molecular weight heparin (68%), although only 12% of all patients had a (suspected or confirmed) thrombotic episode, and the mean highest D-dimer in this study was 1.558 ng/mL. Twenty-two patients (26.83%) met the criteria for intensive care. Eight of them died, but only one was admitted into intensive care. All patients who died had respiratory failure, and 46% of patients with respiratory failure eventually died. Oxygen requirements were also related to mortality, and 73% of patients with high oxygen flow died. Obviously, pneumonia severity was related to a higher risk of death as well as carbapenem treatment, being the most frequent treatment with antibiotics in those situations. The mean number of days of hospitalization was 12. In this series, 27 patients (30.2%) of all neutropenic oncological patients died after SARS-CoV-2 infection, while 69.7% of them were discharged after an improvement. Among the survivors (55 patients), 36 (68.5%) could continue their original treatment after the COVID-19 infection. We can see a trend towards a more severe COVID-19 infection in the G-CSF-treated patients, with higher proportions of severe pneumonia, thrombosis, days of hospitalization, and mortality. Especially striking is the highly significant increased proportion of patients with respiratory failure who require stronger oxygen support in the G-CSF group. In this group, only 13 patients survived and could retain their treatment prior to COVID-19 compared with the 24 no-filgrastim-treated patients (Table 2).

Table 2. COVID-19 features of all patients included: total and split by G-CSF treatment. No attempt was made to impute missing values present in some variables. p value of association with G-CSF treatment is also shown.

COVID-19 Features	Total	Without G-CSF	With G-CSF	p-Value
Respiratory failure				
No	30 (36.6%)	23 (54.8%)	7 (17.5%)	<0.001
Yes	52 (63.4%)	19 (45.2%)	33 (82.5%)	
Oxygen support				
No	21 (25.6%)	16 (38.1%)	5 (12.5%)	
<35%	30 (36.5%)	17 (40.5%)	13 (32.5%)	0.002
35–50%	6 (7.3%)	0	6 (15%)	
>50%	25 (30.5%)	9 (21.4%)	16 (40%)	
Fever				
No	11 (13.4%)	6 (14.3%)	5 (12.5%)	1
Yes	71 (86.6%)	36 (85.7%)	35 (87.5%)	
Pneumonia				
No	19 (23.2%)	12 (28.6%)	7 (17.5%)	
Unilobar	18 (22.4%)	10 (23.8%)	8 (20%)	0.38
Multilobar/bilateral	45 (54.9%)	20 (47.6%)	25 (62.5%)	
Thrombosis				
No	73 (87.9%)	40 (93.02%)	33 (82.5%)	0.18
Suspicious/confirmed	10 (12.1%)	3 (6.98%)	7 (17.5%)	
In-hospital days (mean ± SD)	11.9 ± 9.6	10.6 ± 7	13.6 ± 11.6	0.09
Clinical evolution after neutropenia				
Better/no changes	62 (78.4%)	34 (79.07%)	28 (70%)	0.45
Worse	17 (21.5%)	9 (20.93%)	12 (30%)	
Death				
Yes	27 (32.9%)	10 (23.8%)	17 (42.5%)	0.1
No	55 (67.1%)	32 (76.19%)	26 (57.5%)	
Evolution after discharge *:				
-No change of treatment	37 (68.5%)	24 (75%)	13 (59.1%)	0.25
-Change of treatment	19 (31.5%)	8 (25%)	9 (40.9%)	

* Patient could maintain active treatment or required stopped active treatment and receive only definitive supportive management.

3.3. Descriptive Analysis of Neutropenia Characteristics and G-CSF Administration

Table 3 includes the most relevant parameters collected about neutropenia and G-CSF treatment. All patients recruited had different grades of neutropenia during SARS-CoV-2 infection. Among the initial neutropenic patients, the lowest level of neutrophils reported was 0 cls/mm^3. The mean was 707 cls/mm^3, and the median was 650 cls/mm^3. Around half of all patients (40, 49%) received growth colony stimulating factor (G-CSF) as routine dose of 5 ug/Kg to recover neutrophil counts. The rest of the patients in this series (43) did not receive this treatment for different reasons, mainly related to the uncertainty in its usefulness for patients with this type of cancer and infection with COVID-19: severity of neutropenia, doubts about lung inflammatory effect, and hospital protocols. The G-CSF treatment duration was very variable: from 1 day to 14, with a mean and median number of days on treatment of around 4.5 days. All patients who received G-CSF were on chemotherapy or chemo-immunotherapy treatment (see Table 1). In 26/40 patients (65%), G-CSF was initiated when neutropenia symptoms were detected but in the remaining 14/40 (35%), G-CSF was previously prescribed to prevent febrile neutropenia after a routine chemotherapy administration. After several days of G-CSF administration, the highest level of neutrophil count was 26.100 cls/mm^3. Neutropenia outcome was variable: 21% had a worsening of neutrophil count and 50% improved. However, in 27% of the patients, their neutrophil count remained stable during SARS-CoV-2 infection. In addition, among the patients who were treated with G-CSF with a worsening of neutropenia, 91.6% died versus 0% among patients with total neutrophil recovery after G-CSF treatment. On the other hand, the mean lowest value of lymphocyte counts was 473/L, with no clear differences between G-CSF-treated patients vs. non-treated ones, while the mean of the highest LDH value was 685 U/L. The mean highest D-dimer value was 4513 ng/mL, that of calcitonin was 2.5 ng/dL, and that of C-reactive protein was 115 mg/dL. Again, we can see a trend in the data towards an increase in mortality according to the levels of these variables; in the case of D-dimer, pointing to an increase in thrombosis; while for LDH and the highly significantly increased C-reactive protein, signaling an increase in the number of inflammatory processes.

Table 3. Descriptive analysis of neutropenia variables.

Neutropenia and Inflammation Variables	Total	Without G-CSF	With G-CSF	p-Value
Lowest neutrophils count	616 ± 419	691 ± 369	541 ± 457	0.11
Highest neutrophils count	5423 ± 5078	3409 ± 2973	7538 ± 5940	<0.001
Lowest lymphocyte count	473 ± 310	467 ± 269	469 ± 356	0.77
Highest D-dymer	4513 ± 10134	2401 ± 3180	7456 ± 14880	0.062
Highest LDH	685 ± 1410	585 ± 604	792 ± 1943	0.86
Highest calcitonin	2.5 ± 5.3	2.6 ± 6.2	2.4 ± 3.6	0.06
Highest C-reactive protein	115 ± 143	90 ± 140	143 ± 143	0.001

3.4. Bivariate Analyses of COVID-19 Infection in Patients with Neutropenia: Death Risk Factors

Figure 1 shows a forest plot with the odds ratios (and corresponding 95% confidence intervals) for the association of different factors with mortality in our sample. In it, we could not find a significant association between age, ECOG, cardiovascular disease, type of tumor, or stage and mortality. Diabetes was related to a worse outcome and a higher risk of mortality compared with non-diabetes, although not significant (30.4% vs. 11.3%; p = 0.0533). The intention of treatment (palliative vs. curative) was also related to a trend of higher mortality in those patients with palliative treatment: 19 (83%) versus 4 (18%) patients, but this relation did not reach a statistically significant value (p = 0.064). Regarding oncological treatment, all patients treated with a combination of chemotherapy and immunotherapy died (3, 100%), but we could not find a significant association to a worse prognosis of SARS-CoV-2 infection and type of anti-cancer treatment received. Focusing on infections with COVID-19, in this series, we found that those patients with any type of pneumonia and neutropenia (unilateral, bilateral, unilobed, or multilobed) presented higher mortality compared with those without it: 19 (82.6%) versus 4 (17.3%), p = 0.0027. We also observed that men had more severe pneumonias compared with women, with higher oxygen requirements: 67.5% multilobe or bilateral in men versus 44.3% in women, p = 0.011. Although we did not find a significant relation between the type of tumor and COVID-19 mortality, we observed that 72.9% of lung cancer patients presented more severe infection with COVID-19, followed by colon cancer (41.2%), although this association was not significant (p = 0.064). We found an association between body mass index (BMI) and oxygen requirements when classified as no oxygen requirements vs. any oxygen flow. Oxygen support was needed in 57.2% of patients with BMI < 20, in 68% with BMI 20–25, in 82.6% with BMI 25–30, and in 100% with BMI > 30 (p = 0.0045). Smoking status was also associated with a higher risk for severe pneumonia and worse COVID-19 prognosis: 33 (73.3%) of smokers or former smokers developed some type of pneumonia vs. non-smokers, 12 (26.6%), p = 0.0035. In this series, 23 (27%) of all patients included died due to infections with COVID-19, and respiratory failure was present in all of them (100%). In our series, as we expected, higher oxygen needs were related to a significantly higher risk of mortality. We observed that low counts of neutrophils ($p = 0.001$) and lymphocytes ($p = 0.013$) were related to a higher mortality, and high values for LDH ($p = 0.001$) and Protein C ($p = 0.003$) were also associated with a worse outcome. In our cohort, corticoid administration in our patients with SARS-CoV2 infection and neutropenia was associated with a trend toward a lower mortality rate (52.17%) compared with patients without (67.9%) ($p = 0.08$). Regarding the impact of G-SCF administration, we observed a significant relation to mortality with 60.9% versus 39% in patients who did not receive G-CSF, as described before. There are also different conditions related to G-CSF administration, related as well to worse outcome, such as oxygen ($p = 0.003$) and carbapenems ($p = 0.15$) requirements ($p = 0.003$), pneumonia ($p = 0.0585$), and neutropenia severity ($p = 0.035$). Patients treated with G-CSF received corticoids more frequently compared with those without G-CSF (50% versus 16%).

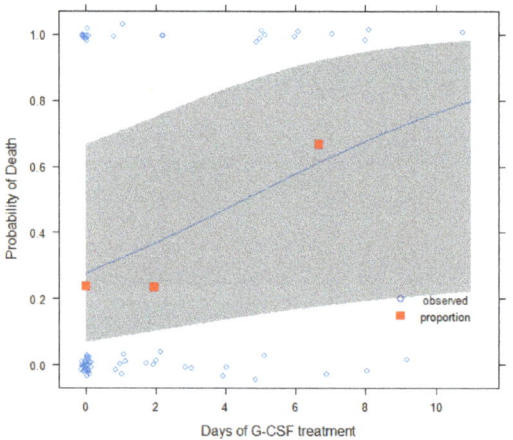

Figure 1. Death probability as a function of G-CSF treatment days: observed data (open circles, fitted to ease visualization), proportions (red squares, in subgroups of <1, 1–4, and >4 days), and fitted logistic model with 95% confidence bands are shown.

3.5. A Multivariable Model to Test the Effect of G-CSF on COVID-19 Severity

We also carried out a multivariable analysis to test the potential effect of G-CSF treatment on COVID-19 mortality. In this analysis, we saw that the administration of G-CSF depends on multiple factors, with the hospital protocol being a very important one among them. For example, in the bivariate analyses, while tumor type; cancer treatment; treatment intention; ECOG; sex; age; and indeed, the lowest level of neutrophils, a proxy for neutropenia severity, are not associated with the hospital, as expected, the G-CSF treatment binary variable is $p < 0.001$. This fact suggests that patients with similar neutropenia conditions were treated in different ways depending on the oncologist criteria considering emergent data about the role of G-CSF in COVID-19 infection outcome. Thus, in some way, G-CSF treatment can be considered approximately randomized, and by adjusting for appropriate covariables, unbalanced in the sample and with a possible influence, the effect of G-CSF treatment on outcomes for these patients could be tested in order to gain insights about its possible beneficial or harmful effects. It would also be expected that the harmful or beneficial effects of G-CSF depend on the number of days it was administered, which has also a protocol-dependent component and is highly variable in this sample. Therefore, after removing a few patients for which G-CSF was administered in a preventive way, a logistic regression model was developed to predict respiratory distress as a function of the number of days of G-CSF treatment (Figures 2 and 3). As adjusted covariates, sex, age, treatment purpose (palliative vs. curative, to adjust for global patient health status), tumor type, the lowest levels of lymphocytes (to adjust for immune status), and the lowest level of neutrophils in the patient (to adjust for neutropenic status) were used. A significant risk effect was obtained for the number of days of G-CSF treatment (OR = 1.40, 95% CI [1,2,05,07], *p*-value = 0.01). In Figure 2, we can see that the proportion of respiratory distress increases as we move from the first to the third intervals of treatment days. Superimposed is the fit of the logistic model. On the other hand, if death was used as a response variable instead, with the same adjusted variables, again, a significant risk effect was obtained for the number of days of G-CSF treatment (OR = 1.24, 95% CI [1,01,1,55], *p*-value = 0.04). Thus, a one-day increment of G-CSF treatment increases the odds ratio for respiratory distress by 1.4 and that of death by 1.24. This is represented in Figure 3, where the proportion of deaths is represented at three intervals for treatment days together with the fit of the logistic model. These results suggest that long neutropenic treatments in cancer patients could be harmful for the treatment of COVID-19 infection, instead of being beneficial.

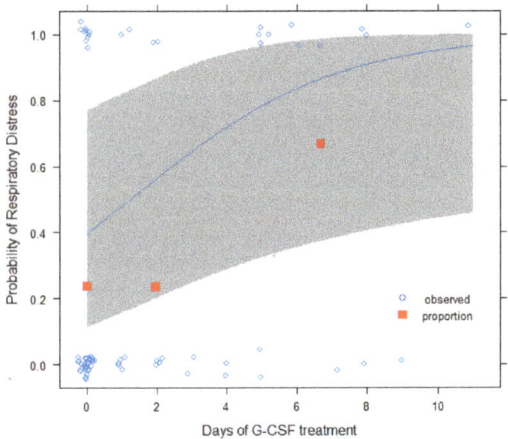

Figure 2. Respiratory distress as a function of G-CSF treatment days: observed data (open circles, fitted to ease visualization), proportions (red squares, in subgroups of <1, 1–4, and >4 days), and fitted logistic model with 95% confidence bands are shown.

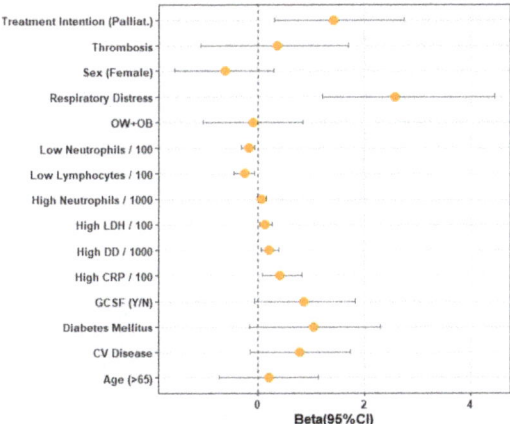

Figure 3. Forest plot showing mortality according to different variables related to neutropenia severity, treatment, and infection with COVID-19.

4. Discussion

The COVID-19 pandemic has made daily oncological clinical care even more challenging. We performed a retrospective study of real-world data (RWD) of neutropenic oncological patients during the first wave of the COVID-19 pandemic in 14 hospitals in Spain. To our knowledge, this is the first analysis of SARS-CoV-2 infection in a significant number of cancer patients with neutropenia. We analyzed the impact of different variables in the SARS-CoV-2 infection outcome, mainly, G-CSF administration, which has been recently related to a probable worsening of SARS-CoV-2 prognosis [18]. Previous reports have reported around 13% of infections with COVID-19 in cancer patients [19], but in our study, this rate was 30.3%, probably due to the added risk of neutropenia, and it reached 60.9% in those treated with G-CSF. Some published studies have shown worse outcomes in patients with SARS-CoV-2 infection and neutropenia after treatment with G-CSF [18,20]. In our work, a direct correlation between G-CSF use and the severity of infection with COVID-19, respiratory failure, and death were found. Several putative confounding factors (sex, age, treatment intention, and lymphocyte and neutrophil counts) are possibly involved in the outcome, but a logistic regression model after adjusting for these covariables still seems significant, increasing the effect of the number of days of G-CSF treatment on death. Different immunological factors have been involved in severe coronavirus disease, associated with high levels of neutrophils and a high neutrophil–lymphocyte ratio (NLR) [4]. In our study, both neutrophilia and lymphocytopenia were correlated with a higher rate of respiratory failure and death, as it has been previously reported [21,22], specifically after G-CSF treatment [19,23]. In addition to the number of days of Filgrastim® treatment, in our series, we found that higher levels of PCR, LDH, D-dimer, and lymphocytopenia have been related to poor prognosis in neutropenic patients with COVID-19, as has been previously described [24]. Before the COVID-19 pandemic, G-CSF use and neutrophil count recovery had been related with lung injury and Acute Respiratory Distress Syndrome (ARDS) [24,25]. In autopsy studies of patients infected with SARS-CoV-2, diffuse alveolar damage with hyaline membranes, hemorrhage, and neutrophilic infiltration have been reported [26–28]. Vascular neutrophilic inflammation and immune thrombosis are characteristics of COVID-19 infection [29] and have been described as being associated with G-CSF treatment. Neutrophil extracellular traps (NETS) may contribute to organ damage and mortality in COVID-19 disease. NETS are web-like structures of DNA and proteins expelled from the neutrophils that ensnare pathogens and have demonstrated a role in both venous and arterial thrombosis in several diseases [30] and can even promote cancer metastasis [31]. The intravascular aggregation of NETs in severe COVID-19 infection leads to immune thrombosis and disturbed microcirculation, organ damage, and ARDS [32,33]. Neutrophilia itself is associated with the release of cytokines, neutrophil activation, and NETs [34,35]. Increased NET formation correlates with ARDS, thrombosis, and cytokine storms, all of which are key in severe COVID-19 infections [36]. Filgrastim is a potent mobilizer of hematopoietic bone marrow cells and has a role activating cytokines to regulate T-cells and dendritic cell activation [37]. Some authors have suggested that we should be very cautious with G-CSF use in neutropenic patients with SARS-CoV-2 infection because there is a risk of triggering inflammation mediators related to severe COVID-19 infection [23,37]. We found a link between G-CSF and parameters of seriousness, a higher failure respiratory rate, higher neutrophil counts, lower lymphocytes, higher thrombosis, ARDS, and death. Although this is a small, non-randomized retrospective study and it was not designed to measure the effect of G-CSF treatment on the disease, a direct correlation of G-CSF treatment with a worse outcome was demonstrated after adjusting for possible confounding variables. This is a multicentric study of RWD describing neutropenic cancer management of patients with SARS-CoV-2 infection and showing a differential outcome for those treated or not with G-CSF under similar circumstances. Interestingly, corticoids have a beneficial effect in reducing mortality, as other authors have previously observed [38]. Morjaria et al. have published a pre-print study of 16 patients with neutropenia and COVID-19 treated with G-CSF. They classified these types of patients as good or poor responders according to the induced neutrophilia the day after G-CSF first dose administration. They found that good responders had a worse outcome, and they concluded that G-CSF treatment should be weighed in neutropenic patients with COVID-19 infections [20]. Moss et al. found that aged rhesus macaques infected by SARS-CoV-2 presented high G-CSF, involving the early release of neutrophils, less maturity, and less functionality compared with younger rhesus macaques, suggesting the potential role of GCSF administration in this mature human sample in worse COVID 19 outcomes [39]. Some authors have also described a link with neutrophil recovery and respiratory deterioration, and some reflections about this observed relation have been made in the literature [40]. According to the evidence as well as presented data, we should be more cautious in neutropenia management concurrent with infections by COVID-19 [41]. Nevertheless, other experiences suggest that G-CSF can counteract lymphocytopenia and could improve the outcome of the coronavirus disease [42]. A fully randomized clinical phase III trial could be designed to find the optimal balance, both in terms of the dose and duration of G-CSF treatment for these neutropenic cancer patients and with a more elaborate design (e.g., stratification) in terms of types of cancer. From this observational study, we have been able to obtain and test these findings about the risk of G-CSF treatment in patients with neutropenic cancer and infected by SARS-CoV-2 by applying appropriate adjustment variables, but further studies are required to confirm these findings and to obtain more information about aspects such as the involvement of cancer therapies, type of tumor, vaccination status, etc.

5. Conclusions

In our retrospective study, we found a potential correlation between G-CSF treatment as well as the duration of G-CSF administration with the development of severe disease and mortality after adjusting for other potential variables that could also impact mortality in these types of patients.

Author Contributions: Conceptualization: M.S. and A.M.J.-G.; methodology, G.C.; formal analysis, G.C.; investigation, M.S. and A.M.J.-G.; resources, M.S., A.M.J.-G., J.B.-E., C.A., X.M., A.P., R.Á.-Á., A.S., J.L.L., R.M., A.L.-A., B.H., L.E.C., A.M.M., A.L.-M., M.D., A.C.-L., E.C. and G.C.; writing—original draft preparation M.S., A.M.J.-G. and G.C.; writing—review and editing, M.S., A.M.J.-G. and G.C.; visualization M.S. and A.M.J.-G.; supervision, E.C. and A.R.d.M.; project administration, M.S. All authors have read and agreed to the published version of the manuscript.

Funding: This research received no external funding.

Institutional Review Board Statement: This study was conducted according to the guidelines of the Declaration of Helsinki and was approved by the Clinical Research Ethics Committee University Hospital of La Paz (HULP: PI-4194).

Informed Consent Statement: This is a retrospective analysis and it was not necessary to obtain Informed consent from subjects alive involved in the study according to Clinical Research Ethics Committee University Hospital of La Paz (HULP: PI-4194).

Acknowledgments: Thanks to all patients and their families included in the study and to all heath workers involved in the fight against the COVID-19 pandemic from our institution and from all over the world.

Conflicts of Interest: The authors declare no conflict of interest.

References

1. Chen, N.; Zhou, M. Epidemiological and clinical characteristics of 99 cases of 2019 novel coronavirus pneumonia in Wuhan, China: A descriptive study. *Lancet* **2020**, *395*, 507–513. [CrossRef]
2. Crisci, C.D.; Ardusso, L.R.F. Precision Medicine Approach to SARS-CoV-2 Pandemic Management. *Curr. Treat. Options Allergy* **2020**, *8*, 1–19. [CrossRef]
3. Vijayvargiya, P.; Esquer Garrigos, Z. Treatment Considerations for COVID-19: A Critical Review of the Evidence (or Lack Thereof). *Mayo Clin. Proc.* **2020**, *95*, 1454–1466. [CrossRef]

4. Qin, C.; Zhou, L.; Hu, Z.; Zhang, S.; Yang, S.; Tao, Y.; Xie, C.; Ma, K.; Shang, K.; Wang, W.; et al. Dysregulation of Immune Response in Patients with Coronavirus 2019 (COVID-19) in Wuhan, China. *Clin. Infect. Dis.* **2020**, *71*, 762–768. [CrossRef]
5. Delang, L.; Neyts, J. Medical treatment options for COVID-19. *Eur. Heart J. Acute Cardiovasc. Care* **2020**, *9*, 209–214. [CrossRef] [PubMed]
6. Zhang, L.; Zhu, F.; Xie, L.; Wang, C.; Wang, J.; Chen, R.; Jia, P.; Guan, H.Q.; Peng, L.; Chen, Y.; et al. Clinical characteristics of COVID-19-infected cancer patients: A retrospective case study in three hospitals within Wuhan, China. *Ann. Oncol.* **2020**, *31*, 894–901. [CrossRef] [PubMed]
7. Yu, J.; Ouyang, W.; Chua, M.L.K.; Xie, C. SARS-CoV-2 Transmission in Patients with Cancer at a Tertiary Care Hospital in Wuhan, China. *JAMA Oncol.* **2020**, *7*, 1108–1110. [CrossRef]
8. Kim, J.S.; Lee, K.H.; Kim, G.E.; Kim, S.; Yang, J.W.; Li, H.; Hong, S.H.; Ghayda, R.A.; Kronbichler, A.; Koyanagi, A.; et al. Clinical characteristics and mortality of patients with hematologic malignancies and COVID-19: A systematic review. *Eur. Rev. Med. Pharmacol. Sci.* **2020**, *24*, 11926–11933. [PubMed]
9. El Gohary, G.M.; Hashmi, S.; Styczynski, J.; Kharfan-Dabaja, M.A.; Alblooshi, R.M.; de la Cámara, R.; Mohamed, S.; Alshaibani, A.; Cesaro, S.; El-Aziz, N.A.; et al. The risk and prognosis of COVID-19 infection in cancer patients: A systematic review and meta-analysis. *Hematol. Stem Cell Ther.* **2020**, *30*, 1206–1213. [CrossRef]
10. Liang, W.; Guan, W. Cancer patients in SARS-CoV-2 infection: A nationwide analysis in China. *Lancet Oncol.* **2020**, *21*, 335–337. [CrossRef]
11. Kasi, P.M.; Grothey, A. Chemotherapy-Induced Neutropenia as a Prognostic and Predictive Marker of Outcomes in Solid-Tumor Patients. *Drugs* **2018**, *78*, 737–745. [CrossRef] [PubMed]
12. Felsenstein, S.; Herbert, J.; McNamara, P.S.; Hedrich, C.M. COVID-19: Immunology and treatment options. *Clin. Immunol.* **2020**, *215*, 108448. [CrossRef]
13. Aapro, M.; Bohlius, J.; Cameron, D.; Lago, L.D.; Donnelly, J.P.; Kearney, N.; Lyman, G.; Pettengell, R.; Tjan-Heijnen, V.; Walewski, J.; et al. 2010 update of EORTC guidelines for the use of granulocyte-colony stimulating factor to reduce the incidence of chemotherapy-induced febrile neutropenia in adult patients with lymphoproliferative disorders and solid tumours. *Eur. J. Cancer* **2011**, *47*, 8–32. [CrossRef] [PubMed]
14. Wiedermann, F.J. Acute lung injury during G-CSF-induced neutropenia recovery: Effect of G-CSF on pro- and anti-inflammatory cytokines. *Bone Marrow Transplant.* **2005**, *36*, 731. [CrossRef]
15. Słomka, A.; Kowalewski, M.; Żekanowska, E. Coronavirus Disease 2019 (COVID–19): A Short Review on Hematological Manifestations. *Pathogens* **2020**, *9*, 493. [CrossRef] [PubMed]
16. Taha, M.; Sharma, A.; Soubani, A. Clinical deterioration during neutropenia recovery after G-CSF therapy in patient with COVID-19. *Respir. Med. Case Rep.* **2020**, *31*, 101231. [CrossRef] [PubMed]
17. R Core Team. *R: A Language and Environment for Statistical Computing*; R Foundation for Statistical Computing: Vienna, Austria, 2019.
18. Kuderer, N.M.; Choueiri, T.K.; Shah, D.P.; Shyr, Y.; Rubinstein, S.M.; Rivera, D.R.; Shete, S.; Hsu, C.-Y.; Desai, A.; de Lima Lopes, G.; et al. Clinical impact of COVID-19 on patients with cancer (CCC19): A cohort study. *Lancet* **2020**, *395*, 1907–1918. [CrossRef]
19. Zhang, A.W.; Morjaria, S.; Kaltsas, A.; Hohl, T.M.; Parameswaran, R.; Patel, D.; Zhou, W.; Predmore, J.; Perez-Johnston, R.; Jee, J.; et al. The Effect of Neutropenia and Filgrastim (G-CSF) in Cancer Patients With COVID-19 Infection. *Clin. Infect. Dis.* **2021**, *15*. [CrossRef]
20. Fu, J.; Kong, J.; Wang, W.; Wu, M.; Yao, L.; Wang, Z.; Jin, J.; Wu, D.; Yu, X. The clinical implication of dynamic neutrophil to lymphocyte ratio and D-dimer in COVID-19: A retrospective study in Suzhou China. *Thromb. Res.* **2020**, *192*, 3–8. [CrossRef]
21. Sun, S.; Cai, X.; Wang, H.; He, G.; Lin, Y.; Lu, B.; Chen, C.; Pan, Y.; Hu, X. Abnormalities of peripheral blood system in patients with COVID-19 in Wenzhou, China. *Clin. Chim. Acta* **2020**, *507*, 174–180. [CrossRef]
22. Nawar, T.; Morjaria, S.; Kaltsas, A.; Patel, D.; Perez-Johnston, R.; Daniyan, A.F.; Mailankody, S.; Parameswaran, R. Granulocyte-colony stimulating factor in COVID-19: Is it stimulating more than just the bone marrow? *Am. J. Hematol.* **2020**, *95*, 210–213. [CrossRef]
23. Guan, W.-J.; Ni, Z.-Y.; Hu, Y.; Liang, W.-H.; Ou, C.-Q.; He, J.-X.; Liu, L.; Shan, H.; Lei, C.-L.; Hui, D.S.; et al. Clinical Characteristics of Coronavirus Disease 2019 in China. *N. Engl. J. Med.* **2020**, *382*, 1708–1720. [CrossRef]
24. Zemans, R.L.; Matthay, M.A. What drives neutrophils to the alveoli in ARDS? *Thorax* **2017**, *72*, 1–3. [CrossRef]
25. Balsat, M.; Xhaard, A.; Lengline, E.; Tavernier, E.; Cornillon, J.; Guyotat, D.; Darmon, M. Worsening of Respiratory Status during Neutropenia Recovery in Noncritically Ill Hematological Patients: Results of a Prospective Multicenter Study. *Respiration* **2015**, *90*, 229–234. [CrossRef]
26. Fox, S.E.; Akmatbekov, A.; Harbert, J.L.; Li, G.; Brown, J.Q.; Heide, R.S.V. Pulmonary and cardiac pathology in African American patients with COVID-19: An autopsy series from New Orleans. *Lancet Respir. Med.* **2020**, *8*, 681–686. [CrossRef]
27. Barnes, B.J.; Adrover, J.M.; Baxter-Stoltzfus, A.; Borczuk, A.; Cools-Lartigue, J.; Crawford, J.M.; Daßler-Plenker, J.; Guerci, P.; Huynh, C.; Knight, J.S.; et al. Targeting potential drivers of COVID-19: Neutrophil extracellular traps. *J. Exp. Med.* **2020**, *217*, e20200652. [CrossRef] [PubMed]
28. Nicolai, L.; Leunig, A.; Brambs, S.; Kaiser, R.; Joppich, M.; Hoffknecht, M.; Gold, C.; Engel, A.; Polewka, V.; Muenchhoff, M.; et al. Vascular neutrophilic inflammation and immunothrombosis distinguish severe COVID-19 from influenza pneumonia. *J. Thromb. Haemost.* **2021**, *19*, 574–581. [CrossRef]

29. Thålin, C.; Hisada, Y. Neutrophil Extracellular Traps: Villains and Targets in Arterial, Venous, and Cancer-Associated Thrombosis. *Arterioscler. Thromb. Vasc. Biol.* **2019**, *39*, 1724–1738. [CrossRef]
30. Yang, L.; Liu, Q.; Zhang, X.; Liu, X.; Zhou, B.; Chen, J.; Huang, D.; Li, J.; Li, H.; Chen, F.; et al. DNA of neutrophil extracellular traps promotes cancer metastasis via CCDC25. *Nature* **2020**, *583*, 133–138. [CrossRef] [PubMed]
31. Leppkes, M.; Knopf, J.; Naschberger, E.; Lindemann, A.; Singh, J.; Herrmann, I.; Stürzl, M.; Staats, L.; Mahajan, A.; Schauer, C.; et al. Vascular occlusion by neutrophil extracellular traps in COVID-19. *EBioMedicine* **2020**, *58*, 102925. [CrossRef] [PubMed]
32. Middleton, E.A.; He, X.-Y.; Denorme, F.; Campbell, R.A.; Ng, D.; Salvatore, S.P.; Mostyka, M.; Baxter-Stoltzfus, A.; Borczuk, A.C.; Loda, M.; et al. Neutrophil extracellular traps contribute to immunothrombosis in COVID-19 acute respiratory distress syndrome. *Blood* **2020**, *136*, 1169–1179. [CrossRef]
33. Wang, J.; Li, Q.; Yin, Y.; Zhang, Y.; Cao, Y.; Lin, X.; Huang, L.; Hoffmann, D.; Lu, M.; Qiu, Y. Excessive Neutrophils and Neutrophil Extracellular Traps in COVID-19. *Front. Immunol.* **2020**, *11*, 2063. [CrossRef]
34. Skendros, P.; Mitsios, A.; Chrysanthopoulou, A.; Mastellos, D.C.; Metallidis, S.; Rafailidis, P.; Ntinopoulou, M.; Sertaridou, E.; Tsironidou, V.; Tsigalou, C.; et al. Complement and tissue factor–enriched neutrophil extracellular traps are key drivers in COVID-19 immunothrombosis. *J. Clin. Investig.* **2020**, *130*, 6151–6157. [CrossRef] [PubMed]
35. Roberts, A.W. G-CSF: A key regulator of neutrophil production, but that's not all! *Growth Factors* **2005**, *23*, 33–41. [CrossRef] [PubMed]
36. Sahu, K.K.; Siddiqui, A.D. From Hematologist's desk: The effect of COVID-19 on the blood system. *Am. J. Hematol.* **2020**, *95*, E213–E215. [CrossRef]
37. Mertens, J.; Laghrib, Y.; Kenyon, C. A Case of Steroid-Responsive, COVID-19 Immune Reconstitution Inflammatory Syndrome Following the Use of Granulocyte Colony-Stimulating Factor. *Open Forum Infect. Dis.* **2020**, *7*, ofaa326. [CrossRef] [PubMed]
38. Moss, D.L.; Rappaport, J. The good, the bad and the ugly: G-CSF, ageing and neutrophils-Implications for severe COVID-19. *J. Leukoc. Biol.* **2021**, *109*, 1017. [CrossRef]
39. Tralongo, A.C.; Danova, M. Granulocyte colony-stimulating factors (G-CSF) and COVID-19: A double-edged sword? *Infez. Med.* **2020**, *28*, 459–460.
40. Lasagna, A.; Zuccaro, V.; Ferraris, E.; Rizzo, G.; Tancredi, R.J.; Pedrazzoli, P. How to Use Prophylactic G-CSF in the Time of COVID-19. *JCO Oncol. Pract.* **2020**, *16*, 771–772. [CrossRef]
41. Lazarus, H.M.; Gale, R.P. Is G-CSF Dangerous in COVID-19: Why Not Use GM-CSF? *Acta Haematol.* **2021**, *144*, 350–351. [CrossRef]
42. Chen, G.-B.; Lin, J.-T.; Zhang, Z.; Liu, L. Effect of recombinant human granulocyte colony-stimulating factor on lymphocyte subsets in patients with COVID-19. *Infect. Dis.* **2020**, *52*, 759–761. [CrossRef] [PubMed]

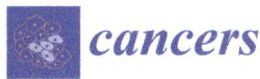 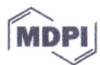

Review

Melanoma Management during the COVID-19 Pandemic Emergency: A Literature Review and Single-Center Experience

Caterina Cariti [1,†], Martina Merli [1,*,†], Gianluca Avallone [1], Marco Rubatto [1], Elena Marra [1], Paolo Fava [1], Virginia Caliendo [2], Franco Picciotto [2], Giulio Gualdi [3], Ignazio Stanganelli [4], Maria Teresa Fierro [1], Simone Ribero [1,‡] and Pietro Quaglino [1,‡]

1. Department of Medical Sciences, Dermatology Clinic, University of Turin, 10126 Turin, Italy; caterina.cariti@gmail.com (C.C.); gianluca.avallone@hotmail.it (G.A.); marco.rubatto@edu.unito.it (M.R.); emarra@cittadellasalute.it (E.M.); fava_paolo@yahoo.it (P.F.); mariateresa.fierro@unito.it (M.T.F.); simone.ribero@unito.it (S.R.); pietro.quaglino@unito.it (P.Q.)
2. Dermatologic Surgery Department, Surgery Department, University Hospital, 10126 Turin, Italy; virginia.caliendo@unito.it (V.C.); fpicciotto@cittadellasalute.to.it (F.P.)
3. Department of Medicine and Ageing Science, Dermatologic Clinic, "G. D'Annunzio" University, 66100 Chieti, Italy; giuliogualdi@libero.it
4. Skin Cancer Unit, IRCCS-IRST Scientific Institute of Romagna for the Study and Treatment of Cancer, Meldola and University of Parma, 43121 Parma, Italy; ignazio.stanganelli@unipr.it
* Correspondence: martina.merli@edu.unito.it; Tel.: +39-011-633-5843
† These authors contributed equally to this paper as first authors.
‡ These authors contributed equally to this paper as senior authors.

Simple Summary: COVID-19 is a highly contagious infection caused by severe acute respiratory syndrome coronavirus 2 (SARS-CoV-2). In March 2020, the World Health Organization (WHO) declared that COVID-19 had become a pandemic; since then, several elective clinical and surgical activities have been postponed to reduce the risk of nosocomial infection. This has influenced the diagnosis and management of many diseases, including melanoma. The aim of our literature review was to evaluate whether the management of melanoma has been changed by the outbreak of COVID-19, and if so, what the consequences of these changes are. The main topics in this literature review are the screening of suspicious lesions, diagnosis of primary melanoma, and the management of early-stage and advanced melanomas in the COVID-19 era. We also reported the experience of our dermatological clinic in Turin, one of the most affected areas in Italy.

Abstract: Background: The current COVID-19 pandemic has influenced the modus operandi of all fields of medicine, significantly impacting patients with oncological diseases and multiple comorbidities. Thus, in recent months, the establishment of melanoma management during the emergency has become a major area of interest. In addition to original articles, case reports and specific guidelines for the period have been developed. Purpose: This article aims to evaluate whether melanoma management has been changed by the outbreak of COVID-19, and if so, what the consequences are. We summarized the main issues concerning the screening of suspicious lesions, the diagnosis of primary melanoma, and the management of early-stage and advanced melanomas during the pandemic. Additionally, we report on the experience of our dermatological clinic in northern Italy. Methods: We performed a literature review evaluating articles on melanomas and COVID-19 published in the last two years on PubMed, as well as considering publications by major healthcare organizations. Concerning oncological practice in our center, we collected data on surgical and therapeutic procedures in patients with a melanoma performed during the first months of the pandemic. Conclusions: During the emergency period, the evaluation of suspicious skin lesions was ensured as much as possible. However, the reduced level of access to medical care led to a documented delay in the diagnosis of new melanomas. When detected, the management of early-stage and advanced melanomas was fully guaranteed, whereas the follow-up visits of disease-free patients have been postponed or replaced with a teleconsultation when possible.

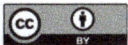

Keywords: melanoma; COVID-19; management; pandemic; teledermatology; diagnostic delay; immunotherapy; vaccination; lymph adenopathy

1. Introduction

The severe acute respiratory syndrome coronavirus 2 (SARS-CoV-2) pandemic has increased the workload of the health system in the last two years, which has also presented a global challenge for dermatologists. Several elective clinical and surgical activities have been postponed to reduce the risk of nosocomial infections in patients and healthcare workers. This does not concern oncological patients, whose medical care has been guaranteed. However, cancer screening programs have clearly been interrupted by the onset of COVID-19 [1].

An early diagnosis is essential for the survival of patients with a melanoma [2]. The position statement issued by the European Academy of Dermatology and Venereology (EADV) affirmed that an in-person physical examination is obligatory for an accurate diagnosis of suspicious new cutaneous lesions, and that dermoscopy remains the gold standard for melanoma diagnosis. Although there have been no reports of COVID-19 transmission via dermatoscopes, the device must be carefully disinfected between patients and adequate personal protective equipment must be worn by physicians and patients [3]. In this context, the reduced level of access to medical care is a problem for dermatologists, due to the potential decrease in diagnoses of thin melanomas and delays in the presentation of patients with thick tumors. A survey conducted by the International Dermoscopy Society (IDS) showed that its members had experienced a 75% reduction in daily work activity since the beginning of pandemic, and remarkably, the number of melanomas diagnosed in these months was practically zero for more than half of them (56.78%) [4]. In addition to the devastating consequences for patients, delays in the treatment of melanomas can have a profound impact on the economic burden of this disease, because advanced melanomas have higher healthcare costs than earlier-stage melanomas [5].

In this paper, we examine the main topics concerning the management of melanomas during this healthcare emergency, focusing on the importance of teledermatology, the diagnostic delay of melanomas, and how daily oncology practice has been impacted by the COVID-19 pandemic (Figure 1). We also report on the experience of our clinical center, which is situated in one of the most affected areas in Italy.

KEY SUMMARY POINTS

The COVID-19 pandemic significantly influenced the management of suspicious skin lesions, leading to a reduction in early diagnoses of primary melanomas
Teledermatology can be used to perform the first triage of suspicious skin lesions and to select those requiring a face-to-face consultation
The follow-up visits of stage 0-I-IIA melanomas can be postponed for up to 3 months in asymptomatic patients
It is essential to maintain the management of early-stage and advanced melanomas during the pandemic, without postponing diagnostic, surgical, and therapeutical procedures
There is no evidence that systemic therapies for melanoma increase the risk of becoming infected with SARS-CoV-2
COVID-19 vaccination is highly recommended for patients undergoing active melanoma therapy and their relatives
A lymphadenopathy should distinguish between a malignant spread and a benign reaction to a recent vaccination

Figure 1. The main topics discussed in the literature review.

2. The Increased Importance of Teledermatology Caused by COVID-19

The role of telemedicine has been discussed at length as a valid medical approach during the COVID-19 era. Telemedicine can be defined as the application of diagnostic and therapeutic tools at a distance from the patient as an alternative to a face-to-face consultation; it can be used in several fields of medicine.

Teledermatology can be classified into real-time teledermatology (VTC—live video consultation) and store-and-forward teledermatology (SAF—image transmission by the patient). Both types of teledermatology have facilitated remote dermatological assistance during the pandemic for chronic diseases and the appearance/modification of skin lesions [6]. The IDS questioned 678 of its members, from 52 different countries, about their activity during the emergency period. In total, 27.73% of respondents affirmed that telemedicine represented an important method of performing consultations; the number of unofficial teleconsultations (e.g., by mail, SMS, Skype®, WhatsApp®, Messenger®, etc.) they were asked to conduct increased by 83.33% during the COVID-19 pandemic [4]. A small-scale, randomized controlled trial comparing all teledermatology modalities and face-to-face consultations found that the diagnosis and recommended course of treatment was the same in 85% and 78% of cases, respectively [7]. Even if teledermatology can correctly identify the majority of malignant lesions, the diagnostic accuracy of face-to-face consultations remains higher than that of remote consultations [8].

Smartphone-based teledermoscopy, an extension of teledermatology, has improved in recent years due to the development of mobile applications and devices. Veronese et al. tested an inexpensive and easy-to-use smartphone microscope device; overall, they obtained an accuracy of 83.9% for the diagnoses of skin lesions based on images acquired through the device [6]. Considering these useful tools, teledermoscopy in association with teledermatology can be used to perform the first triage of skin lesions, helping the clinician to select patients who require a face-to-face consultation [8].

Nahm et al. described an example of telemedicine's usefulness during the COVID-19-enforced lockdown. They reported the case of a 66-year-old man with two biopsy-proven melanomas that were diagnosed in situ before the pandemic. The patient refused the exeresis of the two lesions due to his fear of coronavirus infection. Hence, the patient was treated with a combination of topical imiquimod 5% cream, 5-fluorouracil 2% solution, and tretinoin 0.1% cream every day for a month. The follow-up consultations were conducted exclusively via video consultation, and the histological evaluation completed 3 months after the treatment showed a complete resolution of the lesions [9].

3. The Diagnostic Delay of Melanomas during the Emergency Period

The great concern regarding the diagnostic delay of melanomas, and generally tumors, has been reflected by the large number of studies conducted on this topic during the emergency period.

The number of first diagnoses of malignancy recorded during weeks 11 to 20 of 2020 was compared with the same periods from 2018 and 2019. The data were collected from seven secondary care hospital networks of northern and central Italy. In 2020, there were 2751 new diagnoses, representing a decrease of 44.9% compared to 2018 and 2019 (4991.5 cases on average). The weekly number of diagnoses, considering the beginning of lockdown as the baseline time, constantly decreased during the first 2 weeks. The main reduction in new diagnoses occurred at week 16 (64.6% decrease compared with the same week in 2018–2019) and, during the last 2 weeks, a new increase was observed. Of the total number of all missing cancer diagnoses, melanoma and nonmelanoma skin cancers represented 56.7% [10].

Longo and Peris reported a significant reduction in the diagnoses of primary melanomas between 1 January 2020 and 9 May 2020 in Reggio Emilia and Rome, respectively. The number of new primary melanomas detected during this timeframe in 2019 was 141 and 115 in Rome and Reggio Emilia, respectively, whereas in 2020, there were 62 and 28 new primary melanomas detected [11].

Similarly, a third-level center in northern Italy observed a significant 60% reduction in new melanoma diagnoses between 22 February 2020 and 3 May 2020 compared to the same timeframes in 2018 and 2019. The most frequent histotype analyzed during the lockdown period was in situ melanoma (66.7%), whereas superficial spreading melanoma was the most frequent during 2019 and 2018 (52.4%). This may reflect a loss of thick melanomas in 2020, that conversely had been removed in 2019 and 2018 [12].

Generally, in Italy from February 2020 to April 2020, the Intergruppo Melanoma Italiano (IMI) detected a substantial reduction in the number of first visits (−31.3%) and biopsies (−36.5%), with a decrease of approximately 25% in histological diagnoses, and a 22.9% reduction in wide local excisions in comparison to 2019. As a result, there was a 20.8% reduction in the number of patients starting systemic therapy [13].

The Italian data described above are in agreement with studies in other countries. Lallas et al. compared the observed and expected numbers of new melanomas, basal cell carcinomas (BCCs), and cutaneous squamous cell carcinomas (cSCCs) in 2020 in northern Greece. The expected incidence of each tumor was calculated as the mean of the previous 4 years (2016–2019), considering this figure to be stable in 2020. The total number of these new skin cancers was 30.1% lower than expected, with a 36.4% reduction in the number of expected melanoma diagnoses. The patients with a melanoma were significantly younger than those in previous years, reflecting the greater fear of COVID-19 among elderly individuals. Additionally, a significantly higher proportion of melanomas than expected were diagnosed at stages IIC, III, and IV [14].

A multicenter observational study performed in Spain analyzed all patients who underwent melanoma or cSCC surgery in the period between March and June 2020. The comparison with the same period in 2019 revealed that there was a 41% reduction in treated melanoma during the first lockdown, with fewer melanomas in situ (34.9% vs. 29%) and a slight increase in thick melanomas (>4 mm) (10.2% vs. 18.4%). Similar results were obtained for cSCC. Patient-related factors, such as age, living in a nursing home, and fear of infection with SARS-CoV-2, were associated with a greater Breslow thickness [15].

Conversely, a dermatology department in London reported that a high proportion of early-stage melanomas were diagnosed during the UK's COVID-19 lockdown. There are several factors implicated in this higher melanoma detection-to-referral ratio, including the impact that the setting of anxiety and restricted healthcare services has on patient self-selection [16].

4. Melanoma Surgery and Disease-Free Patient Follow-Up during the Pandemic

According to the European Society for Medical Oncology (ESMO) [17] and National Comprehensive Cancer Network (NCCN) guidelines [18], the position statement of the EADV Melanoma Task Force affirmed that the excision of a suspicious lesion should be performed as soon as possible to remove everything that is clinically visible [3]. In addition, the NCCN suggests that performing a broad-shave biopsy for larger suspected melanomas in situ and lentigo maligna, preventing the need to perform a subsequent radicalization. Wide excision should be postponed for up to 3 months for melanomas in situ and invasive melanomas for which a previous biopsy has showed clear histopathological margins or a peripheral transection of the in situ component [18]. It has been noted that delaying the surgical excision of melanoma by one month or longer increases the proportion of large or thick tumors, resulting in a lower chance of overall survival. In this regard, Tejera-Vaquerizo and Nagore built a model based on melanoma rate of growth (ROG), i.e., the rate of increase in Breslow thickness (millimeters per month) from the time a subject first observes a suspicious lesion to its excision. This predictive model was used to understand how diagnostic delays may impact the prognosis of melanomas [19].

When possible, wide excision and sentinel lymph node biopsy (SLNB—for melanoma thicker than 0.8 mm) should be performed at the same time. Otherwise, SLNB may be delayed by up to 3 months [18], as it has been demonstrated that such an interval of time does not have a negative effect on disease-free and overall survival [20]. Regarding therapeutic lymph node dissection, the EADV's position statement indicated that it should be limited to patients with clinically evident regional lymph node metastases [3]. Conversely, NCCN guidelines affirm that lymphadenectomy should also be delayed in cases of clinically evaluable lymph adenopathy when a systemic neoadjuvant treatment is possible. In such a case, surgery should be performed 8–9 weeks after starting neoadjuvant treatment. This is not applicable when the affected lymph node is adjacent to vital organs and/or there is a contraindication to systemic therapy or a previous neoadjuvant treatment failure [18]. Finally, the guidelines agree that high surgical priority should be given to all invasive primary melanomas, resectable stage III melanomas, and oligo-metastatic disease [3].

Regarding disease-free patients, and according to the EADV's position statement, the clinical and radiological follow-up in stage 0-I-IIA melanoma can be postponed for up to 3 months in asymptomatic patients [3]. Moreover, no clear evidence of an increase in survival in stages IB and IIA has been reported in ultrasound-based follow-ups [21]. High-risk patients should continue to have physical and imaging examinations, particularly during the first 3 years after surgery on the primary tumor [3]. On the other hand, NCCN guidelines suggest a possible deferral of up to 6 months even for stages IIB/IIC. During this delayed time, self-examination once a month is highly recommended [18].

5. Advanced Melanoma Management and Immunotherapy in the COVID-19 Era

For adjuvant therapy and treatment of unresectable stage III or IV melanomas, the indication of EADV is the same in a non-emergency setting; the treatment of melanomas with approved drugs must be started within 12 weeks of surgery. Considering these patients at higher risk for a severe course of COVID-19 infection, antibodies against Programmed Cell Death Protein 1 (PD1) should be administered using the longest approved treatment schedule to decrease hospital admissions: pembrolizumab 400 mg every 6 weeks and nivolumab 480 mg every 4 weeks [3]. Given its favorable safety profile, a monotherapy with anti-PD1 should be preferred in the majority of patients requiring immunotherapy [22]. The addition of ipilimumab, an antibody targeting cytotoxic T-lymphocyte-associated protein 4 (CTLA-4), significantly increases the risk of immune-related adverse events (iRAEs) from 15%–20% to 50%–60% compared to anti-PD1 monotherapy; this often leads to the need for immunosuppressive therapies and hospitalization, which in turn potentially increases the rate of COVID-19 transmission and severe disease [23]. Among the complications caused by immune checkpoint inhibitors (ICIs), immunotherapy-related pneumonitis and COVID-19 pneumonia have overlapping clinical and radiological features, leading to significant challenges in differential diagnosis [24]. Accordingly, the combination of nivolumab and ipilimumab is recommended only in subsets of patients with specific clinical features, including symptomatic and asymptomatic cerebral metastases, elevated LDH levels, bulky disease, PD-L1 negativity, and mucosal and acral melanoma [3,25]. The CheckMate 511 regimen—that is, ipilimumab 1 mg/kg plus nivolumab 3 mg/kg—is the preferred course of treatment due to a significantly lower incidence of treatment-related grade 3–5 AEs [26].

In patients undergoing BRAF and MEK inhibitor treatments, hyperpyrexia must be considered primarily as an adverse event rather than an indicator of COVID-19 infection. For this reason, encorafenib combined with binimetinib is preferred when available compared to other regimens due to its lower fever incidence [27]. In cases of fever associated with grade 2 or higher dyspnea, diarrhea, or neurological symptoms that do not resolve after therapy discontinuation, patients should be tested for a SARS-CoV-2 infection [3].

Concerning intracranial metastases, in cases of neurological deterioration or surgery, such as palliative care following treatment delays, stereotactic radiosurgery should be considered [25].

According to NCCN guidelines, in patients progressing beyond standard immune checkpoint blockade and targeted therapy, hospice care should be considered, because chemotherapy only provides a limited benefit. Oral temozolomide is the preferred option for palliative care cases [28].

As indicated by the EADV's recommendations, all patients undergoing surgery, radiotherapy, chemotherapy, or immunotherapy must be tested for COVID-19 infection, despite studies in real-world settings showing a high safety profile in these patients. Additionally, to date, no clear evidence suggests that ICIs increase the risk of a SARS-CoV-2 infection [3]. Whether the administration of anti-PD1 drugs, by stimulating the immune system, could directly contribute to a more severe course of COVID-19, compared to that observed in patients not receiving immunotherapy, is currently an open question. The potential interplay between COVID-19 infection and treatment with immune-checkpoint inhibitors of patients with a melanoma is still unknown. Nevertheless, preliminary evidence and case reports suggest that anti-PD1 therapy does not worsen the course of COVID-19, allowing patients with cancer to continue their treatment [29]. In this Italian multicenter study by Pala et al., out of 169 patients with unresectable stage III or IV melanomas treated with immunotherapy, 104 continued without modifications, and among 15 patients showing symptoms compatible with COVID-19, only one tested positive on the nasopharyngeal swab [30].

6. Vaccination against COVID-19 in Patients with Cancer Receiving Active Therapy

Most currently authorized trials of vaccines against COVID-19 have not included patients with active malignancies. Hence, data on safety, tolerability, and efficacy in cancer populations are limited. However, these patients represent a high-priority subgroup for vaccination due to their higher risk of death from SARS-CoV-2 infection and, for this reason, vaccination is supported by the ESMO, the Society for Immunotherapy of Cancer (SITC), the Spanish Medical Oncology Society (SEOM), and the NCCN COVID-19 Vaccination Advisory Committee [31–34]. In Israel, a study was conducted on the efficacy of the BNT162b2 vaccine in 102 patients with solid tumors undergoing a systemic therapy. The most frequently used types of therapy were chemotherapy (29%), followed by immunotherapy (22%), and chemotherapy plus biological therapy (20%). Ninety percent of oncological patients tested positive for SARS-CoV-2 anti-spike IgG antibodies after the second vaccine dose. Furthermore, patients undergoing chemotherapy plus immunotherapy presented a median IgG titer that was significantly lower than the control group. Conversely, immune checkpoint inhibitors alone did not interfere with antibody production. To date, there is no evidence of the correlation between the efficacy/duration of protection and IgG titer; therefore, these serology data strongly support the current recommendations for the oncology population. Moreover, as these patients may not be able to develop a sufficient immune response themselves, it has become crucial that their caregivers are also vaccinated [35]. In an Italian center, 131 patients with cancer receiving active therapy (57% had skin cancers) and immunized against SARS-CoV-2 were compared to healthy individuals after two doses of mRNA-1273 (Moderna). The median values of anti-spike IgG were significantly higher for patients receiving immunotherapy compared to those receiving chemotherapy/targeted therapy [36]. Some researchers have hypothesized that the vaccine could hypothetically lead to an exaggerated immune response in immunotherapy recipients. Since vaccination may overload the immune system and trigger an important cytokine response, severe toxicity may damage the organs [24]. However, several studies evaluated that there were no new or exacerbated immune-related side effects in patients undergoing immunotherapy and receiving mRNA COVID-19 vaccines [37,38]. These data are also supported by the experience of the safety of influenza vaccination in the same population [39].

7. Lymph Adenopathy during Pandemic: Malignant Spread versus Benign Reaction to Vaccination

Unilateral axillary adenopathy is a potential side effect following COVID-19 vaccination (specifically the mRNA vaccines) and it was reported to appear 2 to 4 days after administration. During the clinical trials of Moderna, the average duration of lymphadenopathy was 1 to 2 days, whereas the Pfizer-BioNTech clinical trials showed an average duration of approximately 10 days [40,41]. This finding may be present in the staging or routine follow-up imaging of oncologic patients. Indeed, an FDG-avid lymphadenopathy, detected using a PET-CT scan, was described after COVID-19 vaccination and after an influenza vaccination [42,43]. Prieto et al. reported the case of a patient with a history of stage IIIA melanoma in the left deltoid region who underwent an image-guided biopsy of a right axillary lymphadenopathy that was discovered during the initial stage. A histological examination showed a reactive lymphoid tissue. Further investigations revealed that the patient had received the first dose of the Moderna vaccine in the right deltoid muscle 5 days prior to the PET-CT scan [44]. Sonographically detectable lymph node changes after COVID-19 vaccination have been described in patients with skin cancer attending tumor follow-up appointments. These lymphadenopathies resemble lymph node metastases in terms of enlargement, peripheral vascularization, and decreased echogenicity [45]. Given an ever-increasing worldwide vaccinated population, it will be important for oncologists and dermatologists to obtain a vaccination history to better interpret the results of imaging studies and to avoid invasive procedures that are not strictly necessary. Additionally, in tumor patients, the vaccination should be performed contralateral to the primary tumor to ensure the lowest possible chance of misdiagnosis. Ultimately, management should consider the probability of a malignant spread versus a benign reaction to recent vaccination. The factors to consider include the local site of the primary malignancy, common drainage pathways, time since vaccination (within or beyond 6 weeks after vaccination), prognosis, and overall risk profile [46].

8. Experiences in Our Dermatological Clinic

In our dermatological clinic in Turin, Italy, we retrospectively collected data on melanomas excised in May and June of the years 2017, 2018, 2019 and 2020 (Table 1).

Table 1. Demographic and histological features of melanomas excised in the two-month period from May to June in 2017, 2018, 2019, and 2020. MIS: melanoma in situ; SSM: superficial spreading melanoma; LMM: lentigo maligna melanoma; NM: nodular melanoma.

Year	N. of Melanomas Excised	Male	Female	Mean Age (Years)	Histotype	Breslow Thickness (Average)
2017	51	31	20	61	28 MIS 21 SSM 1 LMM 1 NM	1 mm
2018	41	20	21	62	25 MIS 11 SSM 4 LMM 1 NM	0.42 mm
2019	48	31	17	61	27 MIS 18 SSM 2 LMM 1 NM	0.99 mm
2020	32	16	16	55	13 SSM 12 MIS 3 LMM 2 NM 1 nevoid melanoma 1 acral melanoma	1.56 mm

This study aimed to highlight possible differences between the two-month period during the pandemic and the same timeframe in the previous three years, focusing on patient demographics and histological characteristics of melanomas. In the two months of 2020, there was an approximately 32% reduction in melanoma exeresis compared to the previous years. There were no gender-based differences but the average age was lower at 55 years—in the previous three years, the average age was greater than 60. The most frequently excised histotype in 2020 was superficial spreading melanoma (SSM), whereas in previous years it was melanoma in situ. The greatest Breslow index was recorded in 2020 with a thickness of 9 mm and, in the same year, the average thickness was 1.56 mm; although the average thickness was higher than the average in previous years, this difference was not statistically significant.

Concerning the sentinel lymph node (SLN) surgical interventions in our melanoma unit, we performed SLN biopsies in 41 patients in the first two months of the emergency; the average age was 55, four of whom were over 70. All patients received an antibiotic prophylaxis before the surgical procedure, the same treatment that was prescribed before the COVID-19 era. No COVID-19-related complications were observed, supporting the possibility of continuing surgical diagnostic procedures in patients with a melanoma if carefully managed and suspicious symptoms are strictly monitored [47].

At the beginning of the emergency period, 80 patients with a melanoma were receiving immune checkpoint inhibitors (ICIs) in our center (62 nivolumab and 18 pembrolizumab). Adjuvant therapy was administered to 31 subjects for disease-free stages III-IV, whereas 49 patients were treated for advanced metastatic disease. A total of 57 patients (71%) continued treatment without interruptions, whereas 16 postponed their therapy of one (14 patients; 17.5%) or two cycles (two patients; 2.5%). The remaining seven patients (9%) suspended treatment due to progression ($N = 5$), completion of schedule ($N = 1$) or were lost to follow-up ($N = 1$). Moreover, four patients started a new treatment during the pandemic. In our experience, at the time of writing, no patients under ICIs developed COVID-19 infection [48]. In the same period, there were 67 advanced metastatic patients with a melanoma receiving targeted therapy with BRAF and MEK inhibitors at our center: 58 patients were receiving dabrafenib and trametinib, six were receiving vemurafenib and cobimetinib, and three were receiving encorafenib and binimetinib. There were also 23 patients receiving adjuvant treatment for disease-free stage III exclusively with dabrafenib and trametinib. Despite the COVID-19 outbreak, we decided to maintain treatment in all patients due to the available clinical data on the increased relapse risk in subjects discontinuing target therapy. The symptoms of patients were strictly monitored to detect potential COVID-19 infection at an early stage, in addition to maintaining strict triage procedures at the hospital entrance. At the time of writing, no patients developed COVID-19 infection [49].

9. Conclusions

The pandemic significantly influenced dermatological practice and the management of skin tumors. Despite the growing importance of telemedicine, suspicious skin lesions require a face-to-face consultation, which can be completed safely by ensuring that all prevention measures for COVID-19 infection are followed.

Although a decrease in the early diagnoses of melanoma was observed, surgical interventions and systemic treatments for advanced cases were guaranteed, largely following the pre-pandemic-era international guidelines. Unfortunately, all cases with a diagnostic delay caused by the pandemic have a profound impact on healthcare procedures and costs, as well as having devastating consequences for patients.

Considering the high mortality rate of COVID-19 infection among patients with cancer and the safety of vaccines in those also undergoing systemic therapy, vaccination for these patients and their families is a priority.

Based on our experience, the choice to continue all diagnostic and therapeutic procedures in patients with a melanoma has proven to be safe, ensuring that the care these patients require continues during pandemics.

Author Contributions: Conceptualization, C.C., M.M., G.A. and M.R.; methodology, C.C., M.M., and G.A.; investigation, C.C., M.M., G.A., M.R., V.C., F.P., G.G., I.S., S.R. and P.Q.; data curation, C.C., M.M., G.A., M.R., E.M., P.F., I.S. and M.T.F.; writing—original draft preparation, C.C., M.M. and G.A.; writing—review and editing, S.R. and P.Q.; visualization, E.M., P.F., V.C., F.P., G.G., I.S., M.T.F., S.R.

and P.Q.; supervision, S.R. and P.Q. All authors have read and agreed to the published version of the manuscript.

Funding: For this article no external funding was received.

Conflicts of Interest: The authors declare no conflict of interest.

References

1. Alkatout, I.; Biebl, M.; Momenimovahed, Z.; Giovannucci, E.; Hadavandsiri, F.; Salehiniya, H.; Allahqoli, L. Has COVID-19 Affected Cancer Screening Programs? A Systematic Review. *Front. Oncol.* **2021**, *11*, 675038. [CrossRef]
2. Villani, A.; Fabbrocini, G.; Costa, C.; Scalvenzi, M. Melanoma Screening Days during the Coronavirus Disease 2019 (COVID-19) Pandemic: Strategies to Adopt. *Dermatol. Ther. (Heidelb.)* **2020**, *10*, 525–527. [CrossRef] [PubMed]
3. Arenbergerova, M.; Lallas, A.; Nagore, E.; Rudnicka, L.; Forsea, A.M.; Pasek, M.; Meier, F.; Peris, K.; Olah, J.; Posch, C. Position Statement of the EADV Melanoma Task Force on Recommendations for the Management of Cutaneous Melanoma Patients during COVID-19. *J. Eur. Acad. Dermatol. Venereol.* **2021**, *35*, e427–e428. [CrossRef]
4. Conforti, C.; Lallas, A.; Argenziano, G.; Dianzani, C.; di Meo, N.; Giuffrida, R.; Kittler, H.; Malvehy, J.; Marghoob, A.A.; Soyer, H.P.; et al. Impact of the COVID-19 Pandemic on Dermatology Practice Worldwide: Results of a Survey Promoted by the International Dermoscopy Society (IDS). *Dermatol. Pract. Concept.* **2021**, *11*, e2021153. [CrossRef]
5. Gomolin, T.; Cline, A.; Handler, M.Z. The Danger of Neglecting Melanoma during the COVID-19 Pandemic. *J. Dermatol. Treat.* **2020**, *31*, 444–445. [CrossRef]
6. Veronese, F.; Branciforti, F.; Zavattaro, E.; Tarantino, V.; Romano, V.; Meiburger, K.M.; Salvi, M.; Seoni, S.; Savoia, P. The Role in Teledermoscopy of an Inexpensive and Easy-to-Use Smartphone Device for the Classification of Three Types of Skin Lesions Using Convolutional Neural Networks. *Diagnostics* **2021**, *11*, 451. [CrossRef]
7. Romero, G.; Sánchez, P.; García, M.; Cortina, P.; Vera, E.; Garrido, J.A. Randomized Controlled Trial Comparing Store-and-Forward Teledermatology Alone and in Combination with Web-Camera Videoconferencing. *Clin. Exp. Dermatol.* **2010**, *35*, 311–317. [CrossRef]
8. Chuchu, N.; Dinnes, J.; Takwoingi, Y.; Matin, R.N.; Bayliss, S.E.; Davenport, C.; Moreau, J.F.; Bassett, O.; Godfrey, K.; O'Sullivan, C.; et al. Teledermatology for Diagnosing Skin Cancer in Adults. *Cochrane Database Syst. Rev.* **2018**, *2018*, CD013193. [CrossRef]
9. Nahm, W.J.; Gwillim, E.C.; Badiavas, E.V.; Nichols, A.J.; Kirsner, R.S.; Boggeln, L.H.; Shen, J.T. Treating Melanoma in Situ During a Pandemic with Telemedicine and a Combination of Imiquimod, 5-Fluorouracil, and Tretinoin. *Dermatol. Ther. (Heidelb.)* **2021**, *11*, 307–314. [CrossRef] [PubMed]
10. Ferrara, G.; de Vincentiis, L.; Ambrosini-Spaltro, A.; Barbareschi, M.; Bertolini, V.; Contato, E.; Crivelli, F.; Feyles, E.; Mariani, M.P.; Morelli, L.; et al. Cancer Diagnostic Delay in Northern and Central Italy during the 2020 Lockdown Due to the Coronavirus Disease 2019 Pandemic. *Am. J. Clin. Pathol.* **2020**, *155*, aqaa177. [CrossRef] [PubMed]
11. Longo, C.; Pampena, R.; Fossati, B.; Pellacani, G.; Peris, K. Melanoma Diagnosis at the Time of COVID-19. *Int. J. Dermatol.* **2021**, *60*, e29–e30. [CrossRef] [PubMed]
12. Barruscotti, S.; Giorgini, C.; Brazzelli, V.; Vassallo, C.; Michelerio, A.; Klersy, C.; Chiellino, S.; Tomasini, C.F. A Significant Reduction in the Diagnosis of Melanoma during the COVID-19 Lockdown in a Third-Level Center in the Northern Italy. *Dermatol. Ther.* **2020**, *33*, e14074. [CrossRef] [PubMed]
13. Intergruppo Melanoma Italiano. The Effect of COVID-19 Emergency in the Management of Melanoma in Italy. *Dermatol. Rep.* **2021**, *13*, 8972. [CrossRef]
14. Lallas, A.; Kyrgidis, A.; Manoli, S.M.; Papageorgiou, C.; Lallas, K.; Sotiriou, E.; Vakirlis, E.; Sidiropoulos, T.; Ioannides, D.; Apalla, Z. Delayed Skin Cancer Diagnosis in 2020 Because of the COVID-19–Related Restrictions: Data from an Institutional Registry. *J. Am. Acad. Dermatol.* **2021**, *85*, 721–723. [CrossRef]
15. Tejera-Vaquerizo, A.; Paradela, S.; Toll, A.; Santos-Juanes, J.; Jaka, A.; López, A.; Cañueto, J.; Bernal, À.; Villegas-Romero, I.; Fernández-Pulido, C.; et al. Effects of COVID-19 Lockdown on Tumour Burden of Melanoma and Cutaneous Squamous Cell Carcinoma. *Acta Derm. Venereol.* **2021**, *101*, adv00525. [CrossRef]
16. Schauer, A.A.; Kulakov, E.L.; Martyn-Simmons, C.L.; Bunker, C.B.; Edmonds, E. Melanoma Defies 'Lockdown': Ongoing Detection during COVID-19 in Central London. *Clin. Exp. Dermatol.* **2020**, *45*, 900. [CrossRef]
17. ESMO ESMO Management and Treatment Adapted Recommendations in the COVID-19 Era: Melanoma. Available online: https://www.esmo.org/guidelines/cancer-patient-management-during-the-covid-19-pandemic/melanoma-in-the-covid-19-era (accessed on 4 October 2021).
18. NCCN Short-Term Recommendations for Cutaneous Melanoma Management during COVID-19 Pandemic. Available online: https://www.nccn.org/covid-19/pdf/Melanoma.pdf (accessed on 6 May 2020).
19. Tejera-Vaquerizo, A.; Nagore, E. Estimated Effect of COVID-19 Lockdown on Melanoma Thickness and Prognosis: A Rate of Growth Model. *J. Eur. Acad. Dermatol. Venereol.* **2020**, *34*, e351–e353. [CrossRef]
20. Mandalà, M.; Galli, F.; Patuzzo, R.; Maurichi, A.; Mocellin, S.; Rossi, C.R.; Rulli, E.; Montesco, M.; Quaglino, P.; Caliendo, V.; et al. Timing of Sentinel Node Biopsy Independently Predicts Disease-Free and Overall Survival in Clinical Stage I-II Melanoma Patients: A Multicentre Study of the Italian Melanoma Intergroup (IMI). *Eur. J. Cancer* **2020**, *137*, 30–39. [CrossRef] [PubMed]

21. Ribero, S.; Podlipnik, S.; Osella-Abate, S.; Sportoletti-Baduel, E.; Manubens, E.; Barreiro, A.; Caliendo, V.; Chavez-Bourgeois, M.; Carrera, C.; Cassoni, P.; et al. Ultrasound-Based Follow-up Does Not Increase Survival in Early-Stage Melanoma Patients: A Comparative Cohort Study. *Eur. J. Cancer* **2017**, *85*, 59–66. [CrossRef]
22. Rogiers, A.; Pires da Silva, I.; Tentori, C.; Tondini, C.A.; Grimes, J.M.; Trager, M.H.; Nahm, S.; Zubiri, L.; Manos, M.; Bowling, P.; et al. Clinical Impact of COVID-19 on Patients with Cancer Treated with Immune Checkpoint Inhibition. *J. Immunother. Cancer* **2021**, *9*, e001931. [CrossRef]
23. Patrinely, J.R.; Johnson, D.B. Pandemic Medicine: The Management of Advanced Melanoma during COVID-19. *Melanoma Manag.* **2020**, *7*, MMT45. [CrossRef]
24. Abid, M.B. Overlap of Immunotherapy-Related Pneumonitis and COVID-19 Pneumonia: Diagnostic and Vaccine Considerations. *J. Immunother. Cancer* **2021**, *9*, e002307. [CrossRef] [PubMed]
25. Nahm, S.H.; Rembielak, A.; Peach, H.; Lorigan, P.C. Consensus Guidelines for the Management of Melanoma during the COVID-19 Pandemic: Surgery, Systemic Anti-Cancer Therapy, Radiotherapy and Follow-Up. *Clin. Oncol. (R. Coll. Radiol.)* **2021**, *33*, e54–e57. [CrossRef]
26. Lebbé, C.; Meyer, N.; Mortier, L.; Marquez-Rodas, I.; Robert, C.; Rutkowski, P.; Menzies, A.M.; Eigentler, T.; Ascierto, P.A.; Smylie, M.; et al. Evaluation of Two Dosing Regimens for Nivolumab in Combination With Ipilimumab in Patients With Advanced Melanoma: Results From the Phase IIIb/IV CheckMate 511 Trial. *J. Clin. Oncol.* **2019**, *37*, 867–875. [CrossRef] [PubMed]
27. Meirson, T.; Asher, N.; Bomze, D.; Markel, G. Safety of BRAF+MEK Inhibitor Combinations: Severe Adverse Event Evaluation. *Cancers* **2020**, *12*, 1650. [CrossRef]
28. Swetter, S.M.; Thompson, J.A.; Albertini, M.R.; Barker, C.A.; Baumgartner, J.; Boland, G.; Chmielowski, B.; DiMaio, D.; Durham, A.; Fields, R.C.; et al. NCCN Guidelines® Insights: Melanoma: Cutaneous, Version 2.2021: Featured Updates to the NCCN Guidelines. *J. Natl. Compr. Cancer Netw.* **2021**, *19*, 364–376. [CrossRef]
29. Maio, M.; Lahn, M.; di Giacomo, A.M.; Covre, A.; Calabrò, L.; Ibrahim, R.; Fox, B. A Vision of Immuno-Oncology: The Siena Think Tank of the Italian Network for Tumor Biotherapy (NIBIT) Foundation. *J. Exp. Clin. Cancer Res.* **2021**, *40*, 240. [CrossRef]
30. Pala, L.; Conforti, F.; Saponara, M.; de Pas, T.; Giugliano, F.; Omodeo Salè, E.; Jemos, C.; Rubatto, M.; Agostini, A.; Quaglino, P.; et al. Data of Italian Cancer Centers from Two Regions with High Incidence of SARS CoV-2 Infection Provide Evidence for the Successful Management of Patients with Locally Advanced and Metastatic Melanoma Treated with Immunotherapy in the Era of COVID-19. *Semin. Oncol.* **2020**, *47*, 302–304. [CrossRef]
31. SITC Statement on SARS-CoV-2 Vaccination and Cancer Immunotherapy. Available online: https://www.sitcancer.org/aboutsitc/press-releases/2020/sitc-statement-sars-cov-2-vaccination-cancer-immunotherapy (accessed on 4 October 2021).
32. COVID-19 Resources. Available online: https://www.nccn.org/covid-19 (accessed on 4 October 2021).
33. Garassino, M.C.; Vyas, M.; de Vries, E.G.E.; Kanesvaran, R.; Giuliani, R.; Peters, S. The ESMO Call to Action on COVID-19 Vaccinations and Patients with Cancer: Vaccinate. Monitor. Educate. *Ann. Oncol.* **2021**, *32*, 579–581. [CrossRef] [PubMed]
34. SEOM Posicionamiento y Recomendaciones de Seom En Relació n Con La Campaña de Vacunación Frente al COVID-19 En Pacientes Con Cáncer. Available online: https://seom.org/images/Posicionamiento_SEOM_vacunacion_COVID19_pacientes_con_cancer.pdf (accessed on 10 August 2021).
35. Massarweh, A.; Eliakim-Raz, N.; Stemmer, A.; Levy-Barda, A.; Yust-Katz, S.; Zer, A.; Benouaich-Amiel, A.; Ben-Zvi, H.; Moskovits, N.; Brenner, B.; et al. Evaluation of Seropositivity Following BNT162b2 Messenger RNA Vaccination for SARS-CoV-2 in Patients Undergoing Treatment for Cancer. *JAMA Oncol.* **2021**, *7*, 1–8. [CrossRef]
36. Di Giacomo, A.M.; Giacobini, G.; Gandolfo, C.; Lofiego, M.F.; Cusi, M.G.; Maio, M. Severe Acute Respiratory Syndrome Coronavirus 2 Vaccination and Cancer Therapy: A Successful but Mindful Mix. *Eur. J. Cancer* **2021**, *156*, 119–121. [CrossRef] [PubMed]
37. Waissengrin, B.; Agbarya, A.; Safadi, E.; Padova, H.; Wolf, I. Short-Term Safety of the BNT162b2 MRNA COVID-19 Vaccine in Patients with Cancer Treated with Immune Checkpoint Inhibitors. *Lancet Oncol.* **2021**, *22*, 581–583. [CrossRef]
38. Chen, Y.-W.; Tucker, M.D.; Beckermann, K.E.; Iams, W.T.; Rini, B.I.; Johnson, D.B. COVID-19 MRNA Vaccines and Immune-Related Adverse Events in Cancer Patients Treated with Immune Checkpoint Inhibitors. *Eur. J. Cancer* **2021**, *155*, 291–293. [CrossRef]
39. Spagnolo, F.; Boutros, A.; Croce, E.; Cecchi, F.; Arecco, L.; Tanda, E.; Pronzato, P.; Lambertini, M. Influenza Vaccination in Cancer Patients Receiving Immune Checkpoint Inhibitors: A Systematic Review. *Eur. J. Clin. Investig.* **2021**, *51*, e13604. [CrossRef] [PubMed]
40. Centers for Disease Control and Prevention Local Reactions, Systemic Reactions, Adverse Events, and Serious Adverse Events: Moderna COVID-19 Vaccine. Available online: https://www.cdc.gov/vaccines/covid-19/info-by-product/moderna/reactogenicity.html (accessed on 20 August 2021).
41. Centers for Disease Control and Prevention Local Reactions, Systemic Reactions, Adverse Events, and Serious Adverse Events: Pfizer-BioNTech COVID-19 Vaccine. Available online: https://www.cdc.gov/vaccines/covid-19/info-by-product/pfizer/reactogenicity.html (accessed on 20 August 2021).
42. Eifer, M.; Eshet, Y. Imaging of COVID-19 Vaccination at FDG PET/CT. *Radiology* **2021**, *299*, 210030. [CrossRef]
43. Shirone, N.; Shinkai, T.; Yamane, T.; Uto, F.; Yoshimura, H.; Tamai, H.; Imai, T.; Inoue, M.; Kitano, S.; Kichikawa, K.; et al. Axillary Lymph Node Accumulation on FDG-PET/CT after Influenza Vaccination. *Ann. Nucl. Med.* **2012**, *26*, 248–252. [CrossRef]
44. Prieto, P.A.; Mannava, K.; Sahasrabudhe, D.M. COVID-19 MRNA Vaccine-Related Adenopathy Mimicking Metastatic Melanoma. *Lancet Oncol.* **2021**, *22*, e281. [CrossRef]

45. Placke, J.-M.; Reis, H.; Hadaschik, E.; Roesch, A.; Schadendorf, D.; Stoffels, I.; Klode, J. Coronavirus Disease 2019 Vaccine Mimics Lymph Node Metastases in Patients Undergoing Skin Cancer Follow-up: A Monocentre Study. *Eur. J. Cancer* **2021**, *154*, 167–174. [CrossRef] [PubMed]
46. Lehman, C.D.; D'Alessandro, H.A.; Mendoza, D.P.; Succi, M.D.; Kambadakone, A.; Lamb, L.R. Unilateral Lymphadenopathy After COVID-19 Vaccination: A Practical Management Plan for Radiologists Across Specialties. *J. Am. Coll. Radiol.* **2021**, *18*, 843–852. [CrossRef]
47. Caliendo, V.; Picciotto, F.; Quaglino, P.; Ribero, S. COVID Infection and Sentinel Lymph Node Procedure for Melanoma: Management in a Dermato-oncology Center in a High-risk Pandemic Area. *Dermatol. Ther.* **2020**, *33*, e13536. [CrossRef]
48. Quaglino, P.; Fava, P.; Brizio, M.; Marra, E.; Rubatto, M.; Agostini, A.; Tonella, L.; Ribero, S.; Fierro, M.T. Metastatic Melanoma Treatment with Checkpoint Inhibitors in the COVID-19 Era: Experience from an Italian Skin Cancer Unit. *J. Eur. Acad. Dermatol. Venereol.* **2020**, *34*, 1395–1396. [CrossRef] [PubMed]
49. Quaglino, P.; Fava, P.; Brizio, M.; Marra, E.; Rubatto, M.; Merli, M.; Tonella, L.; Ribero, S.; Fierro, M.T. Anti-BRAF/Anti-MEK Targeted Therapies for Metastatic Melanoma Patients during the COVID-19 Outbreak: Experience from an Italian Skin Cancer Unit. *Future Oncol.* **2021**, *17*, 759–761. [CrossRef] [PubMed]

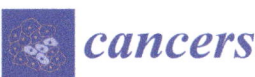 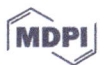

Review

Charting the Unknown Association of COVID-19 with Thyroid Cancer, Focusing on Differentiated Thyroid Cancer: A Call for Caution

Maria V. Deligiorgi [1,*], Gerasimos Siasos [2], Lampros Vakkas [1] and Dimitrios T. Trafalis [1]

1. Clinical Pharmacology Unit–Department of Pharmacology, Faculty of Medicine, National and Kapodistrian University of Athens, 75 Mikras Asias St., 11527 Athens, Greece; smd1700343@med.uoa.gr (L.V.); dtrafal@med.uoa.gr (D.T.T.)
2. First Department of Cardiology, Hippokration General Hospital of Athens, Faculty of Mediine, National and Kapodistrian University of Athens, 11527 Athens, Greece; gsiasos@med.uoa.gr
* Correspondence: mdeligiorgi@yahoo.com; Tel.: +30-210-746-2587; Fax: +30-210-746-2504

Simple Summary: Leveraging lessons learned from the coronavirus disease 2019 (COVID-19) pandemic, resilient health systems focus on the preservation of the continuum of care of chronic diseases, especially of cancer, beyond addressing emergency health requirements. Obesity has a detrimental impact on COVID-19 and affects the epidemic of thyroid cancer (TC). TC, especially differentiated TC (DTC), is a notable paradigm of obesity-related cancers. Thus, obesity–COVID-19–(D)TC interplay can be a constant threat to public health. The present review dissects the COVID-19–(D)TC association in the setting of obesity and beyond, highlighting: (i) the interrelationship between immunity, inflammation, obesity, oxidative stress, and cancer underlying this association; (ii) the challenging management of (D)TC in the COVID-19 era; (iii) the impact of COVID-19 on (D)TC and vice versa; and (iv) the oncogenic potential of SARS-CoV-2. Future perspectives for understanding and harnessing the COVID-19–(D)TC association to inform decision-making are underlined.

Abstract: Background: Conceived of as the "silver lining" of the dark cloud of the coronavirus disease 2019 (COVID-19) pandemic, lessons taught by this catastrophe should be leveraged by medical authorities and policy makers to optimize health care globally. A major lesson is that resilient health systems should absorb sudden shocks incited by overwhelming health emergencies without compromising the continuum of care of chronic diseases, especially of cancer. Methods: The present review dissects the association between COVID-19 and thyroid cancer (TC), especially with differentiated TC (DTC), focusing on available data, knowledge gaps, current challenges, and future perspectives. Results: Obesity has been incriminated in terms of both COVID-19 severity and a rising incidence of TC, especially of DTC. The current conceptualization of the pathophysiological landscape of COVID-19–(D)TC association implicates an interplay between obesity, inflammation, immunity, and oxidative stress. Whether COVID-19 could aggravate the health burden posed by (D)TC or vice versa has yet to be clarified. Improved understanding and harnessing of the pathophysiological landscape of the COVID-19–(D)TC association will empower a mechanism-guided, safe, evidence-based, and risk-stratified management of (D)TC in the COVID-19 era and beyond. Conclusion: A multidisciplinary patient-centered decision-making will ensure high-quality (D)TC care for patients, with or without COVID-19.

Keywords: COVID-19; SARS-CoV-2; thyroid cancer; differentiated thyroid cancer; COVID-19 severity; inflammation; immunity; oxidative stress; obesity

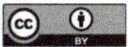

1. Introduction

Globally, as of the writing of this review more than one and a half years after the emergence of the novel severe acute respiratory syndrome (SARS)-associated coronavirus 2

(SARS-CoV-2), and designation of the attendant coronavirus disease 2019 (COVID-19) as a pandemic, there have been more than 200 million confirmed COVID-19 cases, and more than 4 million related deaths reported by the WHO [1]. This situation, while dismal, has taught us several lessons to be leveraged immediately.

Assessment of the responses of health policies worldwide reveal that the resilience of health systems against health crises of this magnitude lies in going beyond boosting hospital capacity and mitigation of the spread of a virus to maintain continuity of care for all [2]. A major priority of strong health systems is optimization of the care of cancer, which is the second leading cause of death globally [3], with a soaring burden, and which is expected to climb to 28.4 million cases in 2040 (a 47% increase compared to 2020) [4].

To forge agile and resilient health systems in the COVID-19 era, it is necessary to reorganize healthcare without compromising the care of cancer [5]. Indeed, the COVID-19–cancer association is bidirectional. On the one hand, cancer care in the COVID-19 era must reconcile conflicting priorities, i.e., mitigation of the risk of SARS-CoV-2 infection and of severe COVID-19 versus prompt cancer diagnosis and treatment despite limited resources and an overwhelmed healthcare system [6]. Delays in diagnosis and treatment, and/or suboptimal treatment of cancer due to the COVID-19 pandemic are clearly acknowledged [4,7–9], but quantification will take long time on account of the lag in the dissemination of population-based surveillance data [4]. On the other hand, cancer has been indicated as a prognostic factor for unfavorable outcomes of COVID-19 [10].

In that respect, a critical mass of scientists has committed to transcending the boundaries of faculties to untangle the COVID-19–cancer association and address emerging challenges in a multidisciplinary way. Central to this initiative is the association of COVID-19 with cancers related to obesity, which is defined as a body mass index (BMI) $\geq$30 kg/m^2 [11]. The rationale for this concept is that obesity—designated as an epidemic by the WHO in 1998 [11]—is the main culprit of the global burden of cancer [12] and of unfavorable outcomes of COVID-19 [13,14]. Additionally, obesity has been suggested as a critical player in the pathophysiological background of the COVID-19–cancer association [15].

Thyroid cancer (TC)—especially differentiated thyroid cancer (DTC), which arises from thyroid follicular epithelial cells, and accounting for the vast majority of TC [16]—is the most common endocrine malignancy [17]. Despite its indolent nature [17], TC poses a rising burden on public health, and is attributed mostly to obesity [18–22]. In fact, TC can be considered as the epitome of obesity-related cancers.

Although thyroid is a well-known target of SARS-CoV-2 [23], the COVID-19–TC association remains terra incognita; however, the COVID-19–TC association is of paramount clinical importance in the context of obesity, and beyond, for many reasons. First, the mounting burden of obesity promotes both an explosion of TC incidence and unfavorable outcomes of COVID-19. Second, obesity may contribute to unfavorable outcome COVID-19 in TC patients. Third, TC provides a prism for investigating the pathophysiological background of the COVID-19–cancer association. Fourth, the oncological strategy for management of TC has been reformed in the COVID-19 era. Finally, TC may worsen COVID-19 outcomes.

Prompted by this, the present review dissects COVID-19–TC association in the context of obesity, and beyond, with a focus on knowledge gaps, current challenges, and future perspectives.

Most available data concerning the association of COVID-19 with TC in the context of obesity and beyond provide no information about distinct histological TC types, or exclusively concern DTC. Herein, this approach is represented by the term "COVID-19–(D)TC association".

2. TC Epitomizes the Obesity-Related Cancers

With 586,202 new cases globally in 2020, TC ranks as the 9th most common cancer type. Although TC most often shows low mortality rates (0.5 per 100,000 in women and 0.3 per 100,000 in men) [17], it constitutes a growing healthcare challenge due to rising incidence, and is nominated as a "TC epidemic". This extends beyond an "epidemic of diagnosis" to reflect the increasing exposure of populations to risk factors, among which obesity prevails [18–22].

TC is included among the 13 cancer types causally associated with obesity, according to the landmark report by the International Agency for Research on Cancer (IARC) [24]. The causality between excess body weight and obesity-related cancers is sustained by accumulating epidemiological and experimental evidence [11,25–27]. A convincing argument favoring the contribution of obesity to cancer risk is the recognition of a decrease in the risk of certain cancer types as a collateral beneficial effect of bariatric surgery [28].

It is acknowledged that obesity has a differential impact on distinct TC types [24]. DTC, which comprises more than 90% of all thyroid malignancies, including papillary thyroid carcinoma (PTC) (the most common histotype) and follicular thyroid carcinoma (FTC) (the 2nd most-common histotype), is the histological TC type that is most often positively associated with obesity. Medullary thyroid cancer (MTC), accounting for less than 5% of all TC types, is a neuroendocrine tumor with a distinct profile [29] and has an inverse association with obesity [24]. Anaplastic TC is another obesity-related TC type [24], but it is rare, accounting for 1.7% of TC in the United States, and for 1.3% to 9.8% (median = 3.6%) of TC geographically [30].

A hallmark systematic analysis of data from the Global Burden of Disease (GBD) 2017 study of 195 countries and territories showed that 11.8% of worldwide TC-related deaths in females was attributable to high a BMI; a percentage that was higher compared to that in males. Interestingly, the highest proportion of TC-related deaths attributable to high BMI occurred in developed countries and in middle-aged individuals [18].

Analysis of the influence of obesity on PTC incidence trends in the US during the period of 1995–2015 showed that, compared to normal weights (18.5–24.9 kg/m^2), overweight (25.0–29.0 kg/m^2) and obesity ($\geq$30.0 kg/m^2) increased the risk of PTC by 1.26-fold (95% confidence interval (CI), 1.05- to 1.52-fold) and 1.30-fold (95% CI, 1.05- to 1.62-fold), respectively, as well as the risk of large (>4 cm) PTC (hazard ratio (HR), 2.93; 95% CI, 1.25–6.87 for overweight; and HR, 5.42; 95% CI, 2.24–13.1 for obesity). Over 1995–2015, an increase in population-attributable fractions (PAF) for overweight and obesity was observed, from 11.4% to 16.2%, for all PTCs, and from 51.4% to 63.2% for large PTCs. Overweight and obesity were responsible for 13.6% and 57.8% of the annual percent changes in all (5.9%/year) and large (4.5%/year) PTC incidences, respectively [22].

There is ample epidemiological evidence sustaining the tumor-promoting role of obesity in TC [21,24,28,31,32]. The underlying mechanisms have not been fully elucidated, but they implicate five different players: thyroid-stimulating hormone (TSH) [28], estrogens [28,33], insulin resistance (IR) [28,31], inflammation [28], and adipokines [28,31].

Adipokines—a subset of cytokines produced by adipose tissue—are considered the orchestrators of the interrelationship between obesity, IR, and inflammation. The main alterations in the secretion of adipokines, which are closely related to the obesity–TC association, are a decrease of adiponectin (APN), an increase of leptin, and an increase of resistin.

A critical link between obesity and TC is a decrease in APN levels, which undermines the tumor-suppressive role of APN [31,34]. Downstream of decreased APN levels are promoted signaling pathways that counteract the APN-mediated tumor-suppressive signaling pathways, fostering tumor initiation and progression through (1) inhibition of the adenosine monophosphate-activated protein kinase (AMPK), which in turn allows the activation of both mitogen-activated protein kinase (MAPK) and phosphoinositide-3 kinase (PI3K)/protein kinase B (PKB) (Akt)/mammalian target of rapamycin (mTOR) pathways, eventually favoring cancer cell proliferation; (2) downregulation of the expression of important factors involved in the arrest of the cell cycle and apoptosis, such as p21 and p53; (3) inflammatory and immunomodulating tumor promoting effects; (4) pro-angiogenetic effects; (5) a decrease in the APN/leptin ratio, favoring the action of excess fat-driven increase of leptin, which exerts a tumor-promoting role mediated by Akt/mTOR/PI3K, extracellular signal-regulated kinases (ERK)/MAPK, and Janus kinase (JAK)/signal transducer and activator of transcription 3 (STAT3) cascades; and (6) the unopposed carcinogenic effect of chronic hyperinsulinemia. The carcinogenic effect of chronic hyperinsulinemia is attributed to (i) stimulation of MAPK and PI3K/Akt pathways; (ii) an increase in the bioavailability and synthesis of insulin-like growth factor 1 (IGF-1); and (iii) overexpression of vascular endothelial growth factor (VEGF), favoring pro-angiogenic pathways [28,31,34–36].

Increased levels of resistin produced by excess body fat can stimulate cancer cell proliferation and survival, as well as pro-inflammatory and pro-angiogenic pathways, which are critical for the promotion of TC [28].

Figure 1 illustrates the main signaling pathways presumed to mediate the tumor-promoting role of obesity in TC.

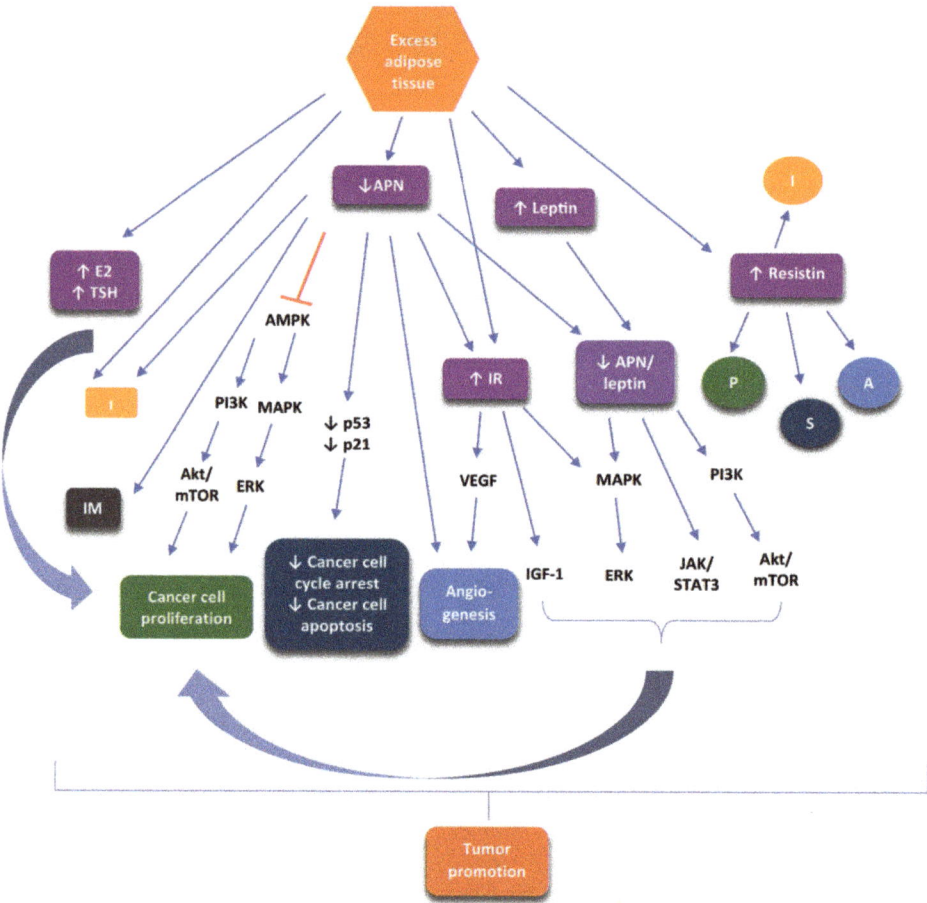

Figure 1. The main signaling pathways presumed to mediate the tumor-promoting role of obesity in TC. Excess adipose tissue causes an increase in TSH and 17-β-estradiol, decrease of adiponectin, insulin resistance, and increase of leptin and resistin. These alterations modulate numerous signaling cascades, which crosstalk and result in tumor promotion. Symbols: increase: ↑; inhibiton: ⊥; stimulation: ↓. Abbreviations: A, angiogenesis; Akt, protein kinase B; AMPK, adenosine monophosphate-activated protein kinase; APN, adiponectin; E2, 17-β-estradiol; ERK, extracellular signal-regulated kinases; I, inflammation; IGF-1, insulin-like growth factor 1; IM, inflammatory-immune responses; IR, insulin resistance; JAK, MAPK; mitogen-activated protein kinase; mTOR, mammalian target of rapamycin; P, proliferation; PI3K, phosphoinositide-3 kinase; S, survival; STAT3, signal transducer and activator of transcription 3; TSH, thyroid-stimulating hormone; VEGF, vascular endothelial growth factor.

The association of obesity with TC is not a consistent finding. Analysis of a retrospective series of 4849 patients with thyroid nodules by Rotondi et al. did not confirm an association between obesity and DTC [37]. Furthermore, analyses from two national data sources—the military recruitment health examinations and the Israel National Cancer Register—totaling 24,389,502 person-years of follow-up, by Farfel et al., revealed 60 incidence cases of TC, but no association between BMI and TC incidence [38]. Additionally, Fussey et al. analyzed data from 1812 participants with benign thyroid nodular disease and 425 with DTCs from the UK Biobank, and demonstrated that higher BMI was positively associated with benign thyroid nodular disease (odds ratio (OR), 1.15; 95% CI, 1.08–1.22) and higher waist-hip ratio (OR, 1.16; 95% CI, 1.09–1.23), but not with TC. Mendelian randomization revealed no causal association between obesity and benign nodular thyroid disease or TC, but an increased risk of TC in the highest quartile of the genetic liability of type 2 diabetes mellitus (DM 2) compared to the lowest quartile (OR, 1.45; CI, 1.11–1.90) [39]. No interpretation of the discordant evidence on the contribution of obesity to TC exists thus far. Table 1 summarizes controversial data on the association between obesity and (D)TC.

Table 1. Controversial data on the association between obesity and (D)TC.

Controversy over the Association of Obesity with (D)TC	
Data Sustaining the Association of Obesity with (D)TC [Ref].	Data Sustaining no Association of Obesity with (D)TC [Ref].

➤ TC is included among the 13 cancer types causally associated with obesity, according to the landmark report of the International Agency for Research on Cancer (IARC) [25].
➤ 1.8% of TC-related deaths in females worldwide is attributable to high BMI, a percentage higher compared to males [18].
➤ Compared to normal weight (18.5–24.9 kg/m^2), overweight (25.0–29.0 kg/m^2) and obesity ($\geq$30.0 kg/m^2) increased:
  • PTC risk by 1.26-fold and 1.30-fold respectively
  • risk of large (>4 cm) PTC (HR, 2.93 and 5.42 for overweight and obesity respectively) [22].
➤ During 1995–2015:
  • Increase of PAF for overweight and obesity: from 11.4% to 16.2% for all PTC and from 51.4% to 63.2% for large PTC.
  • Overweight or obesity were responsible for 13.6% and 57.8% of the annual percent changes in all and large PTC incidence, respectively [22].
➤ The association of obesity with increased TC risk is mediated by mechanisms implicating adipokines and chronic inflammation [31].
➤ Compared to normal-weight and overweight, obese individuals show statistically significant increased TC risk: 25% and 55%, respectively [21].
➤ Association of each 5-unit increase in BMI, 5 kg increase in weight, 5 cm increase in W or H circumference and 0.1-unit increase in W/H ratio with 30%, 5%, 5%, and 14% increased TC risk, respectively [21].
➤ Significant positive association of obesity with PTC, FTC, and anaplastic TC [21].
	➤ No association of obesity with DTC [37].
	➤ No association of BMI with TC [38].
	➤ Positive association of higher BMI with benign thyroid nodular disease (OR, 1.15; 95% CI, 1.08–1.22), higher W/H (OR, 1.16; 95% CI, 1.09–1.23), but not with TC [39].
	➤ Mendelian randomization: no causal association between obesity and benign nodular thyroid disease or TC [39].

Table 1. *Cont.*

Controversy over the Association of Obesity with (D)TC	
Data Sustaining the Association of Obesity with (D)TC [Ref].	Data Sustaining no Association of Obesity with (D)TC [Ref].
➢ Association of both general and abdominal adiposity with TC [21]. ➢ Association of obesity with a significantly increased TC risk (adjusted RR, 1.33) [24]. ➢ Five key players of the link between excessive weight and TC: thyroid hormones, insulin resistance, adipokines, inflammation, and sexual hormones [28].	

Abbreviations: BMI, body mass index; FTC, follicular thyroid carcinoma; H, hip; HR, hazard ratio; PAF, population attributable fractions, PTC, papillary thyroid carcinoma; RR, relative risk; TC, thyroid cancer; Ref, reference, W, waist.

3. Obesity in Relation to the Severity of COVID-19 in Non-Cancer and in Cancer Patients

In the general population, obesity is widely acknowledged as a bona fide risk factor for increased severity of COVID-19, resulting in higher rates of intensive care unit (ICU) admission, mechanical ventilation, and mortality compared to non-obesity [12,13]. This effect can be partially explained by the recognition of chronic non-communicable diseases (NCDs) related to obesity, e.g., DM 2 [40], hypercholesterolemia [41], hypertension, and cardiovascular diseases [42], as risk factors for increased severity of COVID-19. However, obesity has been proven an independent significant factor for unfavorable COVID-19 outcome after adjusting for coexistent NCDs. In fact, several mechanisms increasing the severity of COVID-19 in obese patients have been suggested; a detailed presentation of this is beyond the scope of the present review. First, excess fat can trigger many metabolic disorders, i.e., aberrant fatty acid metabolism, cellular hypertrophy and death, endoplasmic reticulum (ER) stress, hypoxia, and mitochondrial dysfunction, forging a pro-inflammatory milieu that is both local and systemic, which, in turn, can attenuate the immune response. Second, the immune response can be compromised by IR and leptin resistance attributed to excess fat. Third, up-regulation of the expression of angiotensin-converting enzyme 2 (ACE-2) in adipose tissue may cause adipose tissue to be a deposit reservoir of SARS-CoV-2 in the host, given that ACE-2 is co-opted by SARS-CoV-2 in order to enter host cells. Fourth, obesity is correlated with a hypercoagulable state, marked by elevated levels of prothrombin factors and reduced levels of anti-thrombin molecules, which can aggravate COVID-19-related coagulopathy/thrombosis [43–47]. Finally, obese COVID-19 patients may have increased abdominal pressure, limited chest expansion and movement, and insufficient respiratory compensatory function, parameters that can easily drive lung infection to respiratory failure [48].

However, whether obesity is a determinant of increased severity of COVID-19 in cancer patients remains uncertain. A single-center, prospective cohort study conducted in France, enrolling 178 mixed ambulatory and hospitalized patients with cancer, showed that obesity was not a risk factor for clinical worsening and overall survival (HR, 1.16; 95% CI, 0.36–3.69) in a univariable Cox proportional model [49].

A cohort study of 928 patients with COVID-19 and cancer revealed no association between obesity and increased 30-day all-cause mortality (OR, 0.84; 95% CI, 0.50–1.41), even after adjusting for age, sex, and smoking status (OR, 0.99; 95% CI, 0.58–1.71) [50].

A systematic review/meta-analysis of obesity and all-cause mortality in cancer patients with COVID-19 retrieved 3387 studies, and only three retrospective cohort studies reported outcomes according to obesity status. These three studies were multi-national and enrolled 419 obese and 1694 non-obese cancer patients with COVID-19 in both in-patient/outpatient settings. Analysis of these three studies showed no correlation between obesity and all-cause mortality (OR, 0.95; 95% CI, 0.74–1.23) in cancer patients with COVID-19. Heterogeneity was low (I^2 = 33%) and no significant funnel plot asymmetry was identified using Egger's test (p = 0.2273) [51].

The absence of an association of obesity with COVID-19 severity and mortality in cancer patients is difficult to interpret. This notion seems reminiscent of the so-called "obesity paradox", i.e., the association of obesity with a favorable cancer prognosis [46,52]. The "obesity paradox" is observed, not only in head and neck cancers, but also in premenopausal breast cancer, non-small cell lung cancer (NSCLC), renal cell cancer (RCC), and metastatic colorectal cancer (CRC) [52]. Avgerinos et al. suggested that the "obesity paradox" in cancer patients is ascribed, at least partially, to methodologic issues, such as: (i) selection, stratification, and detection biases; (ii) application of BMI as an index of general adiposity; and (iii) confounding factors (age, smoking, physical activity, etc.) [52]. On the other hand, Park et al. assumed that the "obesity paradox" insinuates a greater metabolic reserve favored by abundant adipose tissue, enhancing patient resilience [46]. In that respect, the absence of an association between obesity and COVID-19 severity and mortality in cancer patients may reflect methodological issues or insinuate an enhanced resilience of obese cancer patients against COVID-19 compared to non-obese cancer patients. More studies are needed to confirm or refute this hypothesis. Table 2 summarizes the discordant data regarding the contribution of obesity to COVID-19 outcomes in non-cancer and cancer patients.

Table 2. Discord in the contribution of obesity to COVID-19 outcome in non-cancer and cancer patients.

Discordance about the Contribution of Obesity to Unfavorable COVID-19 Outcome in Non-Cancer and Cancer Patients	
Obesity is Related to Unfavorable COVID-19 Outcome in Non-Cancer Patients	Obesity is Not Related to Unfavorable COVID-19 Outcome in Cancer Patients
➢ Significant association of obesity with increased risk of mortality among patients with COVID-19 (RR_{adjust}: 1.42 (95%CI, 1.24–1.63, $p < 0.001$) [13]. ➢ Inflammatory and immune mechanisms may increase susceptibility of obese individuals to severe COVID-19 and poor COVID-19 clinical outcome [43]. ➢ Inflammation, RAS activation, elevated adipokines and higher ectopic fat may contribute to COVID-19 severity in obese individuals [44]. ➢ Obesity is associated with increased risk of severe COVID-19. Limited data exist on metabolic parameters (such as BMI and levels of glucose and insulin) in patients with COVID-19 [45]. ➢ In general patient population with COVID-19, obesity is a determinant of increased morbidity and mortality [46]. ➢ Metabolic impairments and chronic low-grade systemic inflammation related to obesity create a pro-inflammatory microenvironment, building on SARS-CoV-2 related cytokine storm [47]. ➢ Patients with severe COVID-19 have a higher BMI than patients with no severe COVID-19 (WMD, 2.67; 95% CI, 1.52–3.82) [48]. ➢ COVID-19 patients with obesity have a worse outcome than those without obesity (OR = 2.31; 95% CI, 1.3–4.12) [48].	➢ Obesity is not a determinant of increased COVID-19 related morbidity and mortality in cancer patients [46]. ➢ Obesity is not a risk factor for COVID-19 related clinical worsening and overall survival (HR, 1.16; 95% CI, 0.36–3.69) in cancer patients a univariable Cox proportional model [49]. ➢ No association of obesity with increased 30-day mortality in cancer patients with COVID-19 (OR, 0.84; 95% CI, 0.50–1.41), not even after adjusting for age, sex, and smoking status (OR, 0.99; 95% CI, 0.58–1.71) [50]. ➢ No correlation of obesity with mortality (OR, 0.95, 95% CI, 0.74–1.23) in cancer patients with COVID-19 [51].

Abbreviations: BMI, body mass index; CI, confidence interval; COVID-19, coronavirus disease 2019; HR, hazard ratio; OR, odds ratio; RAS, renin-angiotensin-aldosterone system; Ref, reference; RR_{adjust}, relative risk adjusted; WMD, weighted mean difference.

4. Pursuing the Pathophysiological Landscape of the COVID 19–TC Association

Thus far, the pathophysiological landscape of the COVID-19–cancer association remains elusive. However, an insightful hypothesis was proposed by Derosa et al. Based on accumulating datasets, Derosa et al. assumed that cancer and COVID-19 meet at the crossroad of inflammaging—a state of aberrant tuning of systemic inflammation due to cytokine dysregulation ascribed to remodeling of immune system—and immunosenescence—a state of diminishing functioning of the immune system. Both states are promoted by obesity and risk factors for diminished immunity and stimulation of inflammation (e.g., aging), as well as cancer and poor performance status [15].

In fact, immunosenescence and inflammaging can compromise innate and adaptive immune responses, aggravating both overt inflammation and cancer dissemination, predisposing to SARS-CoV-2 infection, increasing the risk of severe COVID-19, and favoring cancer progression. Additionally, obesity can promote cancer initiation and progression through contribution to the acquisition of all hallmarks of cancer [14], increased insulin resistance resulting in hyperinsulinemia, and altered adipokines. Cancer per se, especially advanced and metastatic cancer, may subvert the fine balance between viral replication and appropriate innate immune responses (for example, type I and III interferon (IFN)), as well as cognate immune responses (for example, memory T helper 1 (Th1) response and antibody-secreting cell cross-reactivity with other beta coronaviruses), favoring virus replication [15].

Furthermore, chemotherapy and radiotherapy can also cause deficits in immune response, interrelated with and critical for long-term protective anticancer and antiviral immune responses, e.g., type I and II IFN responses. Such deficits may favor, not only cancer progression, but also vulnerability to viral infections [15]. Furthermore, major adverse effects of conventional therapies (such as cytotoxic chemotherapy, hormone therapy, and radiotherapy), targeted therapies (such as tyrosine kinase inhibitors (TKI) and mTOR inhibitors) and immunotherapies (such as immune-checkpoint inhibitors and CAR T cells), as well as poor patient performance status, can aggravate the outcome of COVID-19.

Alarmingly, comorbidities that act as trigger points for the COVID-19–cancer association (e.g., obesity, aging) may also undermine the efficacy of immune-based anticancer and antiviral therapies [15].

Another presumptive link between COVID-19 and cancer is oxidative stress—a key player in both COVID-19 [53,54] and cancer [55,56]. Oxidative stress is defined as a relative excess of chemically reactive oxygen species (ROS) compared to antioxidants [55]. Superoxide, the precursor of most ROS, is formed by the univalent reduction of triplet-state molecular oxygen ($^3O_2$), enzymatically (e.g., by NAD(P)H oxidases) or non-enzymatically. ROS stem from endogenous sources (e.g., mitochondria, peroxisomes, lipoxygenases, NADPH oxidases, cytochrome P450), antioxidant defense systems (e.g., enzymatic, and non-enzymatic systems), or exogenous sources (ultraviolet light, ionizing radiation, chemotherapy, and environmental toxins) [57,58]. Although low/moderate levels of ROS are critical for various physiological functions, increased ROS levels undermine genome stability and cellular integrity, contributing to aging and cancer [58–60], including TC [61]. SARS-CoV-2 may promote oxidative stress via downregulation of ACE2, the hallmark protein co-opted by SARS-CoV-2 for its internalization. ACE2 is a key regulator of the renin–angiotensin–aldosterone system (RAS), promoting the conversion of angiotensin II into angiotensin-1,7. The latter is credited with counteracting the negative effects of RAS, exerting anti-hypertensive, anti-inflammatory, anti-fibrotic, and anti-oxidative effects, which are protective for the heart, blood vessels, kidney, and central nervous system. It has been shown that SARS-CoV-2 not only binds to ACE2 via its spike protein (S) to enter host cells, but it can also downregulate ACE2 expression in cells, thereby disrupting the protective effects of angiotensin 1–7 [62]. Accumulating data suggest a key role for oxidative stress in the pathogenesis and severity of COVID-19 [53].

Figure 2 illustrates the interplay between obesity, cancer, immunity, and oxidative stress presumed to underlie the pathophysiological landscape of COVID 19–cancer association.

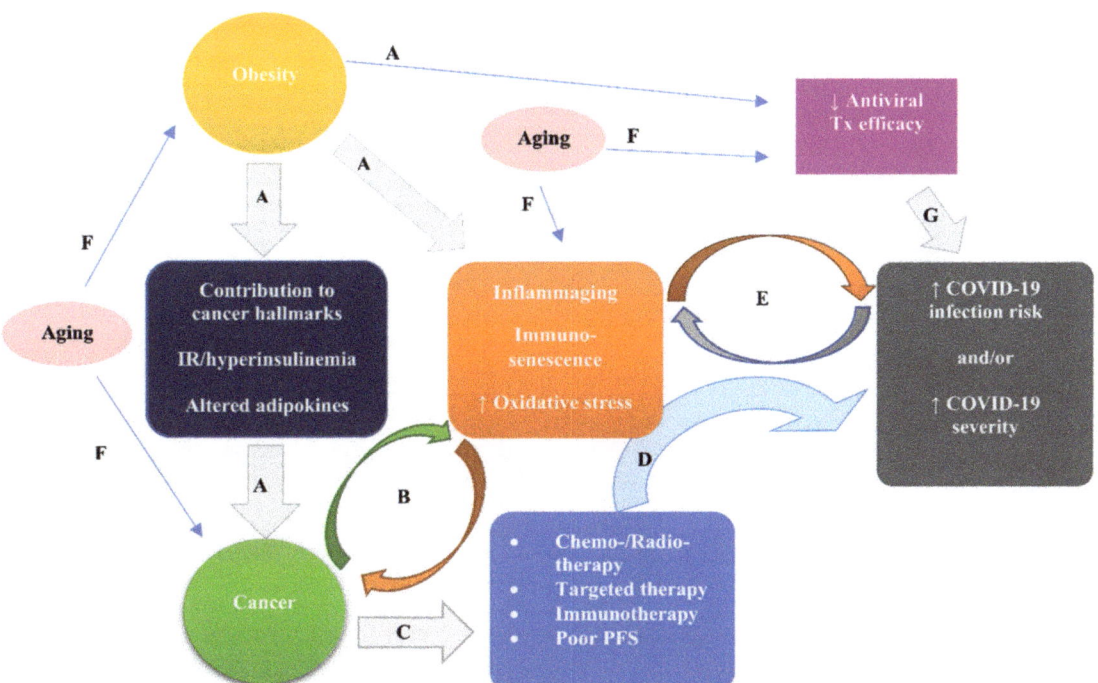

Figure 2. The interplay between obesity, cancer, immunity, and oxidative stress presumed to underlie the pathophysiological landscape of the COVID 19–cancer association. Obesity via contribution to all cancer hallmarks, and stimulation of insulin resistance leading to hyperinsulinemia, and of altered adipokines can promote cancer initiation and progression (A). The obesity-elicited states of inflammaging, immunosenescence, and increased oxidative stress (A) can promote and be promoted by cancer (B). Cancer due to attendant treatments (i.e., chemo-/radio-therapy, targeted therapy, and immunotherapy) and possible poor performance status (C) can increase susceptibility to and severity of COVID-19 (D). COVID-19 risk and/or severity can aggravate and be aggravated by the states of inflammaging, immunosenescence, and increased oxidative stress (E), the latter being elicited by obesity (A) and/or cancer (B). Aging can be a risk factor for obesity, cancer, inflammaging, immunosenescence, and increased oxidative stress (F), leading eventually to increased risk and/or severity of COVID-19 via mechanisms A, B, C, D, and E. Additionally, both aging (F) and obesity (A) may decrease the efficacy of immune-based antiviral treatments, increasing the severity of COVID-19 (G). Abbreviations: COVID-19, coronavirus disease 19; PFS, performance status; Tx, treatment.

The COVID-19–(D)TC association provides a prism for understanding COVID-19–cancer association in many aspects. First, the key host proteins co-opted by SARS-CoV-2 to invade host cells, i.e., ACE2 and transmembrane protease serine 2 (TMPRSS2), are amply expressed in the thyroid [63]. Second, internalization of SARS-CoV-2 in the host's target cells is mediated by integrin $\alpha v \beta 3$ [64], which mediates the non-genomic actions of thyroid hormones, especially of those of thyroxine (T4). Accordingly, T4 binding to integrin $\alpha v \beta 3$ may influence the internalization of SARS-CoV-2. Third, the hypothalamus–pituitary–thyroid axis is a well-documented target of SARS-CoV-2 [65], and of the related cytokine storm, resulting in a wide spectrum alterations to thyroid function [66]. Fourth, the long-pursued, yet not clarified, inflammatory and immunological background of DTC, discussed by two of the authors of this review (M.V.D, D.T.T) elsewhere [67], can interact with the immune-inflammatory reactions triggered by SARS-CoV-2 [68]. Fifth, there are convincing data sustaining the critical role of oxidative stress—a key player of COVID-19—in DTC, namely: (i) the exposure of follicular thyroid cells to a great amount of H_2O_2 (a landmark member of non-radical ROS), which is essential for synthesis of thyroid hormones; (ii) the detection of oxidative stress and DNA damage across the continuum of thyroid carcinogenesis from thyroid adenomas to advanced stages of thyroid cancer; and (iii) the upregulation of two main ROS-generating systems, the NADPH oxidases DUOX1 and NOX4, by ionizing radiation and mutated oncogenes RAS and BRAF—the most well-described carcinogenic factors for DTC [62]. Most importantly, obesity is a common risk factor shared by TC and COVID-19.

Albeit speculative, the conceptualization of the pathophysiological landscape of the COVID 19–TC association discussed herein suggests many actionable pathways, which merit further evaluation.

5. The Impact of COVID-19 on the Oncological Strategy for DTC

In the face of the reorganization of health systems compelled by the COVID-19 pandemic, the oncological strategy for the management of DTC raises many challenges.

5.1. Challenge I: Appropriate Patient Selection for Thyroid Fine-Needle Aspiration (FNA)

Thyroid fine-needle aspiration (FNA) is the cornerstone of the diagnostic procedure of DTC [16]. Appropriate patient selection for FNA of thyroid nodules is based on clinical and ultrasound (US) findings, and constitutes the first step in decision-making concerning the diagnosis and the management of DTC. This step entails constructive crosstalk between endocrinologists and cytopathologists [16]. In general, proper requests of thyroid FNA by endocrinologists, justified by clinical and US features of thyroid nodules suspicious of malignancy, increase the diagnostic efficiency of FNA. On the contrary, improper requests of thyroid FNA undermine the diagnostic efficiency of FNA. In the COVID-19 era, the recommended, due to the pandemic, delay of all non-urgent diagnostic procedures, including thyroid FNA, renders the interaction of endocrinologists and cytopathologists more important than ever.

Indeed, analysis of the thyroid FNA trends at Federico II University of Naples before (1 January 2019 to 13 March 2020), during (14 March to 15 May), and after (16 May to 7 July) the first lockdown in Italy revealed a decrease in the average weekly number (AWN) of FNA, from 62.1 to 23.1. In fact, the weekly proportion of benign diagnoses decreased on average by 12%, while the weekly proportion of high-risk diagnoses increased by 6%. This study sustains that the lockdown urged referring endocrinologists to prioritize thyroid FNA for nodules with US and/or clinical features indicative of high-risk of malignancy [69].

Consistent with this finding, an international survey of cytopathologic laboratories in 23 countries assessing the global impact of the COVID-19 pandemic on cytopathology practice revealed that, overall, the sample volumes collected during four weeks of COVID-19 lockdown were lower compared to those obtained during the corresponding period in 2019 (104,319 samples versus 190,225 samples, respectively), with an average volume decrease of 45.3% (range, 0.1–98.0%). The percentages of samples were either increased or decreased depending on the biopsied organ. The percentage of thyroid samples was significantly decreased, from 5.02% to 3.26% ($p < 0.001$). However, the overall decrease in thyroid FNA cytology volume was less profound for samples that usually reveal a higher rate of malignancy, thanks to appropriate patient selection for thyroid FNA [70].

Analyses of databases from China, South Korea, Iran, and Italy during COVID-19 pandemic phase I (25 January–25 February 2020), phase II (26 February–19 March), and phase III (20 March–20 April), compared to corresponding periods of 2019, revealed a reduction in outpatient FNA by 99.7% in phase I, 62.9% in phase II, and 30.1% in phase III [71].

5.2. Challenge II: Schedule of DTC Surgery in an Overburdened Health System

In view of the urgent need to mitigate the risk of transmission of SARS-CoV-2 and optimize the allocation of limited hospital beds and financial resources, healthcare providers are forced to prioritize the treatment of COVID-19 patients and emergency cases, while postponing elective surgical procedures of all types.

Assessment of global real-world data demonstrated the cancellation of more than 28 million surgeries in the face of the COVID-19 pandemic in March 2020. Data collected through interviews with surgical experts from 190 countries demonstrated that approximately 72% of non-essential surgeries were cancelled, i.e., a total of 28,404,603 surgeries globally. Among the cancelled surgeries, most cases concerned benign pathology (90%), while only 8.2% concerned tumor [72].

DTC surgeries are among the most common elective operations in clinical practice. Nevertheless, given the uncertain end of COVID-19 pandemic, the long-term delay of essential thyroid surgical care can be more detrimental than COVID-19 per se. Confronted with this challenge, several distinct panels of experts recommend alternative treatment algorithms as tangible options for the management of thyroid tumors with a focus on DTC for patients who cannot be operated on under the current circumstances. All expert opinions highlight that COVID-19 guidelines for the management of DTC are not applicable under circumstances where surgical treatment is feasible.

COVID-19 pandemic guidelines suggested by a panel of 67 experts (45 endocrine surgeons and 22 endocrinologists) from a wide array of countries recommend a modified risk-stratified approach to thyroid surgery. Postponement of surgery for 3–6 months and alternative treatment options are recommended for patients who are candidate for surgery due to a twice-confirmed result of FNA indicative of atypia/follicular lesion of undetermined significance (AUS/FLUS) (Bethesda 3), or Hürthle cell neoplasia/follicular neoplasia (Bethesda 4), or papillary microcarcinoma without pathological lymph nodes in the neck, or carcinoma without pathological lymph nodes in the neck. Such alternative treatment options are minimally invasive ablation techniques, including laser, microwave, or radiofrequency ablation, and active surveillance until the end of the pandemic [73].

COVID-19 pandemic guidelines suggested by a panel of experts-members of the French-speaking Association of Endocrine Surgery (AFCE) recommend that, in the absence of signs of locoregional aggressiveness of DTC, delay of thyroid surgery should be tailored according to tumor size and lymph node status. Especially, surgery of tumors ≥ 2 cm with or without lymph node metastases can be postponed until the end of crisis, but then, it should be prioritized with a delay shorter than 3 months. Surgery of tumors <2 cm can be performed after the end of COVID-19 pandemic [74].

COVID-19 pandemic guidelines from the Turkish Association of Endocrine Surgery recommend that indeterminate nodules (classified according to cytopathologic findings of FNA as Bethesda 3 and 4 categories) can be subjected to active surveillance, while the positivity of molecular markers (e.g., BRAF, TERT) does not impose immediate surgical intervention. In case of malignant nodules (classified according to cytopathologic findings of FNA as Bethesda 4 and 5 cytopathologic categories), management is guided by risk stratification. DTC with low and intermediate risk of recurrence according to American Thyroid Association (ATA) classification, and intrathyroidal papillary microcarcinomas (PTMC) can remain under active surveillance if US examination is conducted periodically. In the case of DTC with a high risk of recurrence according to ATA classification, i.e., large compressive or locoregionally aggressive DTC, thyroid surgery should be performed immediately. Cross-sectional imaging (computed tomography (CT), magnetic resonance imaging (MRI)) may help to determine the extension of thyroid surgery [75].

A position statement from the thyroid department of the Brazilian Society of Endocrinology and Metabolism (SBEM) highlighted that most TC cases are at low risk of recurrence, associated with an excellent prognosis, and thus "surgical procedures could and should be postponed safely during the pandemic period". Additionally, this position statement endorsed the possibility to safely postpone radioiodine (RAI) therapy in case or a pertinent indication [76]. All COVID-19 guidelines for the management of thyroid tumors with focus on DTC are depicted in Table 3.

Table 3. COVID-19 pandemic guidelines for management of thyroid tumors with focus on DTC by diverse expert committees.

Committee of 67 experts (45 endocrine surgeons and 22 endocrinologists) from multiple countries [a] [73].	
FNA result	Recommendation
➤ Any of the following: • Atypia or follicular lesion of undetermined significance (Bethesda 3) repeated twice. • Hürthle cell neoplasia or follicular neoplasia (Bethesda 4). • Papillary thyroid microcarcinoma (<1 cm).	➤ Alternative options: • Postponement of surgery for 3–6 months and follow-up with active surveillance until the end of the pandemic. OR • Treatment with minimally invasive ablation techniques including laser, microwave, or radiofrequency ablation.
➤ Papillary thyroid carcinoma without LNM in the neck.	➤ Alternative options: • Postponement of surgery for 3–6 months OR • Treatment with minimally invasive ablation techniques including laser, microwave, or radiofrequency ablation.
➤ Papillary carcinoma with LNM at central or lateral neck.	➤ Postponement of surgery for 3–6 months.
Committee of French-speaking Association of Endocrine Surgery (AFCE) [74].	
FNA result	Recommendation
➤ DTC ≥ 2 cm with or without LNM without signs of locoregional aggressiveness.	➤ Postponement of surgery until the end of crisis, but, thereafter, surgery should be prioritized with a delay <3 months.
➤ DTC < 2 cm with or without LNM without signs of locoregional aggressiveness.	➤ Surgery can be performed long after the end of pandemic.
Committee of Turkish Association of Endocrine Surgery [75].	
FNA result	Recommendation
➤ Indeterminate nodules (Bethesda 3 and 4).	➤ Follow-up. AND ➤ BRAF or TERT positivity does not impose immediate surgery.
➤ Any of the following: • DTC with ATA high risk of recurrence (i.e., large tumors, or tumors with gross extrathyroid extension, or tumors with <3 LNM or any LNM <3 cm, or tumors with distant metastasis) • Rapid growth of tumor	➤ Immediate surgery
➤ DTC with ATA low and intermediate risk of recurrence (i.e., DTC without compressive symptoms and signs, apparent LNM, or voice changes).	➤ Postponement of surgery for 3–6 months. AND ➤ In case of extended observation period, US repeated three months after initial diagnosis may allow further delay of surgery.

Table 3. *Cont.*

Committee of Turkish Association of Endocrine Surgery [75].	
FNA result	Recommendation
➢ Intrathyroidal papillary microcarcinoma	➢ Observation until end of pandemic. Certain patients can remain under active surveillance with repeated US even after end of pandemic.
Committee of Brazilian Society of Endocrinology and Metabolism (SBEM) [76].	
FNA result	Recommendation
➢ TC with low risk of recurrence.	➢ "Surgical procedures could and should be postponed safely during the pandemic period." AND ➢ Safe postponement of RAI.

[a] Austria, Belgium, Bulgaria, Greece, Italy, the Netherlands, Poland, Russia, South Korea, Spain, Sweden, Switzerland, Turkey, Ukraine, the United Kingdom and USA. Abbreviations: ATA, American thyroid association; DTC, differentiated thyroid carcinoma; FNA, fine needle aspiration; LNM, lymph node metastases; RAI, radioiodine; TC, thyroid cancer; US, ultrasound.

Real-world data on the DTC surgery during the COVID-19 pandemic are limited. Analysis of databases from China, South Korea, Iran, and Italy concerning thyroid surgery during COVID-19 pandemic phase I (25 January–25 February 2020), phase II (26 February–19 March), and phase III (20 March–20 April) compared to corresponding periods of 2019 revealed that no thyroid surgeries were performed during phase I. A reduction in surgery of advanced DTC was observed in phase II—concerning DTC of stage T1bN1a—and in phase III—concerning DTC of stage T3bN1b [71]. DTC of stage T1b N1a is between 1 cm and 2 cm completely inside the thyroid (T1b) and has spread to pretracheal, paratracheal, and prelaryngeal lymph nodes (level VI), or to the superior mediastinal nodes (level VII) (N1a). DTC of stage T3bN1b is of any size with extrathyroid extension to one or more of the muscles beside the thyroid (strap muscles) (T3b), and to lateral lymph nodes (levels I, II, III, IV, V) or to retropharyngeal lymph nodes (N1b) [16]. Mean surgical time was reduced to 58.3 ± 11.26 min ($p = 0.000$) in phase II versus 2019 and to 55.3 ± 13.32 min in phase III versus 2019 ($p = 0.000$). Postoperative hospitalization was reduced to 2.8 ± 0.9 days ($p = 0.000$) in phase II versus 2019, and to 3.3 ± 1.0 days ($p = 0.008$) in phase III versus 2019 [71].

5.3. Challenge III: Assessment of Delays and Disruptions in DTC Care Due to COVID-19

To assess delays and disruptions in DTC care due to COVID-19, standardizing the measurement and reporting thereof is required.

A systematic review of 62 studies, wherein head and neck cancer patients represented 11% of enrolled patients, identified interruptions in patient care in terms of facilities (up to 77.5%), supply chain, including everything from drugs to technical support of imaging equipment (up to 79%), and availability (up to 60%). The most common delays or disruptions were reductions in routine activity of cancer services and number of cancer surgeries, delay in radiotherapy, and delay, reschedule, or cancellation of outpatient visits. The result was delay in treatment, diagnosis, or general health service [77].

To date, to the best of our knowledge, large studies addressing this issue in the context of DTC are still lacking. A small relevant retrospective study evaluated the impact of lockdown and restrictive policies in Jordan between 17 March and 20 May 2020, on PTC treatment plans for 12 PTC patients with an average tumor size of 44 mm (range: occult–80 mm). Patients were subjected to thyroid surgery for initial management of PTC (11 patients), or recurrence of PTC (1 patient), without any delay of planned surgery. However, the lockdown across international borders decreased the availability of RAI. Consequently, in cases where RAI was indicated, replacing the usual method for the delivery of RAI after levothyroxine (L-T4) withdrawal with the recombinant human (rh) TSH (rh-TSH)-stimulated method in most patients was required. However, given limited financial resources, patients who were unable to afford the additional cost for the rh-TSH-stimulated method experienced increased stress and were classified to mild-to-moderate anxiety group according to the Hamilton Anxiety rating scale (HAM-A scale) [78]. With the increasing number of studies addressing delays in cancer care due to COVID-19, it would be of interest to separately analyze the relevant data regarding DTC to facilitate the design of policies to mitigate this phenomenon.

5.4. Challenge IV: The Safety of DTC Surgery in the COVID-19 Era

The COVID-19 pandemic has created novel barriers to safe head and neck surgery due to intense SARS-CoV-2 replication in the upper aerodigestive tract and aerosol generating head and neck surgical procedures. Thus, a systematic review on head and neck practice during the COVID-19 pandemic inferred that the cancer should be treated in compliance with specific protection measures for medical staff and specific guidelines for patient management [79].

Fortunately, a systematic review on thyroid surgery during COVID-19 pandemic revealed a relatively low risk of SARS-CoV-2 transmission during thyroid surgery. This review analyzed data from nine studies performed across several countries between January and August 2020, in countries with SARS-CoV-2 prevalence in the community varying from low to high. A total of 2217 patients who underwent thyroid surgery were enrolled. Malignancy was the indication for surgery in 60.8% of patients, 83.4% of whom were subjected to total thyroidectomy, accompanied by lymph node dissection in 38.3% of cases. Cross-infections were reported in 14 out of 721 patients (1.9%), while severe pulmonary complications of COVID-19 occurred in 0.4% of infected patients. Based on four studies, the incidence of complications related to thyroid surgery was 20.2%, with hypoparathyroidism and recurrent laryngeal nerve injury being the most common [80].

The prospective database of the Division of Thyroid Surgery in China-Japan Union Hospital of Jilin University of Changchun searched for patients who underwent thyroid surgery during phases I, II, and III of COVID-19 pandemic in China, South Korea, Iran, and Italy revealed no cases of COVID-19-related adverse events during the perioperative period [71].

An international, observational cohort study of 1137 consecutive head and neck cancer patients who underwent primary surgery in 26 countries indicated the thyroid as the second most common site of surgery (21%) after the oral cavity (38%). The overall 30-day mortality was 1.2%, similar to pre-COVID data; however, percentage of positivity of SARS-CoV-2 tests within 30 days of surgery was the same in patients and in the surgical team (3%, each), pointing to ineffective cross-infection measures or personal protective equipment. Among patients infected by SARS-CoV-2, 44.8% experienced severe respiratory complications, and 10.3% died. Medical and surgical complications were within ranges normally seen for the whole cohort. Advanced tumor stage was significantly associated with admission to critical care. Taken together, the authors highlighted that head and neck cancer surgery in the COVID-19 era is safe, but this fact does not undermine the need for compliance with safety measures [81].

The challenges in the oncological strategy for DTC due to the COVID-19 pandemic and relevant studies are depicted in Table 4.

Figure 3 illustrates the challenges in the oncological strategy for DTC due to the COVID-19 pandemic and the corresponding counteracting initiatives.

Table 4. The challenges in the oncological strategy for DTC due to COVID-19 pandemic.

Challenges in in the Oncological Strategy for DTC Due to COVID-19	
Challenge I: Appropriate patient selection for FNA	
Study type [Ref]	Results
Analysis of thyroid FNA trends at Federico II University of Naples before, during and after first lockdown in Italy [a]. [69]	➢ Decrease of AWN of weekly FNA from 62.1 to 23. ➢ Weekly proportion of benign diagnoses: decreased by 12% ➢ Weekly proportion of high-risk diagnoses: increased by 6%.
International survey of cytopathologic laboratories in 23 countries. [70]	➢ Decrease of percentage of thyroid samples collected during 4 weeks of COVID-19 lockdown versus the corresponding period of 2019: 3.26% versus 5.02% ($p < 0.001$). ➢ Less profound overall decrease in thyroid FNA cytology volume for samples with higher rate of malignancy.
Analysis of databases of China, South Korea, Iran, and Italy concerning thyroid surgery during 3 COVID-19 pandemic phases [b]. [71]	➢ Decreased overall collected sample volume during 4 weeks of COVID-19 lockdown versus the corresponding period of 2019: 104,319 samples versus 190,225 samples. ➢ Reduction in outpatient FNA by: ➢ 99.7% (phase I) ➢ 62.9% (phase II) ➢ 30.1% (phase III)
Challenge II: Reschedule of DTC surgery	
Study type [Ref]	Results
Analysis of databases of China, South Korea, Iran, and Italy concerning thyroid surgery during 3 COVID-19 pandemic phases [b]. [71]	➢ Reduction of thyroid surgeries versus 2019: ➢ Phase I: No thyroid surgery. ➢ Phase II: reduction in surgery of advanced DTC (mainly of stage T1b N1a [c]). ➢ Phase III: reduction in surgery of advanced DTC (mainly of T3bN1b [d]). ➢ Reduction of mean surgical time versus 2019: ➢ to 58.3 ± 11.26 min in phase II ($p = 0.000$). ➢ to 55.3 ± 13.32 min in phase III ($p = 0.000$). ➢ Reduction of postoperative hospitalization versus 2019: ➢ to 2.8 ± 0.9 days in phase II ($p = 0.000$). ➢ to 3.3 ± 1.0 days in phase III ($p = 0.008$).
Challenge III: Assessment of delays and disruptions in DTC care	
Study type [Ref]	Results
Systematic review of 62 studies. [77]	➢ Head and neck cancer patients: 11% of total patients. ➢ Interruptions in patient care occurred in facilities (up to 77.5%), supply chain (up to 79%), and availability (up to 60%). ➢ Reduction in routine activity of cancer services, and number of cancer surgeries. ➢ Delay in radiotherapy. ➢ Delay, reschedule, or cancellation of outpatient visits.
Study on PTC treatment plans of 12 PTC patients. [78]	➢ No delay of planned PTC surgery. ➢ Decreased availability of RAI due to lockdown across international borders. ➢ Replacement of the usual method for the delivery of RAI after L-T4 withdrawal with the rh-TSH-stimulated method in most patients. ➢ Distress for patients who could not afford the rh-TSH-stimulated method.

Table 4. Cont.

Challenges in in the Oncological Strategy for DTC Due to COVID-19	
Challenge IV: The safety of DTC surgery in the COVID-19 era.	
Study type [Ref]	Results
Systematic review on thyroid surgery. [80]	➢ Cross-infections in 14 patients (1.9%). ➢ Severe pulmonary complications of COVID-19 in 0.4% of infected patients. ➢ Complications related to surgery (data from 4 studies): 20.2% of patients (mainly hypoparathyroidism and recurrent laryngeal nerve injury).
Analysis of databases of China, South Korea, Iran, and Italy concerning thyroid surgery during 3 COVID-19 pandemic phases. [71]	➢ No cases of COVID-19 related complications during the perioperative period in phases I, II, and III of lockdown in China, South Korea, Iran, and Italy.
International, observational cohort study of 1137 consecutive head and neck cancer patients subjected to primary surgery in 26 countries. [81]	➢ Thyroid: 2nd most common site of surgery (21%). ➢ Overall 30-day mortality after TC surgery: 1.2% (similar to pre-COVID data). ➢ Incidence of positivity of SARS-CoV-2 tests within 30 days of surgery in patients: 3%. ➢ Incidence of positivity of SARS-CoV-2 tests within 30 days of surgery in the surgical team: 3%. ➢ Severe respiratory complications in 44.8% of infected patients. ➢ Medical and surgical complications within normal ranges. ➢ Significant association of advanced tumor stage with admission to critical care.

[a] before: 1 January 2019 to 13 March 2020; during: 14 March to 15 May; after: 16 May to 7 July first lockdown in Italy. [b] phase I (25 January–25 February 2020); phase II (26 February–19 March); phase III (20 March–20 April). [c] T1b N1a: the tumor is between 1 cm and 2 cm completely inside the thyroid (T1b) and has spread to lymph nodes close to the thyroid in the neck pretracheal, paratracheal, and prelaryngeal lymph nodes) (level VI), or in the upper chest (the superior mediastinal nodes) (level VII) (N1a). [d] T3bN1b: the tumor is any size and has grown into one or more of the muscles beside the thyroid (strap muscles) (T3b), and to lateral lymph nodes (levels I, II, III, IV, and V) or to lymph nodes behind the throat (retropharyngeal) (N1b). Abbreviations: AWN, average weekly number; COVID-19, coronavirus disease 2019; DTC, differentiated thyroid cancer; FNA, fine needle aspiration; PTC, papillary thyroid carcinoma; RAI, radioiodine; Ref, references; rh-TSH, recombinant human thyroid-stimulating hormone.

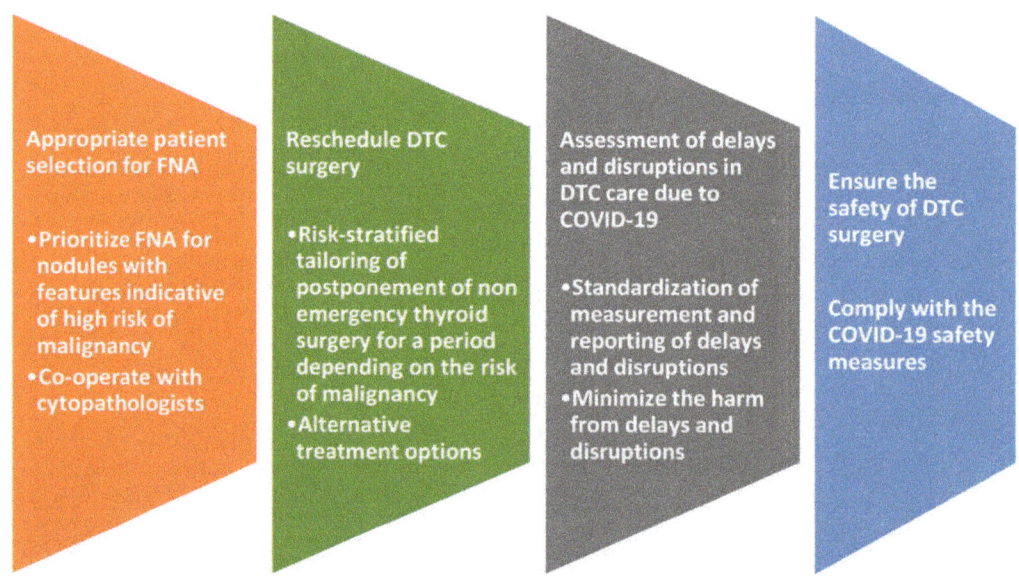

Figure 3. Challenges in the oncological strategy for DTC due to COVID-19 pandemic and the corresponding counteracting initiatives. Abbreviations: COVID-19, coronavirus disease 19; DTC, differentiated thyroid carcinoma; FNA, fine needle aspiration.

6. Discordant Data on the Impact of TC on COVID-19 Severity between Cancer Patients in General and (D)TC Patients

The first estimation of the probability of COVID-19 related death in a large sample of cancer patients with COVID-19 came from China and showed that the COVID-19-related mortality rate in cancer patients was 28.6%, more than ten times higher than that reported in all COVID-19 patients in China [82]. Thus far, it has been constantly reported that cancer patients are more vulnerable to COVID-19 and to unfavorable outcomes of COVID-19 compared to patients without cancer [50,83–85]. Metastatic lung cancer and hematological cancer confer the greatest risk of severe complications of COVID-19 and related mortality [86]. The interrelationship between SARS-CoV-2 and cancer has been reviewed by van Dam et al. [87] and is beyond the scope of the present review. Herein, we discuss some representative data.

The largest study to date addressing the impact of cancer on COVID-19 risk and outcome is a retrospective case-control analysis of patient electronic health records enrolling 73.4 million patients from 360 hospitals and 317,000 clinicians across the 50 US states. Evaluation of the odds ratio of COVID-19 infections for 13 common cancer types revealed that cancer patients before and after adjusting for COVID-19 risk factors had significantly increased risk for COVID-19 infection compared to patients without cancer after adjusting for COVID-19 risk factors.

The death rate of 670 adult patients with COVID-19 and cancer (14.93%) was higher compared to that of 14,840 adult patients with COVID-19 without cancer (5.26%) and compared to that of 270,380 adult and senior patients with cancer but no COVID-19 (4.03%). Hospitalization rate of patients with a recent cancer diagnosis and COVID-19 (47.76%) was higher compared to that of patients with COVID-19 but no recent cancer diagnosis (4.26%) ($p < 0.001$) and higher compared to that of patients with recent cancer diagnosis but no COVID-19 (12.39%) ($p < 0.001$). Overall, COVID-19 and cancer had a synergistic effect on death rate and on hospitalization rate. In this analysis, patients with TC were at significantly increased risk for COVID-19 infection (adjusted odds ratio (aOR), 3.94; 95% CI, 2.88–5.40). The odds ratio of COVID-19 infection for patients with TC decreased after adjusting for COVID-19 risk factors, indicating that these factors contributed to the risk for COVID-19 infections (aOR, 3.10; 95% CI, 2.47–3.87; $p < 0.001$). No analysis of outcomes according to specific cancer was conducted in this study [85].

Cancer patients are considered at increased risk for getting infections due to compromised immune system. Other factors, such as socio-economic status and behavioral and lifestyle factors, may also increase the risk of COVID-19 infection in cancer patients. However, due to limited relevant information in most databases, evaluation of the impact of these factors on the risk of COVID-19 infection among patients with cancer is not often feasible [85].

The outcome of COVID-19 in patients with TC was evaluated in a nationwide retrospective study leveraging the Turkish Ministry of Health database. The authors compared a cohort of 388 COVID-19 patients with TC to 388 gender-matched COVID-19 patients without TC from 11 March to 30 May 2020 in terms of mortality and morbidity. This study showed that the mortality ratio was similar in the TC and the non-TC group. In the TC group, factors correlated with mortality in univariate analysis were age ($p < 0.001$), DM 2 ($p = 0.016$), asthma/chronic obstructive pulmonary disease (COPD) ($p = 0.041$), heart failure ($p = 0.021$), chronic kidney disease ($p < 0.001$), prior coronary artery disease ($p = 0.039$), RAS blocker ($p = 0.036$), and lymphopenia ($p < 0.001$). No impact of RAI treatment and cumulative RAI dose on the severity and mortality of COVID-19 was observed; however, TC diagnosis was an independent risk factor of hospitalization (OR, 0.38; 95% CI, 0.27–0.54; $p < 0.001$). Additional independent risk factors of hospitalization were age (OR, 1.03; 95% CI, 1.01–1.05; $p = 0.001$), and positivity of CT findings of COVID-19 (OR, 3.14; 95% CI, 2.08–4.76; $p < 0.001$) [88].

Kathuria-Prakash et al. analyzed the COVID-19 outcomes in relation to demographic, DTC, and treatment data in a retrospective cohort study of patients with DTC and

COVID-19 from 2 academic Los Angeles healthcare systems. Among 21 patients with DTC and COVID-19, the incidence of hospitalization was 38.1%, and the incidence of COVID-19 related death was 9.5%, the latter being comparable to that of patients with non-thyroid malignancy (7.6%; p = non-significant). No parameter related to DTC (i.e., primary tumor size, risk of recurrence according to ATA classification, DTC status, and response to therapy near the time of COVID-19 diagnosis) was significantly associated with the severity of COVID-19 in DTC patients. Notably, administration of a cumulative RAI dose of ≥100 mCi led to higher rate of hospitalization for COVID-19 compared to no administration of RAI or administration of lower RAI doses, but this association did not reach statistical significance. Evaluation of non-DTC clinical parameters recognized as risk factors for unfavorable COVID-19 outcomes, including older age, male sex, and medical comorbidities, showed that older age and one comorbidity other than DTC were significantly associated with COVID-19 hospitalization (p = 0.047 and p = 0.024, respectively). Among patients with DTC, hospitalization related to COVID-19 was more common in patients with DM 2, lung disease, or cardiovascular disease [89].

Overall, current data on the impact of (D)TC on COVID-19 severity are limited and show no impact of (D)TC on COVID-19-related mortality, contrary to the designation of cancer as prognostic factor for unfavorable outcome of COVID-19 [10]. However, current data in terms of the impact of DTC on COVID-19 hospitalization are conflicting. No explanation for these discordant and inconclusive data exists so far. Table 5 lists the varying, occasionally discordant data on the impact of cancer on COVID-19 severity between cancer patients in general and (D)TC patients.

Table 5. Varying, occasionally discordant, data on the impact of cancer on COVID-19 severity between cancer patients in general and (D)TC patients.

Impact of Cancer in General on COVID-19 Severity	Impact of (D)TC on COVID-19 Severity

➢ Cancer —especially the active one—was indicated as independent factor associated with increased 30-day mortality in COVID-19 patients in logistic regression analysis, after partial adjustment [50].
➢ COVID-19 related mortality rate in cancer patients was 28.6%, more than ten times higher than that reported in all COVID-19 patients [82].
➢ Patients with solid or hematological malignancies and SARS-CoV-2 infection have a high probability of mortality [83].
➢ COVID-19 patients with cancer had higher risks in terms of all severe outcomes [84].
➢ Patients with COVID-19 and cancer versus patients with COVID-19 without cancer versus patients with cancer but no COVID-19 (4.03%):
  • Mortality: 14.93% versus 5.26% versus 4.03%
  • Hospitalization: 47.76% versus 4.26% versus 12.39% [85].
➢ Metastatic lung cancer and hematological cancer confer the greatest risk of severe complications of COVID-19 and related mortality [87].
	➢ Similar COVID-19 related mortality in the TC and the non-TC group [88].
	➢ TC is an independent risk factor of COVID-19 related hospitalization (OR, 0.38; 95% CI, 0.27–0.54; p <0.001) [88].
	➢ In DTC patients, the incidence of COVID-19 related hospitalization was 38.1%, and the incidence of COVID-19 related death was 9.5%, the latter being comparable to that of patients with nonthyroid malignancy (7.6% p = non-significant) [89].

Abbreviations: CI, confidence interval; COVID-19, coronavirus disease 2019; (D)TC, differentiated thyroid cancer; OR, odds ratio; Ref, reference.

From a critical viewpoint, data that show the absence of a detrimental impact of (D)TC on COVID-19 outcome, contrary to the designation of other cancers as prognostic factor for unfavorable outcome of COVID-19, may be attributed to the indolent nature and the favorable prognosis of most cases of PTC—the most common histologic type of TC.

Are Obese Patients with (D)TC at Increased Risk for Unfavorable COVID-19 Outcomes?

Interestingly, in the retrospective cohort study of 21 patients with DTC and COVID-19 from two academic Los Angeles healthcare systems conducted by Kathuria-Prakash et al., hospitalization was required for more than half of patients (4/7, 57.1%) with a BMI > 30 kg/m^2 as opposed to only 28.6% (4/14) of patients with a lower BMI [89]. This finding is in consistence with the association of obesity with increased COVID-19 severity in non-cancer COVID-19 patients compared to no obesity [12,13], but contradicts the constantly reported absence of impact of obesity on COVID-19 severity in cancer patients [49–51]. Nevertheless, the small sample size of the study of Kathuria-Prakash et al. hampers the generalization of this finding, indicating the need for further research. From a critical viewpoint, the indolent nature, and the favorable prognosis of most cases of PTC—the commonest histologic type of TC—may account for the absence of a postulated protective effect of obesity on COVID-19 outcome for TC patients, contrary to what is reported for other tumors.

7. The Hypothesis of the Oncogenic Potential of SARS-CoV-2

The hypothesis of the oncogenic potential of SARS-CoV-2 is discussed herein as the rationale behind the pending question of whether SARS-CoV-2 can cause (D)TC.

Confronted with "long-haul COVID-19", COVID-19 survivors are increasingly reported to experience a constellation of clinical symptoms that synthesize the post-acute COVID-19 syndromes, an issue beyond the scope of the present review [90–92]. Herein, we focus on the alarming hypothesis of post-acute COVID-19 increased risk of development of malignant neoplasms [90].

The rationale for this hypothesis is the identification of a causative link between viral infections and cancer, which dates back to the advent of 20th century [93,94]. So far, advances in research on cancer virology have indicated certain viruses as a causative factor of 12–20% of cancer worldwide, mainly via harnessing host's proteins, hijacking proliferating human cells, and triggering genetic and epigenetic alterations. Seven viruses have been causally associated with human oncogenesis: Epstein Barr virus (EBV), high-risk human papillomaviruses (HPV16/18), hepatitis B and C viruses (HBV, HCV respectively), human T-cell lymphotropic virus-1 (HTLV-1), Kaposi's sarcoma herpesvirus (KSHV), and Merkel cell polyomavirus [95].

The criteria for official assignment of causality between virus and cancer are long-term consistency of association between virus and cancer at the epidemiological and/or molecular level, and demonstration of the tumorigenicity of the virus in animal models, or demonstration of the transforming ability of the virus in cell culture [96].

Whether SARS-CoV-2 has an oncogenic potential can be answered only after years of epidemiological surveillance [97], and concomitant verification of two conditions: persistence of infection in the host, and identification of a pathogenetic link between oncogenesis and infection.

The persistence of SARS-CoV-2 is a new paradigm of COVID-19, yet not confirmed. Some indicative data are: (i) persistent shedding of viral genetic material long after recovery of the acute disease accompanied by a negative RT-PCR test result for SARS-CoV-2, raising concern about re-infection or reactivation of latent infection; (ii) tropism of SARS-CoV-2 towards endothelium, which may foster its persistence in tissues other than those associated with the known symptoms of COVID-19; (iii) involvement of central nervous system in the COVID-19, as indicated by positivity of RT-PCR in cerebrospinal fluid, a site with a known immune privilege, which could provide protection to SARS-CoV-2 and foster its latency [98,99].

As regards the mechanisms underlying the potential oncogenic effect of SARS-CoV-2, little evidence exists so far. A relevant speculative mechanism has been suggested by Stingi et al. [99], according to which SARS-CoV-2 counteracts the tumor suppressor proteins pRb and p53 [100–103]. This hypothesis is based on data derived from SARS-CoV-1. The interaction between the non-structural protein (Nsp) 15 (Nsp 15) of SARS-CoV-1 and the pRB of infected cells via a LXCXE motif has been shown to induce the nuclear export and ubiquitination of pRB, allowing its proteasomal degradation. Additionally, the Nsp3 protein of SARS-CoV-1 has been shown to stabilize the E3 ubiquitin ligase ring-finger and CHY zinc-finger domain-containing 1 (RCHY1), promoting the degradation of p53, and decreasing the levels thereof. Similar effects may be exerted by the Nsp15 and Nsp3 nucleases of the SARS-CoV-2 genome, which share, respectively, 88.7% and 76% sequence similarity with their counterparts of the SARS-CoV1 genome [100].

On the other hand, an argument against the oncogenic effect of SARS-CoV-2 is its cytotoxic effect, which reduces the chances for cell transformation. Although some cells survive following SARS-CoV-2 infection, a decreased possibility of cell transformation is expected due to virus-induced cell cycle arrest and activation of the cascade of apoptosis. However, whether cell transformation could occur in certain infected cell types in case of abortive cycles of the virus and of diminished cytopathic effects of virus remains unknown [100].

To explore a potential direct mutagenic effect of SARS-CoV-2, further in vitro and animal studies are needed; however, interpretation of relevant results will be daunting due to the genotoxic effect of sustained immune/inflammatory response per se. A potential synergistic oncogenic effect between SARS-CoV-2 and obesity is insinuated by the in vitro ability of the downregulation of p53 protein to mediate the obesity-driven tumor progression attributed to increased levels of C1q/TNF-related protein 1 (CTRP1), an adiponectin paralog [103].

8. Future Perspectives

To ensure the continuity of (D)TC care amid the rapidly evolving, multifaceted, challenges posed by the COVID-19 pandemic, concerted efforts should be directed towards filling current knowledge gaps in the COVID-19-DTC association and informing the decision-making.

Primarily, an interesting future perspective is to devise new mechanism-guided, tailored, therapeutic and preventive strategies for the management of (D)TC in these demanding times and beyond. To this end, more research is needed to understand and harness the pathophysiological landscape of the COVID-19–(D)TC association. In that respect, leveraging huge high-throughput "multi-omics" datasets could untangle the molecular basis of the interplay between inflammation, immunity, and obesity that governs the COVID-19–(D)TC association. Such information may lead to validation of patient-specific and cancer-specific biomarkers of this association and development of dual targeted treatments.

Especially, improved understanding of the immune-inflammatory mechanisms underlying the COVID-19–(D)TC association may provide the rationale for the development of novel treatments or the repurposing of existing treatments to combat concomitantly COVID-19 and cancer. For instance, a phase II expanded access trial is ongoing evaluating tocilizumab—a recombinant humanized anti-interleukin-6 receptor (IL-6R) monoclonal antibody—in cancer patients with COVID-19 [104]. The rationale of this trial is that preliminary data show efficacy of tocilizumab as anticancer agent [105,106] and as agent to reduce the risk of mechanical ventilation in hospitalized COVID-19 patients [107]. Furthermore, the dual effects of certain phosphodiesterase (PDE) inhibitors, anti-inflammatory [108] and anticancer [109,110], merit further evaluation in the setting of the COVID-19–(D)TC association.

Given the presumed role of the oxidative stress in the molecular background of the COVID-19-cancer association, it would be of interest to investigate a potential anticancer efficacy of antioxidant therapies that are currently under evaluation as a strategy to reduce the severity of COVID-19 [111]. A pitfall to this perspective is the differential regulation of pro-oxidant and antioxidant systems according to cancer stage. ROS promote cancer initiation at early precancerous and neoplastic stages. At advanced cancer stages, ROS promote the apoptosis of cancer cells, but cancer cells hijack antioxidant systems to evade apoptosis. Consequently, antioxidant therapies may be beneficial for the host only at initial stages of cancer [112].

Deciphering the role of obesity in the molecular background of the COVID-19–(D)TC association should be prioritized considering its modifiable nature. A barrier to this perspective is the significant heterogeneity of the metabolic profile of obese individuals, integrating genetic, epigenetic, socio-economic, and environmental factors [11]. Establishment of a universal terminology of distinct subgroups of obese patients, and validation of corresponding classification markers and indices is mandatory to identify differences between metabolically healthy and metabolically unhealthy obese individuals [113–115]. To combat the growing rates of obesity worldwide, nominated as "globesity" [116], medical authorities and policy makers need to intensify their coordinated actions to implement integrated and intersectoral health strategies [117,118]. Racial and ethnic disparities influencing not only the incidence of obesity, and of (D)TC, but also the severity of COVID-19 [119,120] should be considered.

Another promising area of future research is to evaluate the impact of (D)TC, especially of distinct patient-specific and cancer-specific factors, on COVID-19 outcome. Several issues concerning the impact of DTC treatment on COVID-19 outcome await clarification. First, a cautious patient selection for RAI treatment might be essential in the COVID-19 era due to the potential RAI-driven attenuation of immune responses in parallel with the concern about the safety/efficacy balance of RAI for most intermediate-risk and low-risk subgroups of (D)TC [121–123]. Second, whether L-T4 binding to integrin $\alpha v \beta 3$ can diminish the integrin $\alpha v \beta 3$-mediated internalization of the SARS-CoV-2 is yet to be investigated. Third, as kinases are involved in the virus-induced cytokine storm, tyrosine kinases inhibitors (TKI)—used for treatment of advanced (D)TC—are under evaluation as antiviral agents against SARS-CoV-2 [124,125]. Fourth, L-T4 titration after (D)TC surgery in patients with COVID-19 may be hampered by TSH suppression due to non-thyroidal illness syndrome (NTIS) caused by COVID-19, or due to exogenous corticosteroids used for treatment of severe COVID-19 [126].

Given the increasing recognition of subacute thyroiditis (SAT) as manifestation of COVID-19 [127–130] and the higher than initially presumed prevalence of PTC in SAT patients (4.4%), COVID-19 pandemic may provide the opportunity to revisit the SAT-PTC association [131].

To counteract the pitfalls that are intrinsic in the "sci-infodemic" (i.e., the publishing pandemic) during the COVID-19 pandemic [132], several methodological issues concerning COVID-19 research need to be further addressed, namely (i) sampling errors resulting in non-representative sample, producing non-generalizable results; (ii) variety of diagnostic criteria of COVID-19; (iii) heterogeneity of inclusion criteria of COVID-19 patients between studies; (iv) incomplete reporting of COVID-19 outcomes hampering subgroup analyses; (v) lack of standardized definitions of COVID-19 outcomes; (vi) inadequate follow-up.

Future health strategies for the management of (D)TC should be customized according to different pandemic phases. Additionally, more data are required to determine the impact of telemedicine on (D)TC management [133].

From an holistic viewpoint, COVID-19 pandemic has incited a novel social-economic and cultural landscape, causing a lot of distress due to altered lifestyle, generalized fear, pervasive community anxiety, and financial consequences [134]. In this psychosocial context, specialized health professionals, telephone helplines, active social networks, and dedicated forums are required to support the psychologically vulnerable individuals to deal with (D)TC diagnosis and treatment [135]. Finally, thyroid is interrelated with the psychological, mental, and physiological principals of our being, all threatened by the novel socio-economic and cultural landscape. It is presumed that the coming years will mandate more than ever an holistic approach to thyroid diseases, including (D)TC, because the psychosocial aspects of our being have already been correlated with thyroid function through research in a new realm of interest called Psychoneuroendocrinology. Psychoneuroendocrinology—a complex blend of psychiatry, psychology, neurology, biochemistry, and endocrinology—addresses, among others things, the psychobiological factors that influence the thyroid function in the context of the response to stress. Thus far, hypothalamus–pituitary–thyroid (HPT) axis dysfunction has been associated with major depression [136], post-traumatic stress disorder (PTSD) [137], anxiety disorders [138,139], and suicide risk related to major depressive disorder [140]. Critical life events often precede the onset of autoimmune thyroid diseases, and exposure to psychosocial stress triggers an immediate activation of HPT axis [141]. The activity of TRH neurons is inhibited by negative energy balance situations such as fasting, inflammation or chronic stress [142]. Indeed, very recently, Keestra et al. suggested an evolutionary ecology framework according to which HPT axis is considered a dynamic, adaptive system with a key role in "mediating life-history trade-offs between the functions of reproduction, growth, immunity and basal metabolic rate" [143] in the setting of demanding situations, including depression, psychosocial stress, and traumatic stress [144,145]. The absence of a causality between the psychosocial stress and the thyroid disorders in the setting of COVID-19 pandemic does not undermine the magnitude of an holistic approach to this issue, which will enable an integrated patient-oriented management of thyroid disorders, including DTC, during the challenging COVID-19 pandemic and beyond.

Figure 4 illustrates the main future perspectives in understanding and harnessing the COVID-19–(D)TC association.

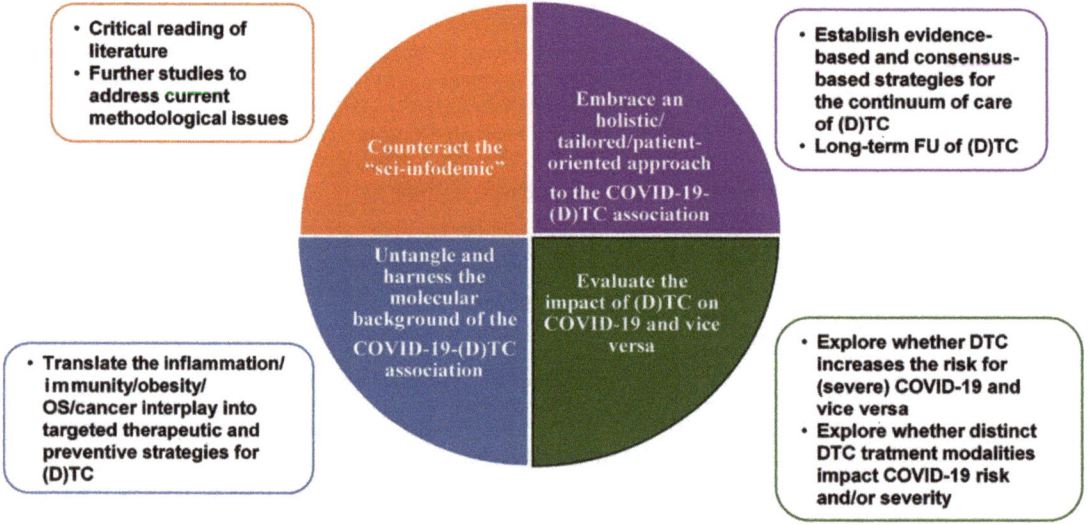

Figure 4. The main future perspectives in understanding and harnessing the COVID-19–(D)TC association. Abbreviations: COVID-19, coronavirus disease 19; (D)TC, (differentiated) thyroid cancer; FU, follow-up.

9. Conclusions

In response to call for caution regarding the COVID-19–(D)TC association, the scientific world acknowledges that there is still more to learn about the underlying interplay between obesity, inflammation, immunity, and cancer. Capitalizing on the COVID-19–(D)TC association may not be far away provided that improved understanding of the molecular background thereof will be translated into therapeutic and preventive strategies. Meanwhile, an evidence-based, risk-stratified, and consensus-based decision-making is embraced to provide consistent, safe, and high-quality care for (D)TC patients. From an optimistic standpoint, the "silver lining" in the dark cloud of COVID-19 is to leverage it as a catalyst for innovative patient-oriented health strategies integrating new knowledge with breakthrough technologies. A hopeful path forward is to entwine cancer care with the COVID-19 care in the setting of strengthened health systems.

Author Contributions: Conceptualization, M.V.D., G.S. and D.T.T.; methodology, M.V.D., L.V. and D.T.T.; investigation, M.V.D. and L.V.; writing—original draft Preparation, M.V.D.; review and editing, M.V.D., G.S. and D.T.T.; supervision and funding acquisition, D.T.T. Final approval of the version to be submitted, M.V.D., G.S., L.V. and D.T.T. All authors have read and agreed to the published version of the manuscript.

Funding: This manuscript was funded by the ATHENA Institute of Biomedical Sciences and EnergonBio Technologies S.A., Greece that cover the publication costs.

Conflicts of Interest: The funders had no role in the design of the study; in the collection, analyses, or interpretation of data; in the writing of the manuscript, or in the decision to publish the results.

References

1. WHO. Available online: https://www.who.int/emergencies/diseases/novel-coronavirus-2019 (accessed on 6 August 2021).
2. Barasa, E.; Mbau, R.; Gilson, L. What Is Resilience and How Can It Be Nurtured? A Systematic Review of Empirical Literature on Organizational Resilience. *Int. J. Health Policy Manag.* **2018**, *7*, 491–503. [CrossRef] [PubMed]
3. Nagai, H.; Kim, Y.H. Cancer prevention from the perspective of global cancer burden patterns. *J. Thorac Dis.* **2017**, *9*, 448–451. [CrossRef] [PubMed]
4. Siegel, R.L.; Miller, K.D.; Fuchs, H.E.; Jemal, A. Cancer Statistics, 2021. *CA Cancer J. Clin.* **2021**, *71*, 7–33. [CrossRef] [PubMed]
5. Knaul, F.M.; Garcia, P.J.; Gospodarowicz, M.; Essue, B.M.; Lee, N.; Horton, R. The Lancet Commission on cancer and health systems: Harnessing synergies to achieve solutions. *Lancet* **2021**, *6736*, 19–21. [CrossRef]
6. Jazieh, A.R.; Akbulut, H.; Curigliano, G.; Rogado, A.; Alsharm, A.A.; Razis, E.D.; Mula-Hussain, L.; Errihani, H.; Khattak, A.; De Guzman, R.B.; et al. Impact of the COVID-19 Pandemic on Cancer Care: A Global Collaborative Study. *JCO Glob. Oncol.* **2020**, *6*, 1428–1438. [CrossRef]
7. Patt, D.; Gordan, L.; Diaz, M.; Okon, T.; Grady, L.; Harmison, M.; Markward, N.; Sullivan, M.; Peng, J.; Zhou, A. Impact of COVID-19 on Cancer Care: How the Pandemic Is Delaying Cancer Diagnosis and Treatment for American Seniors. *JCO Clin. Cancer Inform.* **2020**, *4*, 1059–1071. [CrossRef]
8. London, J.W.; Fazio-Eynullayeva, E.; Palchuk, M.B.; Sankey, P.; McNair, C. Effects of the COVID-19 Pandemic on Cancer-Related Patient Encounters. *JCO Clin. Cancer Inform.* **2020**, *4*, 657–665. [CrossRef]
9. Greenwood, E.; Swanton, C. Consequences of COVID-19 for cancer care a CRUK perspective. *Nat. Rev. Clin. Oncol.* **2021**, *18*, 3–4. [CrossRef]
10. Bellou, V.; Tzoulaki, I.; van Smeden, M.; Moons, K.G.M.; Evangelou, E.; Belbasis, L. Prognostic factors for adverse outcomes in patients with COVID-19: A field-wide systematic review and meta-analysis. *Eur. Respir. J.* **2021**, *2002964*. [CrossRef]
11. Caballero, B. Humans against Obesity: Who Will Win? *Adv. Nutr.* **2019**, *10*, S4–S9. [CrossRef]
12. Colditz, G.A.; Lindsay, L. Obesity and cancer: Evidence, impact, and future directions. *Clin. Chem.* **2018**, *64*, 154–162. [CrossRef]
13. Poly, T.N.; Islam, M.M.; Yang, H.C.; Lin, M.C.; Jian, W.S.; Hsu, M.H.; Jack Li, Y.C. Obesity and Mortality Among Patients Diagnosed With COVID-19: A Systematic Review and Meta-Analysis. *Front. Med.* **2021**, *8*, 620044. [CrossRef]
14. Wichmann, I.A.; Cuello, M.A. Obesity and gynecological cancers: A toxic relationship. *Int. J. Gynaecol. Obstet.* **2021**, *155*, 123–134. [CrossRef]
15. Derosa, L.; Melenotte, C.; Griscelli, F.; Gachot, B.; Marabelle, A.; Kroemer, G.; Zitvogel, L. The immuno-oncological challenge of COVID-19. *Nat. Cancer* **2020**, *1*, 946–964. [CrossRef]
16. Haugen, B.R.; Alexander, E.K.; Bible, K.C.; Doherty, G.M.; Mandel, S.J.; Nikiforov, Y.E.; Pacini, F.; Randolph, G.W.; Sawka, A.M.; Schlumberger, M.; et al. 2015 American Thyroid Association Management Guidelines for Adult Patients with Thyroid Nodules and Differentiated Thyroid Cancer: The American Thyroid Association Guidelines Task Force on Thyroid Nodules and Differentiated Thyroid Cancer. *Thyroid* **2016**, *26*, 1–133. [CrossRef]
17. Sung, H.; Ferlay, J.; Siegel, R.L.; Laversanne, M.; Soerjomataram, I.; Jemal, A.; Bray, F. Global Cancer Statistics 2020: GLOBOCAN Estimates of Incidence and Mortality Worldwide for 36 Cancers in 185 Countries. *CA Cancer J. Clin.* **2021**, *71*, 209–249. [CrossRef]
18. Zhai, M.; Zhang, D.; Long, J.; Gong, Y.; Ye, F.; Liu, S.; Li, Y. The global burden of thyroid cancer and its attributable risk factor in 195 countries and territories: A systematic analysis for the Global Burden of Disease Study. *Cancer Med.* **2021**, *10*, 4542–4554. [CrossRef]
19. Pellegriti, G.; Frasca, F.; Regalbuto, C.; Squatrito, S.; Vigneri, R. Worldwide increasing incidence of thyroid cancer: Update on epidemiology and risk factors. *J. Cancer Epidemiol.* **2013**, *2013*, 65212. [CrossRef]
20. Morris, L.G.; Myssiorek, D. Improved detection does not fully explain the rising incidence of well-differentiated thyroid cancer: A population-based analysis. *Am. J. Surg.* **2010**, *200*, 454–461. [CrossRef]
21. Schmid, D.; Ricci, C.; Behrens, G.; Leitzmann, M.F. Adiposity and risk of thyroid cancer: A systematic review and meta-analysis. *Obes. Rev.* **2015**, *16*, 1042–1054. [CrossRef]
22. Kitahara, C.M.; Pfeiffer, R.M.; Sosa, J.A.; Shiels, M.S. Impact of overweight and obesity on US papillary thyroid cancer incidence trends (1995–2015). *J. Nat. Cancer Inst.* **2020**, *112*, 810–817. [CrossRef]
23. Trimboli, P.; Camponovo, C.; Scappaticcio, L.; Bellastella, G.; Piccardo, A.; Rotondi, M. Thyroid sequelae of COVID-19: A systematic review of reviews. *Rev. Endocr. Metab. Disord.* **2021**, *22*, 485–491. [CrossRef]

24. Ma, J.; Huang, M.; Wang, L.; Ye, W.; Tong, Y.; Wang, H. Obesity and risk of thyroid cancer: Evidence from a meta-analysis of 21 observational studies. *Med. Sci. Monit.* **2015**, *21*, 283–291.
25. Lauby-Secretan, B.; Scoccianti, C.; Loomis, D.; Grosse, Y.; Bianchini, F.; Straif, K. Body Fatness and Cancer Viewpoint of the IARC Working Group. *N. Engl. J. Med.* **2016**, *375*, 794–798. [CrossRef]
26. Sung, H.; Siegel, R.L.; Torre, L.A.; Pearson-Stuttard, J.; Islami, F.; Fedewa, S.A.; Goding Sauer, A.; Shuval, K.; Gapstur, S.M.; Jacobs, E.J.; et al. Global patterns in excess body weight and the associated cancer burden. *CA Cancer J. Clin.* **2019**, *69*, 88–112. [CrossRef]
27. Bruno, D.S.; Berger, N.A. Impact of bariatric surgery on cancer risk reduction. *Ann. Ttransl. Med.* **2020**, *8*, S13. [CrossRef]
28. Marcello, M.A.; Cunha, L.L.; Batista, F.A.; Ward, L.S. Obesity and thyroid cancer. *Endocr. Relat. Cancer* **2014**, *21*, T255–T271. [CrossRef]
29. Zhao, Z.; Yin, X.D.; Zhang, X.H.; Li, Z.W.; Wang, D.W. Comparison of pediatric and adult medullary thyroid carcinoma based on SEER program. *Sci. Rep.* **2020**, *10*, 13310. [CrossRef]
30. Bible, K.C.; Kebebew, E.; Brierley, J.; Brito, J.P.; Cabanillas, M.E.; Clark, T.J., Jr.; Di Cristofano, A.; Foote, R.; Giordano, T.; Kasperbauer, J.; et al. American Thyroid Association Guidelines for Management of Patients with Anaplastic Thyroid Cancer. *Thyroid* **2021**, *31*, 337–386. [CrossRef]
31. Masone, S.; Velotti, N.; Savastano, S.; Filice, E.; Serao, R.; Vitiello, A.; Berardi, G.; Schiavone, V.; Musella, M. Morbid Obesity and Thyroid Cancer Rate. A Review of Literature. *J. Clin. Med.* **2021**, *10*, 1894. [CrossRef]
32. Zhao, Z.G.; Guo, X.G.; Ba, C.X.; Wang, W.; Yang, Y.Y.; Wang, J.; Cao, H.Y. Overweight, obesity and thyroid cancer risk: A meta-analysis of cohort studies. *J. Int. Med. Res.* **2012**, *40*, 2041–2050. [CrossRef] [PubMed]
33. Zane, M.; Parello, C.; Pennelli, G.; Townsend, D.M.; Merigliano, S.; Boscaro, M.; Toniato, A.; Baggio, G.; Pelizzo, M.R.; Rubello, D.; et al. Estrogen and thyroid cancer is a stem affair: A preliminary study. *Biomed. Pharmacother.* **2017**, *85*, 399–411. [CrossRef] [PubMed]
34. Obeid, S.; Hebbard, L. Role of adiponectin and its receptors in cancer. *Cancer Biol. Med.* **2012**, *9*, 213–220. [PubMed]
35. Taylor, E.B. The complex role of adipokines in obesity, inflammation, and autoimmunity. *Clin. Sci.* **2021**, *135*, 731–752. [CrossRef]
36. Ouchi, N.; Walsh, K. Adiponectin as an anti-inflammatory factor. *Clin. Chim. Acta* **2007**, *380*, 24–30. [CrossRef]
37. Rotondi, M.; Castagna, M.G.; Cappelli, C.; Ciuoli, C.; Coperchini, F.; Chiofalo, F.; Maino, F.; Palmitesta, P.; Chiovato, L.; Pacini, F. Obesity Does Not Modify the Risk of Differentiated Thyroid Cancer in a Cytological Series of Thyroid Nodules. *Eur. Thyroid J.* **2016**, *5*, 125–131. [CrossRef]
38. Farfel, A.; Kark, J.D.; Derazne, E.; Tzur, D.; Barchana, M.; Lazar, L.; Afek, A.; Shamiss, A. Predictors for thyroid carcinoma in Israel: A national cohort of 1,624,310 adolescents followed up for up to 40 years. *Thyroid* **2014**, *24*, 987–993. [CrossRef]
39. Fussey, J.M.; Beaumont, R.N.; Wood, A.R.; Vaidya, B.; Smith, J.; Tyrrell, J. Does Obesity Cause Thyroid Cancer? A Mendelian Randomization Study. *J. Clin. Endocrinol. Metab.* **2020**, *105*, e2398–e2407. [CrossRef]
40. Kumar, A.; Arora, A.; Sharma, P.; Anikhindi, S.A.; Bansal, N.; Singla, V.; Khare, S.; Srivastava, A. Is diabetes mellitus associated with mortality and severity of COVID-19? A meta-analysis. *Diabetes Metab. Syndr.* **2020**, *14*, 535–545. [CrossRef]
41. Vuorio, A.; Watts, G.F.; Kovanen, P.T. Familial hypercholesterolaemia and COVID-19: Triggering of increased sustained cardiovascular risk. *J. Intern. Med.* **2020**, *287*, 746–747. [CrossRef]
42. Mehra, M.R.; Desai, S.S.; Kuy, S.; Henry, T.D.; Patel, A.N. Cardiovascular Disease, Drug Therapy, and Mortality in COVID-19. *N. Engl. J. Med.* **2020**, *382*, e102. [CrossRef]
43. Mohammad, S.; Aziz, R.; Al Mahri, S.; Malik, S.S.; Haji, E.; Khan, A.H.; Khatlani, T.S.; Bouchama, A. Obesity and COVID-19: What makes obese host so vulnerable? *Immun. Ageing* **2021**, *18*, 1. [CrossRef]
44. Bhattacharya, I.; Ghayor, C.; Pérez Dominguez, A.; Weber, F.E. From Influenza Virus to Novel Corona Virus (SARS-CoV-2)—The Contribution of Obesity. *Front. Endocrinol.* **2020**, *11*, 556962. [CrossRef]
45. Stefan, N.; Birkenfeld, A.L.; Schulze, M.B.; Ludwig, D.S. Obesity and impaired metabolic health in patients with COVID-19. *Nat. Rev. Endocrinol.* **2020**, *16*, 341–342. [CrossRef]
46. Park, R.; Wulff-Burchfield, E.; Sun, W.; Kasi, A. Is obesity a risk factor in cancer patients with COVID-19? *Future Oncol.* **2021**, *17*, 3541–3544. [CrossRef]
47. Cava, E.; Neri, B.; Carbonelli, M.G.; Riso, S.; Carbone, S. Obesity pandemic during COVID-19 outbreak: Narrative review and future considerations. *Clin. Nutr.* **2021**, *40*, 1637–1643. [CrossRef]
48. Yang, J.; Hu, J.; Zhu, C. Obesity aggravates COVID-19: A systematic review and meta-analysis. *J. Med. Virol.* **2021**, *93*, 257–261. [CrossRef]
49. Albiges, L.; Foulon, S.; Bayle, A.; Gachot, B.; Pommeret, F.; Willekens, C.; Stoclin, A.; Merad, M.; Griscelli, F.; Lacroix, L.; et al. Determinants of the outcomes of patients with cancer infected with SARS-CoV-2: Results from the Gustave Roussy cohort. *Nat. Cancer* **2020**, *1*, 965–975. [CrossRef]
50. Kuderer, N.M.; Choueiri, T.K.; Shah, D.P.; Shyr, Y.; Rubinstein, S.M.; Rivera, D.R.; Shete, S.; Hsu, C.Y.; Desai, A.; de Lima Lopes, G.; et al. COVID-19 and Cancer Consortium. Clinical impact of COVID-19 on patients with cancer (CCC19): A cohort study. *Lancet* **2020**, *395*, 1907–1918. [CrossRef]
51. Park, R.; Wulff-Burchfield, E.M.; Mehta, K.; Sun, W.; Kasi, A. Prognostic impact of obesity in cancer patients with COVID-19 infection: A systematic review and meta-analysis. *J. Clin. Oncol.* **2021**, *39*, e18578. [CrossRef]

52. Avgerinos, K.I.; Spyrou, N.; Mantzoros, C.S.; Dalamaga, M. Obesity and cancer risk: Emerging biological mechanisms and perspectives. *Metabolism* **2019**, *92*, 121–135. [CrossRef] [PubMed]
53. Delgado-Roche, L.; Mesta, F. Oxidative Stress as Key Player in Severe Acute Respiratory Syndrome Coronavirus (SARS-CoV) Infection. *Arch. Med. Res.* **2020**, *51*, 384–387. [CrossRef] [PubMed]
54. Ntyonga-Pono, M.P. COVID-19 infection and oxidative stress: An under-explored approach for prevention and treatment? *Pan Afr. Med. J.* **2020**, *35*, 12. [CrossRef] [PubMed]
55. Hayes, J.D.; Dinkova-Kostova, A.T.; Tew, K.D. Oxidative Stress in Cancer. *Cancer Cell* **2020**, *38*, 167–197. [CrossRef] [PubMed]
56. Arfin, S.; Jha, N.K.; Jha, S.K.; Kesari, K.K.; Ruokolainen, J.; Roychoudhury, S.; Rathi, B.; Kumar, D. Oxidative stress in cancer cell metabolism. *Antioxidants* **2021**, *10*, 642. [CrossRef] [PubMed]
57. Dröge, W. Free radicals in the physiological control of cell function. *Physiol. Rev.* **2002**, *82*, 47–95. [CrossRef] [PubMed]
58. Santos, A.L.; Sinha, S.; Lindner, A.B. The good, the bad, and the ugly of ROS: New insights on aging and aging-related diseases from eukaryotic and prokaryotic model organisms. *Oxidative Med. Cell. Longev.* **2018**, *2018*, 1941285. [CrossRef]
59. Liao, Z.; Damien, C.; Tan, N. Reactive oxygen species: A volatile driver of field cancerization and metastasis. *Mol. Cancer* **2019**, *18*, 65. [CrossRef]
60. Deligiorgi, M.V.; Liapi, C.; Trafalis, D.T. How Far Are We from Prescribing Fasting as Anticancer Medicine? *Int. J. Mol. Sci.* **2020**, *21*, 9175. [CrossRef]
61. Ameziane El Hassani, R.; Buffet, C.; Leboulleux, S.; Dupuy, C. Oxidative stress in thyroid carcinomas: Biological and clinical significance. *Endocr. Relat. Cancer* **2019**, *26*, R131–R143. [CrossRef]
62. Ni, W.; Yang, X.; Yang, D.; Bao, J.; Li, R.; Xiao, Y.; Hou, C.; Wang, H.; Liu, J.; Yang, D.; et al. Role of angiotensin-converting enzyme 2 (ACE2) in COVID-19. *Crit. Care* **2020**, *24*, 422. [CrossRef]
63. Scappaticcio, L.; Pitoia, F.; Esposito, K.; Piccardo, A.; Trimboli, P. Impact of COVID-19 on the thyroid gland: An update. *Rev. Endocr. Metab. Disord.* **2020**, *2020*, 1–13. [CrossRef]
64. Davis, P.J.; Lin, H.Y.; Hercbergs, A.; Keating, K.A.; Mousa, S.A. Coronaviruses and Integrin αvβ3: Does Thyroid Hormone Modify the Relationship? *Endocr. Res.* **2020**, *45*, 210–215. [CrossRef]
65. McFadyen, J.D.; Stevens, H.; Peter, K. The Emerging Threat of (Micro)Thrombosis in COVID-19 and Its Therapeutic Implications. *Circ. Res.* **2020**, *127*, 571–587. [CrossRef]
66. Croce, L.; Gangemi, D.; Ancona, G.; Liboà, F.; Bendotti, G.; Minelli, L.; Chiovato, L. The cytokine storm and thyroid hormone changes in COVID-19. *J. Endocrinol. Invest.* **2021**, *44*, 891–904. [CrossRef]
67. Deligiorgi, M.V.; Trafalis, D.T. Papillary Thyroid Carcinoma Intertwined with Hashimoto's Thyroiditis: An Intriguing Correlation, Knowledges on Thyroid Cancer, Omer Engin, IntechOpen. Available online: https://www.intechopen.com/chapters/66252 (accessed on 17 August 2021).
68. Ruggeri, R.M.; Campennì, A.; Deandreis, D.; Siracusa, M.; Tozzoli, R.; Petranović Ovčariček, P.; Giovanella, L. SARS-COV-2-related immune-inflammatory thyroid disorders: Facts and perspectives. *Expert Rev. Clin. Immunol.* **2021**, *17*, 737–759. [CrossRef]
69. Palladino, R.; Migliatico, I.; Sgariglia, R.; Nacchio, M.; Iaccarino, A.; Malapelle, U.; Vigliar, E.; Salvatore, D.; Troncone, G.; Bellevicine, C. Thyroid fine-needle aspiration trends before, during, and after the lockdown: What we have learned so far from the COVID-19 pandemic. *Endocrine* **2021**, *71*, 20–25. [CrossRef]
70. Vigliar, E.; Cepurnaite, R.; Alcaraz-Mateos, E.; Ali, S.Z.; Baloch, Z.W.; Bellevicine, C.; Bongiovanni, M.; Botsun, P.; Bruzzese, D.; Bubendorf, L.; et al. Global impact of the COVID-19 pandemic on cytopathology practice: Results from an international survey of laboratories in 23 countries. *Cancer Cytopathol.* **2020**, *128*, 885–894. [CrossRef]
71. Zhang, D.; Fu, Y.; Zhou, L.; Liang, N.; Wang, T.; Del Rio, P.; Rausei, S.; Boni, L.; Park, D.; Jafari, J.; et al. Thyroid surgery during coronavirus-19 pandemic phases I, II and III: Lessons learned in China, South Korea, Iran and Italy. *J. Endocrinol. Investig.* **2021**, *44*, 1065–1073. [CrossRef]
72. COVIDSurg Collaborative. Elective surgery cancellations due to the COVID-19 pandemic: Global predictive modelling to inform surgical recovery plans. *Br. J. Surg.* **2020**, *107*, 1440–1449.
73. Agcaoglu, O.; Sezer, A.; Makay, O.; Erdogan, M.F.; Bayram, F.; Guldiken, S.; Raffaelli, M.; Sonmez, Y.A.; Lee, Y.S.; Vamvakidis, K.; et al. Management of endocrine surgical disorders during COVID-19 pandemic: Expert opinion for non-surgical options. *Updates Surg.* **2021**, 1–11. [CrossRef] [PubMed]
74. Baud, G.; Brunaud, L.; Lifante, J.C.; Tresallet, C.; Sebag, F.; Bizard, J.P.; Mathonnet, M.; Menegaux, F.; Caiazzo, R.; Mirallié, É.; et al. Endocrine surgery during and after the COVID-19 epidemic: Expert guidelines from AFCE. *J. Visc. Surg.* **2020**, *157*, S44–S51. [CrossRef] [PubMed]
75. Aygun, N.; Iscan, Y.; Ozdemir, M.; Soylu, S.; Aydin, O.U.; Sormaz, I.C.; Dural, A.C.; Sahbaz, N.A.; Teksoz, S.; Makay, O.; et al. Endocrine Surgery during the COVID-19 Pandemic: Recommendations from the Turkish Association of Endocrine Surgery. *Sisli Etfal Hastan. Tip Bul.* **2020**, *54*, 117–131. [PubMed]
76. Martins, J.; Villagelin, D.; Carvalho, G.A.; Vaisman, F.; Teixeira, P.; Scheffel, R.S.; Sgarbi, J.A. Management of thyroid disorders during the COVID-19 outbreak: A position statement from the Thyroid Department of the Brazilian Society of Endocrinology and Metabolism (SBEM). *Arch. Endocrinol. Metab.* **2021**, *65*, 368–375. [CrossRef]
77. Riera, R.; Bagattini, Â.M.; Pacheco, R.L.; Pachito, D.V.; Roitberg, F.; Ilbawi, A. Delays and Disruptions in Cancer Health Care Due to COVID-19 Pandemic: Systematic Review. *JCO Glob. Oncol.* **2021**, *7*, 311–323. [CrossRef]

78. Bakkar, S.; Al-Omar, K.; Aljarrah, Q.; Al-Dabbas, M.; Al-Dabbas, N.; Samara, S.; Miccoli, P. Impact of COVID-19 on thyroid cancer surgery and adjunct therapy. *Updates Surg.* **2020**, *72*, 867–869. [CrossRef]
79. Hojaij, F.C.; Chinelatto, L.A.; Boog, G.H.P.; Kasmirski, J.A.; Lopes, J.V.Z.; Medeiros, V.M.B. Head and Neck Practice in the COVID-19 Pandemics Today: A Rapid Systematic Review. *Int. Arch. Otorhinolaryngol.* **2020**, *24*, 518–526. [CrossRef]
80. Scappaticcio, L.; Maiorino, M.I.; Iorio, S.; Camponovo, C.; Piccardo, A.; Bellastella, G.; Docimo, G.; Esposito, K.; Trimboli, P. Thyroid surgery during the COVID-19 pandemic: Results from a systematic review. *J. Endocrinolog. Investig.* **2021**, *Jul 19*, 1–8. [CrossRef]
81. COVIDSurg Collaborative. Head and neck cancer surgery during the COVID-19 pandemic: An international, multicenter, observational cohort study. *Cancer* **2021**, *127*, 2476–2488. [CrossRef]
82. Zhang, L.; Zhu, F.; Xie, L.; Wang, C.; Wang, J.; Chen, R.; Jia, P.; Guan, H.Q.; Peng, L.; Chen, Y.; et al. Clinical characteristics of COVID-19-infected cancer patients: A retrospective case study in three hospitals within Wuhan, China. *Ann. Oncol.* **2020**, *31*, 894–901. [CrossRef]
83. Tagliamento, M.; Agostinetto, E.; Bruzzone, M.; Ceppi, M.; Saini, K.S.; de Azambuja, E.; Punie, K.; Westphalen, C.B.; Morgan, G.; Pronzato, P.; et al. Mortality in adult patients with solid or hematological malignancies and SARS-CoV-2 infection with a specific focus on lung and breast cancers: A systematic review and meta-analysis. *Crit. Rev. Oncol. Hematol.* **2021**, *163*, 103365. [CrossRef]
84. Dai, M.; Liu, D.; Liu, M.; Zhou, F.; Li, G.; Chen, Z.; Zhang, Z.; You, H.; Wu, M.; Zheng, Q.; et al. Patients with cancer appear more vulnerable to SARS-CoV-2: A multicenter study during the COVID-19 outbreak. *Cancer Discov.* **2020**, *10*, 783.
85. Wang, Q.; Berger, N.A.; Xu, R. Analyses of Risk, Racial Disparity, and Outcomes among US Patients with Cancer and COVID-19 Infection. *JAMA Oncol.* **2021**, *7*, 220–227. [CrossRef]
86. Addeo, A.; Friedlaender, A. Cancer and COVID-19: Unmasking their ties. *Cancer Treat. Rev.* **2020**, *88*, 102041. [CrossRef]
87. Van Dam, P.A.; Huizing, M.; Mestach, G.; Dierckxsens, S.; Tjalma, W.; Trinh, X.B.; Papadimitriou, K.; Altintas, S.; Vermorken, J.; Vulsteke, C.; et al. SARS-CoV-2 and cancer: Are they really partners in crime? *Cancer Treat. Rev.* **2020**, *89*, 102068. [CrossRef]
88. Sahin, M.; Haymana, C.; Demirci, I.; Tasci, I.; Rıfat, E.; Unluturk, U.; Satman, I.; Demir, T.; Cakal, E.; Ata, N.; et al. The clinical outcomes of COVID-19 infection in patients with a history of thyroid cancer: A nationwide study. *Clin. Endocrinol.* **2021**, *95*, 628–637. [CrossRef]
89. Kathuria-Prakash, N.; Mosaferi, T.; Xie, M.; Antrim, L.; Angell, T.E.; In, G.K.; Su, M.A.; Lechner, M.G. COVID-19 Outcomes of Patients with Differentiated Thyroid Cancer: A Multicenter Los Angeles Cohort Study. *Endocr. Pract.* **2021**, *27*, 90–94. [CrossRef]
90. Walitt, B.; Bartrum, E. A clinical primer for the expected and potential post-COVID-19 syndromes. *Pain Rep.* **2021**, *6*, e887. [CrossRef]
91. Proal, A.D.; VanElzakker, M.B. Long COVID or Post-acute Sequelae of COVID-19 (PASC): An Overview of Biological Factors That May Contribute to Persistent Symptoms. *Front. Microbiol.* **2021**, *12*, 1494. [CrossRef]
92. Chippa, V.; Aleem, A.; Anjum, F. Post Acute Coronavirus (COVID-19) Syndrome. In *StatPearls*; StatPearls Publishing: Treasure Island, FL, USA, 2021.
93. Ciuffo, G. Innesto positivo con filtrato di verruca volgare. *Giorn. Italy Mal. Venereol.* **1907**, *48*, 12–17.
94. Rous, P. A transmissible avian neoplasm. (Sarcoma of the common fowl.). *J. Exp. Med.* **1910**, *12*, 696–705. [CrossRef] [PubMed]
95. Mesri, E.A.; Feitelson, M.A.; Munger, K. Human viral oncogenesis: A cancer hallmarks analysis. *Cell Host Microbe* **2014**, *15*, 266–282. [CrossRef] [PubMed]
96. Pagano, J.S.; Blaser, M.; Buendia, M.A.; Damania, B.; Khalili, K.; Raab-Traub, N.; Roizman, B. Infectious agents and cancer: Criteria for a causal relation. *Semin. Cancer Biol.* **2004**, *14*, 453–471. [CrossRef] [PubMed]
97. Evans, A.S.; Mueller, N.E. Viruses and cancer. Causal associations. *Ann. Epidemiol.* **1990**, *1*, 71–92. [CrossRef]
98. Alhusseini, L.B.; Yassen, L.T.; Kouhsari, E.; Al Marjani, M.F. Persistence of SARS-CoV-2: A new paradigm of COVID-19 management. *Ann. Ig.* **2021**, *33*, 426–432.
99. Stingi, A.; Cirillo, L. SARS-CoV-2 infection and cancer: Evidence for and against a role of SARS-CoV-2 in cancer onset. *BioEssays* **2021**, *43*, 16–21. [CrossRef]
100. Alpalhão, M.; Ferreira, J.A.; Filipe, P. Persistent SARS-CoV-2 infection and the risk for cancer. *Med. Hypotheses* **2020**, *14*, 109882. [CrossRef]
101. Dyson, N.J. RB1: A prototype tumor suppressor and an enigma. *Genes Dev.* **2016**, *30*, 1492–1502. [CrossRef]
102. Anwar, F.; Emond, M.J.; Schmidt, R.A.; Hwang, H.C.; Bronner, M.P. Retinoblastoma expression in thyroid neoplasms. *Modern Pathol.* **2000**, *13*, 562–569. [CrossRef]
103. Park, R.; Jang, M.; Park, Y.I.; Park, Y.; Namkoong, S.; Lee, J.I.; Park, J. Elevated Levels of CTRP1 in Obesity Contribute to Tumor Progression in a p53-Dependent Manner. *Cancers* **2021**, *13*, 3619. [CrossRef]
104. ClinicalTrials.gov Identifier. Available online: https://clinicaltrials.gov/NCT04370834 (accessed on 14 September 2021).
105. Weng, Y.S.; Tseng, H.Y.; Chen, Y.A.; Shen, P.C.; Al Haq, A.T.; Chen, L.M.; Tung, Y.C.; Hsu, H.L. MCT-1/miR-34a/IL-6/IL-6R signaling axis promotes EMT progression, cancer stemness and M2 macrophage polarization in triple-negative breast cancer. *Mol. Cancer* **2019**, *18*, 42. [CrossRef]
106. Alraouji, N.N.; Al-Mohanna, F.H.; Ghebeh, H.; Arafah, M.; Almeer, R.; Al-Tweigeri, T.; Aboussekhra, A. Tocilizumab potentiates cisplatin cytotoxicity and targets cancer stem cells in triple-negative breast cancer. *Mol. Carcinog.* **2020**, *59*, 1041–1051. [CrossRef]

107. Tleyjeh, I.M.; Kashour, Z.; Damlaj, M.; Riaz, M.; Tlayjeh, H.; Altannir, M.; Altannir, Y.; Al-Tannir, M.; Tleyjeh, R.; Hassett, L.; et al. Efficacy and safety of tocilizumab in COVID-19 patients: A living systematic review and meta-analysis. *Clin. Microbiol. Infect.* **2021**, *27*, 215–227. [CrossRef]
108. Dalamaga, M.; Karampela, I.; Mantzoros, C.S. Commentary: Phosphodiesterase 4 inhibitors as potential adjunct treatment targeting the cytokine storm in COVID-19. *Metabolism* **2020**, *109*, 154282. [CrossRef]
109. Peng, T.; Gong, J.; Jin, Y.; Zhou, Y.; Tong, R.; Wei, X.; Bai, L.; Shi, J. Inhibitors of phosphodiesterase as cancer therapeutics. *Eur. J. Med. Chem.* **2018**, *150*, 742–756. [CrossRef]
110. Sponziello, M.; Verrienti, A.; Rosignolo, F.; De Rose, R.F.; Pecce, V.; Maggisano, V.; Durante, C.; Bulotta, S.; Damante, G.; Giacomelli, L.; et al. PDE5 expression in human thyroid tumors and effects of PDE5 inhibitors on growth and migration of cancer cells. *Endocrine* **2015**, *50*, 434–441. [CrossRef]
111. Beltrán-García, J.; Osca-Verdegal, R.; Pallardó, F.V.; Ferreres, J.; Rodríguez, M.; Mulet, S.; Sanchis-Gomar, F.; Carbonell, N.; García-Giménez, J.L. Oxidative Stress and Inflammation in COVID-19-Associated Sepsis: The Potential Role of Anti-Oxidant Therapy in Avoiding Disease Progression. *Antioxidants* **2020**, *9*, 936. [CrossRef]
112. Assi, M. The differential role of reactive oxygen species in early and late stages of cancer. *Am. J. Physiol. Regul. Integr. Comp. Physiol.* **2017**, *313*, R646–R653. [CrossRef]
113. Kramer, C.K.; Zinman, B.; Retnakaran, R. Are metabolically healthy overweight and obesity benign conditions? A systematic review and meta-analysis. *Ann. Intern. Med.* **2013**, *159*, 758–769. [CrossRef]
114. Kwon, H.; Chang, Y.; Cho, A.; Ahn, J.; Park, S.E.; Park, C.Y.; Lee, W.Y.; Oh, K.W.; Park, S.W.; Shin, H.; et al. Metabolic Obesity Phenotypes and Thyroid Cancer Risk: A Cohort Study. *Thyroid* **2019**, *29*, 349–358. [CrossRef]
115. Mayoral, L.P.; Andrade, G.M.; Mayoral, E.P.; Huerta, T.H.; Canseco, S.P.; Rodal Canales, F.J.; Cabrera-Fuentes, H.A.; Cruz, M.M.; Pérez Santiago, A.D.; Alpuche, J.J.; et al. Obesity subtypes, related biomarkers & heterogeneity. *Indian J. Med. Res.* **2020**, *151*, 11–21.
116. Vasileva, L.V.; Marchev, A.S.; Georgiev, M.I. Causes and solutions to "globesity": The new fa(s)t alarming global epidemic. *Food Chem. Toxicol.* **2018**, *121*, 173–193. [CrossRef]
117. Blüher, M. Obesity: Global epidemiology and pathogenesis. *Nat. Rev. Endocrinol.* **2019**, *15*, 288–298. [CrossRef]
118. Chooi, Y.C.; Ding, C.; Magkos, F. The epidemiology of obesity. *Metabolism* **2019**, *92*, 6–10. [CrossRef]
119. Available online: https://www.cdc.gov/obesity/data/obesity-and-covid-19.html (accessed on 13 September 2021).
120. Magreni, A.; Bann, D.V.; Schubart, J.R.; Goldenberg, D. The effects of race and ethnicity on thyroid cancer incidence. *JAMA Otolaryngol. Head Neck Surg.* **2015**, *141*, 319–323. [CrossRef]
121. Orosco, R.K.; Hussain, T.; Noel, J.E.; Chang, D.C.; Dosiou, C.; Mittra, E.; Divi, V.; Orloff, L.A. Radioactive iodine in differentiated thyroid cancer: A national database perspective. *Endocr. Relat. Cancer* **2019**, *26*, 795–802. [CrossRef]
122. Du, W.; Dong, Q.; Lu, X.; Liu, X.; Wang, Y.; Li, W.; Pan, Z.; Gong, Q.; Liang, C.; Gao, G. Iodine-131 therapy alters the immune/inflammatory responses in the thyroids of patients with Graves' disease. *Exp. Ther. Med.* **2017**, *13*, 1155–1159. [CrossRef]
123. Riley, A.S.; McKenzie, G.; Green, V.; Schettino, G.; England, R.; Greenman, J. The effect of radioiodine treatment on the diseased thyroid gland. *Int. J. Radiat. Biol.* **2019**, *95*, 1718–1727. [CrossRef]
124. Galimberti, S.; Petrini, M.; Baratè, C.; Ricci, F.; Balducci, S.; Grassi, S.; Guerrini, F.; Ciabatti, E.; Mechelli, S.; Di Paolo, A.; et al. Tyrosine Kinase Inhibitors Play an Antiviral Action in Patients Affected by Chronic Myeloid Leukemia: A Possible Model Supporting Their Use in the Fight Against SARS-CoV-2. *Front. Oncol.* **2020**, *10*, 1428. [CrossRef]
125. Pillaiyar, T.; Laufer, S. Kinases as Potential Therapeutic Targets for Anti-coronaviral Therapy. *J. Med. Chem.* **2021**. [CrossRef]
126. Haugen, B.R. Drugs that suppress TSH or cause central hypothyroidism. *Best Pract. Res. Clin. Endocrinol. Metab.* **2009**, *23*, 793–800. [CrossRef] [PubMed]
127. Sohrabpour, S.; Heidari, F.; Karimi, E.; Ansari, R.; Tajdini, A.; Heidari, F. Subacute Thyroiditis in COVID-19 Patients. *Eur. Thyroid J.* **2021**, *9*, 321–323. [CrossRef] [PubMed]
128. Brancatella, A.; Ricci, D.; Cappellani, D.; Viola, N.; Sgrò, D.; Santini, F.; Latrofa, F. Is subacute thyroiditis an underestimated manifestation of SARS-CoV-2 infection? Insights from a case series. *J. Clin. Endocrinol. Metab.* **2020**, *105*, e3742–e3746. [CrossRef] [PubMed]
129. Ucan, B.; Delibasi, T.; Cakal, E.; Arslan, M.S.; Bozkurt, N.C.; Demirci, T.; Ozbek, M.; Sahin, M. Caso de carcinoma papilar de tiroide mascarado por tireoidite subaguda. *Arq. Bras. Endocrinol. Metab.* **2014**, *58*, 851–854. [CrossRef]
130. Azer, P.; Zhai, J.; Yu, R. Atypical de Quervain's thyroiditis masquerading as papillary thyroid cancer. *Endocrinol. Nutr.* **2013**, *60*, 158–159. [CrossRef]
131. Gül, N.; Üzüm, A.K.; Selçukbiricik, Ö.S.; Yegen, G.; Tanakol, R.; Aral, F. Prevalence of papillary thyroid cancer in subacute thyroiditis patients may be higher than it is presumed: Retrospective analysis of 137 patients. *Radiol. Oncol.* **2018**, *52*, 257–262. [CrossRef]
132. Škorić, L.; Glasnović, A.; Petrak, J. A publishing pandemic during the COVID-19 pandemic: How challenging can it become? *Croat. Med. J.* **2020**, *61*, 79–81. [CrossRef]
133. Chablani, S.V.; Sabra, M.M. Thyroid cancer and telemedicine during the COVID-19 pandemic. *J. Endocr. Soc.* **2021**, *5*, bvab059. [CrossRef]
134. Serafini, G.; Parmigiani, B.; Amerio, A.; Aguglia, A.; Sher, L.; Amore, M. The psychological impact of COVID-19 on the mental health in the general population. *QJM* **2020**, *113*, 229–235. [CrossRef]

135. Graves, C.E.; Goyal, N.; Levin, A.; Nuno, M.A.; Kim, J.; Campbell, M.J.; Shen, W.T.; Gosnell, J.E.D.; Roman, S.; Sosa, J.A.; et al. Anxiety and Fear During the Covid-19 Pandemic: A Web-Based Survey of Thyroid Cancer Survivors. *J. Endocr. Soc.* **2021**, *5*, A836. [CrossRef]
136. Stipcević, T.; Pivac, N.; Kozarić-Kovacić, D.; Mück-Seler, D. Thyroid activity in patients with major depression. *Coll. Antropol.* **2008**, *32*, 973–976.
137. Olff, M.; Güzelcan, Y.; de Vries, G.J.; Assies, J.; Gersons, B.P. HPA- and HPT-axis alterations in chronic posttraumatic stress disorder. *Psychoneuroendocrinology* **2006**, *31*, 1220–1230. [CrossRef]
138. Siegmann, E.M.; Müller, H.; Luecke, C.; Philipsen, A.; Kornhuber, J.; Grömer, T.W. Association of Depression and Anxiety Disorders With Autoimmune Thyroiditis: A Systematic Review and Meta-analysis. *JAMA Psychiatry* **2018**, *75*, 577–584. [CrossRef]
139. Feng, G.; Kang, C.; Yuan, J.; Zhang, Y.; Wei, Y.; Xu, L.; Zhou, F.; Fan, X.; Yang, J. Neuroendocrine abnormalities associated with untreated first episode patients with major depressive disorder and bipolar disorder. *Psychoneuroendocrinology* **2019**, *107*, 119–123. [CrossRef]
140. Shen, Y.; Wu, F.; Zhou, Y.; Ma, Y.; Huang, X.; Ning, Y.; Lang, X.; Luo, X.; Zhang, X. Association of thyroid dysfunction with suicide attempts in first-episode and drug naïve patients with major depressive disorder. *J. Affect. Disord.* **2019**, *259*, 180–185. [CrossRef]
141. Fischer, S.; Strahler, J.; Markert, C.; Skoluda, N.; Doerr, J.M.; Kappert, M.; Nater, U.M. Effects of acute psychosocial stress on the hypothalamic-pituitary-thyroid (HPT) axis in healthy women. *Psychoneuroendocrinology* **2019**, *110*, 104438. [CrossRef]
142. Joseph-Bravo, P.; Jaimes-Hoy, L.; Uribe, R.M.; Charli, J.L. 60 Years of Neuroendocrinology: TRH, the first hypophysiotropic releasing hormone isolated: Control of the pituitary-thyroid axis. *J. Endocrinol.* **2015**, *226*, T85–T100. [CrossRef]
143. Keestra, S.; Högqvist Tabor, V.; Alvergne, A. Reinterpreting patterns of variation in human thyroid function: An evolutionary ecology perspective. *Evol. Med. Public Health* **2020**, *9*, 93–112. [CrossRef]
144. Dietrich, J.W.; Midgley, J.; Hoermann, R. Editorial: "Homeostasis and Allostasis of Thyroid Function". *Front. Endocrinol.* **2018**, *9*, 287. [CrossRef]
145. Chatzitomaris, A.; Hoermann, R.; Midgley, J.E.; Hering, S.; Urban, A.; Dietrich, B.; Abood, A.; Klein, H.H.; Dietrich, J.W. Thyroid Allostasis-Adaptive Responses of Thyrotropic Feedback Control to Conditions of Strain, Stress, and Developmental Programming. *Front. Endocrinol.* **2017**, *8*, 163. [CrossRef]

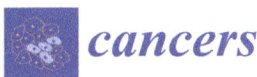

Review

Management of Hematologic Malignancies in the Era of COVID-19 Pandemic: Pathogenetic Mechanisms, Impact of Obesity, Perspectives, and Challenges

Dimitrios Tsilingiris [1,*], Narjes Nasiri-Ansari [2], Nikolaos Spyrou [3], Faidon Magkos [4] and Maria Dalamaga [2]

1. First Department of Propaedeutic Internal Medicine, School of Medicine, National and Kapodistrian University of Athens, Laiko General Hospital, 17 St Thomas Street, 11527 Athens, Greece
2. Department of Biological Chemistry, School of Medicine, National and Kapodistrian University of Athens, 75 Mikras Asias, 11527 Athens, Greece; nnasiri@med.uoa.gr (N.N.-A.); madalamaga@med.uoa.gr (M.D.)
3. Tisch Cancer Institute, Icahn School of Medicine at Mount Sinai, New York, NY 10029, USA; nikolaos.spyrou@mssm.edu
4. Department of Nutrition, Exercise, and Sports, University of Copenhagen, DK-2200 Frederiksberg, Denmark; fma@nexs.ku.dk
* Correspondence: tsilingirisd@gmail.com

Simple Summary: Obesity is epidemiologically and likely, causally related to various hematological cancers, while both conditions may predispose to severe SARS-CoV-2 infection. The COVID-19 pandemic brought about a variety of obstacles with respect to numerous aspects in the management of hematological malignancies. In the present overview, the evidence linking obesity with the development of hematological cancers and their role as risk factors for severe COVID-19 is critically appraised. Furthermore, the various challenges which emerged during the the pandemic are reviewed, regarding not only the treatment of the underlying hematological malignancies themselves, but also the prevention and therapeutic management of SARS-CoV-2 infection in this patient group. Lastly, we discuss further unresolved issues which need to be addressed in order to optimize the management of patients with hematologic cancers in the course of ongoing COVID-19 pandemic.

Abstract: The COVID-19 pandemic brought about an unprecedented societal and healthcare system crisis, considerably affecting healthcare workers and patients, particularly those with chronic diseases. Patients with hematologic malignancies faced a variety of challenges, pertinent to the nature of an underlying hematologic disorder itself as well as its therapy as a risk factor for severe SARS-CoV-2 infection, suboptimal vaccine efficacy and the need for uninterrupted medical observation and continued therapy. Obesity constitutes another factor which was acknowledged since the early days of the pandemic that predisposed people to severe COVID-19, and shares a likely causal link with the pathogenesis of a broad spectrum of hematologic cancers. We review here the epidemiologic and pathogenetic features that obesity and hematologic malignancies share, as well as potential mutual pathophysiological links predisposing people to a more severe SARS-CoV-2 course. Additionally, we attempt to present the existing evidence on the multi-faceted crucial challenges that had to be overcome in this diverse patient group and discuss further unresolved questions and future challenges for the management of hematologic malignancies in the era of COVID-19.

Keywords: blood cancer; COVID-19; hematologic malignancy; leukemia; lymphoma; multiple myeloma; myelodysplasia; obesity; SARS-CoV-2

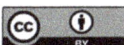

1. Introduction

The outbreak of the COVID-19 pandemic in December 2019 brought about an unprecedented global crisis at health care, societal and economical levels. The subsequent allocation of personnel- and material-related resources towards countering COVID-19 endangered the uninterrupted care of patients with a large variety of chronic health conditions, potentially compromising the overall prognosis, particularly of those in danger of severe SARS-CoV-2 infection [1,2].

Since early in the course of the pandemic, the presence of obesity or hematologic malignancy, among others, were identified as important risk factors for SARS-CoV-2 acquisition and severe infection [3–6]. Interestingly, an epidemiologic and probably pathogenetic connection between these two entities has long been established [7–9].

The inherent pathophysiological features of a variety of hematologic neoplasms, the associated changes in the number and/or function of various immune cells and occasionally, the effects of therapy, all have a profound impact on underlying immune mechanisms. As a result, affected individuals form a patient group particularly susceptible to infectious complications including COVID-19. Additionally, although highly variable depending on hematologic diagnosis, the initial and long-term management of several hematologic cancers exhibits numerous challenges regarding many aspects and demands a meticulous adherence to a strict treatment regimen and follow-up schedule, as well as a collaboration of different medical disciplines at various levels of the health care system. Not surprisingly, the combination of these features has made the management of patients with hematologic malignancies a particularly demanding task during the course of the pandemic.

In the present narrative review, the proposed mechanisms linking obesity with hematologic carcinogenesis and the spectrum of related diagnoses are discussed. Furthermore, the obstacles and challenges that emerged during COVID-19 regarding the management of these patients, and the corresponding measures to meet them, are discussed along with a review of open questions and aspects necessitating optimization.

2. Overview of Obesity-Related Hematologic Neoplasms

A relationship between increased body adiposity and elevated risk of a variety of hematologic neoplasms has long been established, expanding the knowledge linking obesity to the development of solid neoplasms [7,8]. Relevant evidence has derived primarily from a considerable number of population-based cohorts subjected to long-term epidemiologic observation (Table 1).

Table 1. Overview of obesity-related hematologic neoplasms.

Hematologic Malignancies	Study (Design, Reference)	Collective Main Findings
Hodgkin Disease	Meta-analysis [10] Population-based cohort study [11]	HR 1.41 (95% CI, 1.14–1.75) for BMI > 30 kg/m^2 J-shaped association with BMI with ↑ incidence above 24.2 kg/m^2 ↑ 10% HR per 5 kg/m^2 increase
Acute Leukemias Lymphocytic Myeloid	Meta-analysis [12] Retrospective cohort study [13]	RR 1.65 (1.16–2.35) for BMI > 30 kg/m^2 RR 1.52 (1.19–1.95) for BMI > 30 kg/m^2
Plasma cell disorders MGUS Waldenström's Makroglobulinemia Multiple Myeloma	Systematic Review [14] Population-based cohort study [15] Population-based cohort study [16] Prospective cohort study Prospective cohort study [17] Prospective cohort [18] Systematic review [19]	BMI associated MGUS development and progression to MM BMI > 30 kg/m^2 associated with MGUS risk Obesity associated with MGUS progression to MM Viseral fat associated with LC-MGUS HR 1.41 (1.01–1.95) per 4 kg/m^2 increase in BMI HR 1.41 (1.01–1.95) per 4 kg/m^2 increase in BMI RR for MM mortality 1.71 ♂/1.44 ♀ for BMI > 35 kg/m^2 vs. <25 kg/m^2
Non-Hodgkin's Lymphoma/CLL	Prospective cohort study [18] Meta-analysis [10] Population-based cohort study [20]	RR for NHL mortality 1.49 ♂/1.95 ♀ for BMI > 35 kg/m^2 vs. <25 kg/m^2 ↑ NHL incidence 1.07 (1.04–1.10)/1.14 (1.04–1.26) mortality per 5 kg/m^2 increase in BMI, driven chiefly by ↑ risk of DLBCL CLL RR 1.25 (1.11–1.41) for BMI > 30 kg/m^2
Myelodysplastic syndromes	Population-based cohort study [21] Retrospective cohort [22]	RR 2.18 (1.51–3.17) for BMI > 30 kg/m^2 vs. <25 kg/m^2 Higher BMI associated with lower overall survival, particularly in lower-risk MDS

Table 1. Cont.

Hematologic Malignancies	Study (Design, Reference)	Collective Main Findings
Chronic myeloproliferative disorders Polycythemia Vera Chronic Myelogenous Leukemia Essential Thrombocythemia	Retrospective cohort study [23] Case–control study [24] Case–control study [25] Prospective cohort study [26]	BMI > 95th percentile among adolescents: aHR for PV 1.81 (1.13–2.92). Independent dose–response effect between adiposity and risk of CML OR for ET among obese 2.59 (1.02–6.58) RR for ET: 1.52 (0.97, 2.38) for BMI > 29.3 vs. <23.4 kg/m^2

Abbreviations: ALL: acute lymphocytic leukemia; AML: acute myeloid leukemia; BMI: body mass index; CLL: chronic lymphocytic leukemia; CML: chronic myelogenous leukemia; DLBCL: diffuse large B-cell lymphoma; ET; essential thrombocytopenia; LC: light chain; NHL: non-Hodgkin lymphoma; HM: hematologic malignancy; aHR; (adjusted) hazard ratio; MGUS: monoclonal gammopathy of undetermined significance; MDS: myelodysplastic syndrome; MM: multiple myeloma; OR: odds ratio; PV: polycythemia vera; RR: relative risk.

The risk extends to an abundance of difference hematologic malignancies, including non-Hodgkin lymphomas (NHL) [10,18,20], Hodgkin's disease [10,11], multiple myeloma [18,19], and acute leukemia [20] lymphocytic (ALL) and myeloid (AML) [12,13] (Table 1). The impact of obesity on the risk of NHL may not be homogenous across different histological subtypes, and the increased risk appears to concern primarily the more aggressive diffuse large B-cell lymphoma and, to a much lesser extent, the more indolent subtypes, such as follicular lymphoma or small lymphocytic lymphoma/chronic lymphocytic leukemia [27,28].

Furthermore, there is an increased prevalence of pre-malignant hematologic conditions among individuals with obesity, such as the spectrum of myelodysplastic syndromes (MDS), for which obesity is also associated with a worse prognosis regarding overall survival [21,29]; chronic myeloproliferative disorders, especially chronic myeloid leukemia and essential thrombocytosis [23–26]; and monoclonal gammopathy of unknown significance (MGUS) [14]. The probability of progression of monoclonal gammopathy of unknown significance to multiple myeloma also appears to be strongly affected by the presence of overweight and obesity [14,30].

The fact that the bulk of available data has been generated in fairly well-characterized cohorts, which enables their extraction to be independent of potential confounding factors, does not by itself conclusively prove a causal role of obesity and related systemic perturbations in hematologic oncogenesis. On the contrary, it could be argued that these observations may be at least partly attributable to unaccounted dietary or other lifestyle factors, or other genetic and environmental factors that promote both conditions. The major counterargument against this hypothesis stems from the decrease in total and histologic type-specific malignancy risks following conservative or surgical weight loss [31–33]. In the frame of the current discussion, it should be noted that evidence on an incidence reduction specific of hematologic (pre-)malignancies is, to date, extremely scarce, although a reduction in NHL occurrence among females with obesity undergoing bariatric surgery has been reported [33].

Not surprisingly, in most available clinical studies that have verified the association between obesity and hematologic (pre)malignancies, the body mass index (BMI) has been used to characterize and quantify the degree of adiposity among participants. Both the universally accepted cutoffs for overweight (25 kg/m^2) and obesity (30 kg/m^2) and the BMI itself as a continuous parameter have been used to quantify the relationship between the severity of obesity and malignancy risk. Despite its simplicity, BMI is an imperfect tool for the assessment of the qualitative features of adiposity. BMI values do not distinguish between lean and fat mass, while they do not take into consideration differences in fat distribution (including the fractions of visceral and subcutaneous adipose tissue) and the age-related decline of lean mass [34,35]. Although data on other body composition markers are scarce, indices of visceral adiposity, such as waist circumference and body-shape-index as well as waist-to-hip ratio, have been shown be better predictors of the development of any hematologic malignancy and multiple myeloma, respectively [36]. The stronger implication of clinical markers typically associated with an "unhealthier" obese phenotype may imply that the already well-characterized adverse metabolic and overall consequences of increased total obesity and particularly central obesity might be causally implicated in hematologic carcinogenesis [36].

On the other hand, the obesity-related hematologic malignancies and premalignant conditions constitute an extreme diverse collective with respect to their cell line of origin, other risk factors for their development, clinical presentation, prognosis and therapy. Consequently, a unified hypothesis linking their pathogenesis to obesity would be challenging to establish. Among the mechanisms that have been proposed to link obesity with carcinogenesis, the most predominant include aberrant cytokine and adipokine production from the expanded and dysfunctional adipose tissue, increased circulating levels of peptide hormones with growth-factor properties (e.g., insulin, IGF-1) and the development of a systemic oxidative-stress environment promoting DNA-damage and tumor genesis [8,37–45]. The chronic immune stimulation in the frame of the low-grade inflammatory milieu of the obese states may be of particular significance in the case of hematologic neoplasms. Adipose tissue-derived proinflammatory cytokines (e.g., intereukin-6, TNF-alpha) have prominent direct effects on hematopoietic cell proliferation, evasion of apoptosis, kinetics and function [46–50]. Furthermore, altered secretion of members of the adipokine family, most predominantly increased leptin secretion and function and decreased adiponectin, may play a distinct role in obesity-related hematologic carcinogenesis. Leptin partakes in the normal hematopoietic function [51], while exerting antiapoptotic and/or proliferating effects on lymphocytes [52] and myeloblasts through binding to its receptors on the aforementioned cell types [53]. On the other hand, lower adiponectin levels are independently associated with a higher risk of myelodysplastic syndrome, acute myelogenous leukemia and multiple myeloma, among others [8,41,42,44,54]. It is likely that not all obesity-related hematologic malignancies are influenced to the same degree by specific mechanisms; rather, potential combined effects of these factors may be decisive for the oncogenesis of specific hematologic neoplasms.

3. Association between Obesity and Hematologic Cancers with COVID-19 Outcomes

3.1. COVID-19 and Obesity

Since the beginning of the pandemic, obesity was recognized as a major factor associated with SARS-CoV-2 infection adverse outcomes [55,56]. From a meta-analysis of 30 early studies that reported specific outcomes with respect to measures of adiposity, an overall adjusted odds ratio (OR) of 2.09 (1.67, 2.62) for severe COVID-19 among patients with a "high" compared with those with a low BMI was noted. The adjusted ORs for individual outcomes were 2.36 for hospitalization, 2.32 for intensive care unit (ICU) admission, 2.63 for mechanical ventilation and 1.49 for death [5]. Additionally, a considerably higher visceral adipose tissue (VAT) accumulation was ascertained among those experiencing adverse outcomes compared with those with mild disease by three studies [57–59]. It should be noted that even though most included studies used the conventional cut off of 30 kg/m^2, there were others that deviated from this criterion to discriminate between patients with high and low BMI, whereas no clear definition was given in six studies [5]. Later studies confirmed these findings, further highlighting a dose-dependent relationship between the severity of obesity and risk for most adverse COVID-19 outcomes [60–62]. Interestingly, the overall relationship of BMI with serious SARS-CoV-2 infection conforms to a J-shaped curve, with those at the lowest adiposity extreme being more prone to an adverse course, hence, highlighting another manifestation of the "Obesity paradox" in the frame of COVID-19 [60,61].

3.2. COVID-19 Outcomes in Obesity-Related Hematologic Malignancies

An overview of the studies on the impact of hematologic malignancies on SARS-CoV-2 outcomes is presented in Table 2.

Table 2. Overview of key studies addressing the impact of hematologic malignancies on COVID-19 outcomes.

Data Source, Reference	Population of Interest	Main Outcomes
Hematologic cancer registry of India [63]	565 reports of patients of all ages from tertiary Indian centers with HM and laboratory-confirmed COVID-19 between 21 March 2020–20 March 2021	↑ mortality (aHR 2.85, 1.58–5.13) and severe disease (aOR 2.73, 1.45–5.12 for AML vs. ALL) No differences between AML and other hematologic diagnoses ↑ mortality among those not in remission (aOR 1.85, 1.18–2.89) No effects of corticosteroid treatment or exposure to monoclonal antibodies
European Hematology Association Survey [64]	3,801 patients with HM and laboratory-confirmed COVID-19 from 132 hematology centers across Europe between March 2020–December 2020	Highest death rates in AML (40%) and MDS (42.3%) Active malignancy associated with ↑mortality (aHR 1.86, 1.62–2.14) Among different HL diagnoses, only AML independently associated with ↑mortality (aHR 2.046, 1.18–3.56 vs. NHL)
Nationwide retrospective study in Israel [65]	313 patients with HM and COVID-19 from 16 medical centers	Age > 70 years, arterial hypertension, active treatment associated with adverse outcomes Remdesivir treatment linked to ↓ mortality no effects of other treatment modalities (corticosteroids, enoxaparin, convalescent plasma)
Data from population-based registry in Madrid, Spain [66]	833 patients with HM and COVID-19 from 27 medical centers between 28 February 2020 and 25 May 2020	Overall, 62% severe/critical disease, 33% mortality (highest among AML and MDS patients, 40% and 42.3%, respectively) ↑ risk of death > 60 years, no effect of gender ↑ mortality for AML (aHR 2.22, 1.31–3.74 vs. NHL), Monoclonal antibody treatment and conventional chemotherapy (aHRs vs. nontreatment (aHRs 2.02, 1.14–3.60 and 1.50, 0.99–2.29 vs. no treatment, respectively) ↓ mortality for Ph-negative myeloproliferative disorders and treatment with hypomethylating agents (aHRs 0.33, 0.14–0.81 vs. NHL and 0.47, 0.23–0.94 vs. no treatment, respectively)
Case–control study from 2 Hospital in Wuhan province, China [4]	13 cases among 128 hospitalized patients with HM and 16 HCWs with COVID-19	↑ mortality for those with HM vs. controls (62% vs. 0, $p = 0.002$)
Meta-analysis of 34 studies in adult and 5 in pediatric populations [67]	3377 patients with HM from 39 studies in total	No effects of recent systemic overall antineoplastic or cytotoxic therapy (RRs 1.17, 0.83–1.64 and 1.29, 0.78–2.15 vs. no treatment, respectively) on COVID-19 mortality
Case control study from a nationwide database of patient electronic health records in the US [68]	73 million patients, 517.580 with 8 types of HMs, 420 with SARS-CoV-2 infection up to 1 September 2020	Significantly ↑ SARS-CoV-2 acquisition rates for HM vs. controls (overall aOR 11.9, 11.3–12.5 for diagnosis < 1 year, 2.3, 2.2–2.4 for prior diagnosis), highest among ALL, ET, MM, AML and lowest for PV ↑ Higher hospitalization and death rates for HM vs. non-HM
Prospective cohort study among patients enrolled UK Coronavirus Cancer Monitoring project [69]	227 patients with HM (Leukemia, Lymphoma, MM, others) among 1044 with active cancer and documented SARS-CoV-2 infection between 18 March 2020–8 May 2020	↑ risk for adverse outcomes for HM vs. solid tumor patients (aORs for high flow oxygen therapy 1.82, 1.11–2.94, NIV 2.10, 1.14–3.76, ICU 2.73, 1.43–5.11, severe/critical disease 1.57, 1.15–2.15) ↑ in-hospital mortality for HM patients who recently received chemotherapy (1.57, 1.15–2.15 vs. no recent chemotherapy)

Abbreviations: ALL: acute lymphocytic leukemia; AML: acute myeloid leukemia; ET; essential thrombocytopenia; NHL: non-Hodgkin lymphoma; HM: hematologic malignancy; HR; hazard ratio; MDS: myelodysplastic syndrome; MM: multiple myeloma; NIV: non-invasive ventilation; OR: odds ratio; PV: polycythemia vera; RR: relative risk.

The earliest evidence regarding SARS-CoV-2 infection in patients with hematologic malignancies originated from a small cohort study among hospitalized patients in hematologic wards at the time of the initial outbreak in Wuhan, China (Table 2). There were similar

SARS-CoV-2 acquisition rates among patients compared with a matched controlled group of health care workers, but a higher incidence of severe disease and death [4].

Furthermore, an analysis of the data of the openSAFELY platform in the United Kingdom pointed towards increased mortality among patients with hematologic malignancies. The risk was highest (2.5-fold) among those who had received the diagnosis in the last 1–5 years and slightly decreased thereafter, either reflecting the acute detrimental effects of treatment or resulting from survivalist bias among patients with greater survival rates [70]. A subsequent meta-analysis of 39 reports (5 pediatric and 34 among adults) attempted a more comprehensive evaluation of the effects of age, treatment and specific diagnosis on the risk of death from COVID-19. The risk of death in adults was found to be higher than in pediatric hematologic patients (34% vs. 4%), and among those, higher for those aged >60 (relative risk: RR 1.8) as well as lower among white compared to non-white patients (RR 2.2). The pooled risk was substantially higher than this observed in the general population. The decisive effect of age on COVID-19 outcomes observed in this study is in agreement with the vast majority of available reports in diverse populations. The relationship between age and the risk of hospitalization or death due to SARS-CoV-2 infection appears to be linear, without distinct age cut-offs, above which an additional risk for severe disease is conferred [71]. Furthermore, it is likely that the effect of age is not mediated by the increased co-morbidity burden in the elderly population [72]. Although the factors that drive this relationship are not fully elucidated, a crucial role of the age-related immune senescence may be hypothesized [73]. Likewise, an increased risk for severe disease among black patients and racial minorities compared to white patients has been also observed in numerous cohorts. There are likely to be numerous and diverse factors that could explain the racial disparities regarding COVID-19 outcomes. These include a compromised socioeconomic status and poorer living/working conditions, limited or delayed access to health care services, higher prevalence of relevant comorbidities, poor nutritional habits, more frequent smoking and increased psychosocial stress [74,75]. Interestingly, the presence of any or solely cytotoxic recent anticancer therapy was not shown to have an effect on mortality compared to the absence of treatment. It is also noteworthy that, excluding patients with acquired bone marrow failure syndrome (commonly in the frame of MDS or aplastic anemia) which showed a peak mortality rate of 53%, the risk of death was relatively homogenous for the rest of the diagnosis, ranging from 31–33% for those with CLL, lymphomas and MM to 41% for those with acute leukemias [67].

In a more recent report from a nationwide database from the USA, SARS-CoV-2 acquisition, hospitalization and death rates were investigated across a broad spectrum of malignant and premalignant hematologic conditions and were compared to patients without haemato-oncologic diagnoses [68]. Notably, the sum of investigated conditions concerned predominantly obesity-related hematologic malignancies (Table 1). Acquisition rates were substantially higher among patients within a broad spectrum of diagnoses, especially among those who had received a hematologic diagnosis within the last year (pooled adjusted OR 11.9 [11.3–12.5]). Maximal rates were observed in patients with ALL (aOR 31.0) but they were also substantially high across the sum of studied conditions. It cannot be definitely concluded whether, and to which degree, this finding reflects a truly increased risk of viral acquisition or a greater probability of developing symptoms, hence, more frequently diagnosed SARS-CoV-2 infections. Likewise, hospitalization rates and mortality among recently diagnosed hematologic patients with COVID-19 were higher than those without a diagnosis and those with a recent hematologic diagnosis without COVID-19 (51.9% vs. 23.5% and 15% and 14.8% vs. 5.1% and 4.1%, respectively). Findings were comparable when accounting for any time of hematologic diagnosis. Similar to previous reports, patients of African-American origin exhibited generally higher rates of adverse outcomes in comparison with Caucasians.

4. Obesity, Related Hematologic Malignancies and Severe COVID-19: Pathogenetic Considerations

It may not come as a surprise that two epidemiologically- and possibly causally-related conditions—obesity and hematologic malignancies—both belong to the known factors predisposing individuals to adverse COVID-19 prognoses (Figure 1). The organ-specific, obesity-related comorbidities—such as diabetes mellitus and arterial hypertension—that established cardiovascular and restrictive pulmonary disease on one hand, and the overall frailty that characterizes certain groups of individuals affected with hematologic cancers on the other, predispose people to adverse outcomes in acute illnesses of various causes, including sepsis [76–80]. Nonetheless, specific features of the systemic immune response in the frame of SARS-CoV-2 infection can be hypothesized to influence the course of the disease among individuals affected with obesity and/or hematologic malignancies.

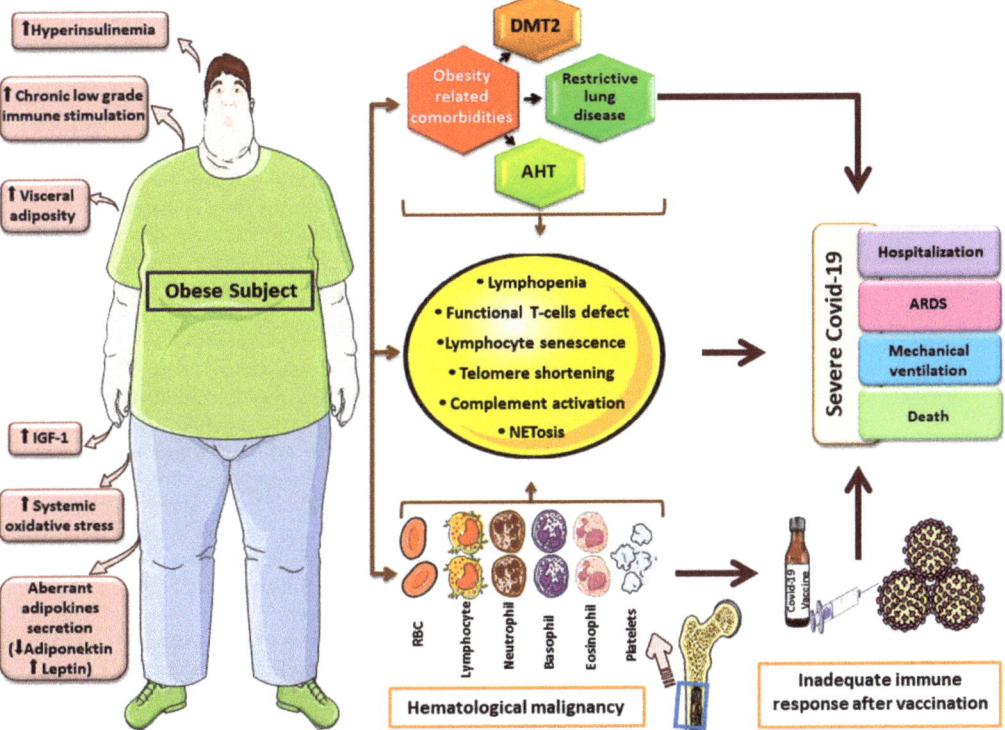

Figure 1. Graphical overview of factors and mechanisms linking obesity, hematologic malignancy and severe COVID-19 course. Obesity has been linked to carcinogenesis through aberrant cytokine and adipokine production, hyperinsulinemia, increase growth-factor levels (IGF-1), elevated oxidative-stress and chronic low-grade inflammation. Obesity-related comorbidities, along with features accompanying hematologic malignancies, such as quantitative and qualitative immune system defects and telomere shortening, may lead to an inadequate immune response after COVID-19 vaccination and severe clinical outcomes. * This image was derived from the free medical site http://smart.servier.com/ (accessed on 31 March 2022) by Servier, licensed under a Creative Commons Attribution 3.0 Unported License.

Successful host defense and viral clearance requires a multifaceted innate and acquired cellular immune response, orchestrated by a complex variety of cellular and humoral components. Of crucial importance are a timely pro- and anti-inflammatory cytokine cascade and the balanced involvement of CD4+/CD8+ and B lymphocytes. An aberrantly exaggerated, uncoordinated immune response may drive the elusive manifestation of the hyperinflammation syndrome [81].

Quantitative and qualitative defects of the immune system are most prominent in hematologic malignancies but are encountered in obesity as well [82]. Lymphopenia is a prominent feature of a broad variety of hematologic malignancies such as MDS [83], Hodgkin disease, NHL [84] and MM [85], and can complicate therapy. ALL can be viewed as a state of "functional" lymphopenia despite the occasionally extremely high lymphocyte counts. Quantitative and qualitative T-lymphocyte defects have also been described in obesity and may be partially reversible following successful weight loss [86]. Interestingly, the association between lymphopenia and adverse SARS-CoV-2 outcomes, including hospitalization, ARDS, mechanical ventilation, and death, has been observed in numerous studies [87–89]. Besides being a consequence of SARS-CoV-2 infection itself [90], which may imply a component of reverse causality for this observation, pre-existing lymphopenia has also been shown to predispose people to severe COVID-19 [91], which advocates for a crucial role of T cell-mediated immune response for successful viral clearance and infection resolution. Furthermore, lymphopenia, either preceding or developing in the course of SARS-CoV-2 infection, may facilitate the development and/or increase the severity of secondary bacterial and/or fungal infections that may further adversely affect prognosis [92,93]. Alternatively, a prominent reduction in regulatory T cells could predispose people to an exaggerated immune response and cytokine storm which are major features of the COVID-19-related hyperinflammation syndrome [94]. A state of systemic chronic low-grade inflammation is a feature of both obesity and various hematologic malignant states, such as MDS, acute leukemias, MM and NHL [95–98]. This feature can promote or be inherent in "inflammaging", which refers to a state of immune cell senescence and dysregulation [99], predisposing to adverse COVID-19-related outcomes [99,100]. Lymphocyte telomere shortening constitutes an important component of lymphocyte senescence and dysfunction, which is typically encountered in hematologic malignancies, occasionally in conjunction with an adverse prognosis [101]. Telomere length has been also shown to inversely associate with BMI [102] and correlates with the negative metabolic consequences of excess adiposity [103], while weight loss causes a dose-dependent elongation [99]. A shorter telomere length has been suggested as the epidemiologic link between known clinical and epidemiologic risk factors for severe COVID-19, implicating impaired lymphocyte replication and recruitment capacity as well as the senescence-associated pro-inflammatory lymphocyte phenotype in severe disease pathogenesis [104,105]. Indeed, a shorter telomere length has been associated with poor SARS-CoV-2 infection outcomes [106,107], while the infection itself may have an accelerating impact on telomere shortening [108].

The release of extracellular traps (NETs) by neutrophils is increased in certain hematologic cancers such as DLBCL [109] or CLL [110] as well as in severe obesity [111]. NETosis has been shown to be a prominent feature of COVID-19 immunothrombosis, which is implicated in target organ damage [112]. Likewise, aberrant complement activation constitutes another common feature of the three entities [112–114].

5. Vaccination against SARS-CoV-2 in Patients with Hematologic Malignancy

Upon the market release of COVID-19 vaccines in December 2020 and in the face of initial relative shortages, there was an urgent need for a rationalized prioritization of vaccine supplies. The aim was to maximize the efficacy of vaccination strategies with respect to maximal prevention of COVID-19-related deaths, reduction in hospitalization burden and societal and economic disruption. The World Health Organization issued corresponding guidance to direct available vaccine resources to the most vulnerable patient groups [115]. Patients with comorbidities rendering them vulnerable to severe disease were categorized in the second priority group; hence, these patients were scheduled to be vaccinated in the first 11–20% of the population. Although individual national programs occasionally deviated from this scheme, both obesity as well as hematologic malignancy fell into this category, the latter corresponding to "cancer" as well as to "conditions or therapies associated with immune suppression" in the issued document [115]. Similar approaches were used for the prioritization of booster vaccinations and are likely to be repeated in the future updated versions of vaccination programs as the pandemic continues.

The vaccines critically altered the course of the pandemic, being highly efficacious against symptomatic SARS-CoV-2 infection and, even after the appearance of altered viral variants, for the prevention of severe course, hospitalization and death. Despite initial considerations, vaccine efficacy was shown to be essentially unaffected by the presence of obesity [116,117]. Vaccine efficacy among those with obesity-related hematologic cancers is inherently more challenging since it is expected that the disturbed immune function originating from the conditions themselves or their therapies may hinder the development of adequate immunity. Indeed, inadequate antibody and/or T-cellular responses have been documented after the vaccination of patients with monoclonal gammopathies (particularly for MM rather than smoldering myeloma [118]), acute leukemias, Hodgkin disease and NHL, MDS, acute leukemias and chronic myeloproliferative disorders [118–120]. Seroconversion rates appear substantially lower among hematologic cancer patients compared with those affected by solid neoplasms [120,121], and may be particularly low in specific diseases, depending on their pathophysiological and cytogenetic characteristics as well as mode of therapy. Greenberger et al. investigated the antibody responses following two mRNA-based platform doses in 1445 hematologic patients from the USA, approximately 40 days following the second dose. Seropositivity rates were found to be minimal across a variety of NHL histological subtypes or CLL and, in contrast, were satisfactory in Hodgkin disease, acute leukemias, monoclonal gammopathies and myeloproliferative disorders [122]. Unsurprisingly, B-cell-targeted therapies such as anti CD20-monoclonal antibodies, chimeric antigen receptor (CAR) T cells against CD19, or Bruton's tyrosine kinase (BTK) inhibitors have been associated with diminished antibody responses [120–122]. Regarding receivers of allogeneic hematopoietic stem cell transplantation (HSCT) and despite some concerns [121], in a cohort of 117 patients vaccinated with BNT162b2, antibody response rates were satisfactory among patients who had received the transplantation more than one or two years ago, compared with less than 12 months. Response rates after two doses were 89%, 96%, 52%, respectively, and were greater among those with lymphocyte counts of >1000/µL compared with those with a lower lymphocyte count (91% vs. 64%, respectively) and those who were not under ongoing treatment (91% vs. 64%, respectively) [123]. Likewise, a study among 67 lymphoma or MM patients who received autologous HSCT showed that 56 (87%) developed humoral [124] immunity following the vaccination of the BNT162b2 mRNA vaccine. Similar findings have been ascertained in a case series of scleroderma patients who received autologous stem cell transplantation [125]. Apart from diagnosis and mode of therapy, other factors acknowledged to positively affect the immune response include vaccination outside the frame of active therapy, a longer time interval since the last anti-CD20 antibody administration, and vaccination during a complete remission status [120,126].

Regarding vaccine type, there have been occasional reports of favorable efficacy profiles of specific platforms; between the two available mRNA-based preparations, higher antibody titers may be observed among patients with monoclonal gammopathies after receiving the mRNA-1273 than the BNT162b2 vaccine [118]. Likewise, in the study by Greenberger et al., the vaccination with mRNA-1273 was associated with greater odds of seropositivity status compared with BNT162b2, independent of multiple confounders, including the type of hematologic malignancy [122]. Although there is a limited number of studies to address specific vaccines among hematologic patients and available reports vary with respect to participant composition and studied circumstances, there were no significant differences in seropositivity rates across the different available vaccine platforms according to a recent meta-analysis [120]. Subsequently, although it does not seem justified based on the current data to prioritize one vaccine platform over another for its use among hematologic patients, more information in hematologic populations according to specific underlying diagnosis and treatment is needed to optimize vaccination strategies. In any case, adherence to a timely vaccination schedule irrespective of a specific platform for all affected patients is strongly warranted.

It should be noted that most available data regarding vaccine immunogenicity have been based on induced neutralizing antibody titers. Undoubtfully, even among individuals who show suboptimal or even negative antibody levels following vaccination or SARS-CoV-2 infection, a certain cellular immunity-mediated protection against symptomatic infection and severe disease may be assumed. However, based on available evidence, it seems likely that neutralizing antibody responses themselves correlate satisfactorily with the probability of SARS-CoV-2 infection [127,128].

At least a third (booster) vaccine dose is recommended in most countries for individuals who have successfully undergone a full vaccination course to overcome the waning of immunity and prevent breakthrough infections, especially by new variants. Immunocompromised individuals are to be prioritized in this strategy, while local guidelines occasionally advise in favor of a second booster (fourth) dose for these patients [129], despite the extremely scarce currently available evidence to support the effectiveness of this recommendation [130,131]. Patients with hematologic malignancy would fall into this category of high-risk patients. Available data on booster dosing demonstrate that despite the fact that a third dose of BNT162b2 strengthens humoral immunity among antibody-positive hematologic patients, it does not alter the serological status among those that remained seronegative despite prior immunization; nevertheless, it does seem to augment T cell-mediated cellular immunity irrespective of antibody status [132], thus, demonstrating a potential benefit of booster immunization even among those with a prior insufficient humoral response.

6. Blood Product Transfusion in the Era of COVID-19

Individuals with hematologic malignancies constitute a pool of patients with urgent and frequent dependency on the transfusion of blood products. Voluminal requirements greatly vary depending on underlying diagnosis, type of treatment and local standard operating procedures of hematology oncology units; nonetheless, transfusion of erythrocytes and/or platelets is frequently necessary in the setting of active cytotoxic therapy, while in the case of certain background diagnoses (e.g., particularly low-risk MDS), erythrocyte and/or platelet transfusions constitute the core of long-term maintenance therapy [133].

Concerns regarding the potential infectivity of blood units from asymptomatic or pre-symptomatic infected donors originate from the ascertainment of viral RNAemia in hospitalized patients in some reports, although this finding is not universal among available studies [134]. Nevertheless, in a broad screening of plasma minipools from 258,000 blood donations between March and September 2020 in the US, positive SARS-CoV-2 PCRs were remarkably uncommon and generally in very low titers [134]. Real-world data from cases of blood product transfusion donated by pre-symptomatic infected patients also support the notion that even though transfusion as a mode of SARS-CoV-2 transmission may be theoretically plausible, it is extremely rare [135–139].

Particularly during the initial outbreak of the pandemic, but also during every subsequent accelerated phase leading to a new surge in infections, there was a visible danger of blood supply shortages. Shortages may develop depending on geographical region, hospital level of care and resource availability as a result of reduced donation rates due to a fear of donors being in contact with healthcare services, attending transfusions, physician concerns in the face of the presence of COVID-19-suspicious donor symptoms, increased demand for blood products to cover the needs of hospitalized COVID-19 patients, or an overall reassignment of personnel- and material-related resources to counter the pandemic waves. In the case of a development of extreme shortages, it is likely that updated guidelines by competent authorities would be necessary regarding a re-evaluation of transfusion intervals and/or thresholds [140,141] with the aim of rationalizing the use of available resources.

Despite initial concerns [141,142], and even though the collective volume of blood donations and success of donor recruitment campaigns reduced during the first pandemic waves [143–146], this was counterbalanced by a reduction in blood product demand, chiefly through a reduction in elective surgical procedures and medical transfusions [147]. Although some blood product supply shortage did develop in some regions [148,149], there is no available evidence that this phenomenon had a significant impact on planned or acute transfusions among patients with hematologic disease [143].

Nevertheless, the degree of shortages and resulting initial uncertainties brought about by COVID-19 have provided further reasons for the reappraisal and optimization of current transfusion strategies. This would concern not only the regular transfusion programs among hematologic patients, but also the transfusions for practically any medical indication in a variety of, at least non-acute, circumstances. With respect to chronic hematologic diseases, caution should be taken in the detection of reversible causes of anemia, such as iron, folic acid, or vitamin B12 deficiency, as well as their treatment through adequate oral or parenteral substitution. Furthermore, the indications for erythropoietin therapy should be meticulously followed or even broadened in the face of emerging new evidence in the long term, since its administration may reduce volume requirements in transfusion-dependent patients [150]. Importantly, lower transfusion thresholds than commonly utilized seem to be safe and well-tolerated among asymptomatic patients [151], thus, restrictive rather than liberal transfusion strategies may be preferred in order to optimally portion erythrocyte supplies. A similar strategy could also apply for stable, non-bleeding patients with chronic thrombocytopenia dependent on thrombocyte transfusions. Furthermore, accessory measures could apply to transfusions for surgical indications, such as the correction of disorders of hemostasis prior to elective surgical procedures, intra- or postoperative use of coagulation factor concentrates, antifibrinolytic agents such as tranexamic acid and utilization of autologous blood transfusion where indicated. Lastly, frequency and volume of blood draws in blood supply storage should be limited to the absolute minimum that may affect clinical decision making, both in the acute and chronic setting.

7. Medical Therapy against COVID-19 among Individuals with Hematologic Malignancies

Although broadly applied vaccination programs have been and continue to constitute the mainstay of strategies to counter the COVID-19 pandemic, there has been a continuing worldwide effort for the development of drug therapies against the SARS-CoV-2 infection, either through the development of new agents or through repurposing already available drugs marketed for other indications [152,153]. Certain national recommendations for the treatment of the SARS-CoV-2 infection according to its severity take into account the comorbidity background of affected patients to guide and possibly escalate medical management [154,155]. Accordingly, patients with hematologic malignancies, particularly those receiving specific therapies, among others, are to be prioritized under the conditions of logistical or supply constraints which may preclude the universal use of anti-SARS-CoV-2 therapies; these patients are at an increased risk of severe disease, as well as they are not able to mount an inadequate immune response after vaccination [154].

The already available and constantly evolving body of relevant evidence contributes to the World Health Organization's living guideline on drugs for COVID-19 [156]. In this guideline, recommendations for medical therapy are formed based on evidence from clinical studies and are escalated according to disease severity (characterized based on clinical criteria as mild, severe or critical). Although there is no specific reference to hematologic cancers or any other specific patient group for that matter, certain recommendations are shaped based on a perceived underlying higher risk for hospitalization based on coexisting medical conditions, a case that arguably also concerns patients with HMs. According to the living guideline of the World Health Organization, as of May 2022, viral protease inhibitors Nirmatrelvir/Ritonavir and conditionally Molnupiravir, monoclonal antibodies such as Sotrovimab and Casirivimab/Imdevimab, and Remdesivir are recommended therapies for patients with non-severe disease; for those with severe or critical COVID-19, corticosteroids, Janus kinase inhibitor Baricitinib, interleukin-6 inhibitors and conditionally Casirivimab/Imdevimab are indicated [156]. In contrast, the use of ivermectin or convalescent plasma outside the context of clinical trials are now discouraged [156].

In the absence of specific recommendations for this population, COVID-19 therapy in hematologic cancer patients is to be guided based on available general recommendations. However, there are points that pertain to the unique characteristics of these patients that may ought to be taken into account, including current and cumulative glucocorticoid doses, presence of hypogammaglobulinemia, perceived degree of immune suppression due to the illness or its therapy, cytopenic status due to the underlying condition or the risk of cytopenia from certain COVID-19 medical treatments (e.g., Remdesivir, Molnupiravir). Various therapies or combinations have been successfully used among hematologic patients [157–160]. In a series of 313 patients with hematologic malignancies from Israel, Remdesivir administration was associated with decreased mortality [65]. Furthermore, in a subgroup of 216 patients with very severe disease from an initial sample of 367 pediatric and adult patients with hematologic malignancies, azithromycin and corticosteroid administration were associated with lower 45-day mortality (OR 0.42 (95% CI 0.2–0.89) and 0.31 (0.11–0.87), respectively). In addition, three cohort studies have demonstrated potential benefits including duration of hospitalization, course severity and survival after administration of convalescent plasma in patients with hematologic malignancies [161–163]. In the largest of those, Thomson et al. investigated a sample of 966 hospitalized hemato-oncologic patients, 143 of whom received convalescent plasma therapy. Even after adjustment for confounders or propensity score matching, 30-day mortality was lower among receivers (HRs 0.60 (0.37–0.97) and 0.52 (0.29–0.92), respectively), while the effects were even more pronounced among patients admitted to the ICU or receiving mechanical ventilation (HRs 0.40 (0.20–0.80) and 0.32 (0.14–0.72), respectively) [163]. These findings contradict the neutral results of convalescent plasma therapy in other populations, most strikingly in the Randomized Evaluation of COVID-19 Therapy (RECOVERY) trial [164]. Although limited by their non-randomized design, cohort studies should be taken into account, and it could be postulated that this discrepancy may reflect the benefit of exogenous immunoglobulin administration in the setting of hypogammaglobulinemia, which often occurs as a result of certain hematologic malignancies such as CLL or MM or their therapies [165].

Despite scarce evidence regarding potential benefits from specific therapies in hemato-oncologic patients, most available recommendations do not offer specific guidance for the treatment of the SARS-CoV-2 infection in this patient group. Nevertheless, given the strongly immune-suppressing nature of many of the conditions themselves or their treatments, additional caution is warranted regarding the use of therapies against COVID-19 with further immune-modulating modes of action (i.e., corticosteroids, intereukin-6 antagonists, interleukin-1 antagonists-anakinra [166]).

8. Influence of the COVID-19 Pandemic on the Treatment of Malignant Hematologic Disease

The outbreak of COVID-19 introduced significant challenges for the care of patients with actively managed hematologic malignancies. Particularly during the initial stages of the pandemic, uncertainties with respect to factors that predispose people to SARS-CoV-2 acquisition and severe course, as well as the lack of effective treatments and vaccines, were added to concerns arising from the frail immune and general poor clinical condition of a large proportion of acutely treated hematologic patients. These may confer increased susceptibility to respiratory viral infections, whereas lymphopenia, as well as specific modes of therapy such as purine analogs anti-CD20 or CD52 and allogeneic HSCT, may pose a particularly increased risk [167]. Additionally, a common adverse event of CAR T-cell therapy is the cytokine release syndrome, attributed to the abrupt secretion of inflammatory mediators by CAR T cells and other cell types [168]. The presence of a similar physiological state of cytokine hypersecretion has been reported to predispose people to a severe SARS-CoV-2 infection course [169]. Interestingly, therapy with tocilizumab, which is an integral component of COVID-19 therapeutic regimens, is also used to treat CAR T cell-related cytokine release syndrome [170].

These concerns, among others, led to initial considerations of delaying non-urgent hematologic malignancy treatment, including autologous HSCT among standard-risk individuals, in order to avoid exposing patients not only to the risks of therapy, but also to reduce the frequency of non-urgent contacts with the healthcare system for treatment and monitoring blood draws [171]. A similar approach has been generally adopted and generalized by numerous national and international hematologic societies. Guidelines vary according to issuing authorities and on the basis of hematologic diagnosis.

A detailed overview of the sum of specific treatment recommendations in the frame of COVID-19 is beyond the scope of the current review. Testing for SARS-CoV-2 and, occasionally, chest computed tomography, is indicated for patients before the initiation of each therapy cycle, in donors and recipients before HSCT as well as in the presence of COVID-19-suspicious clinical symptoms [172–175]. A general pattern of treatment initiation or continuation without delay exists for patients who are considered high risk/high priority within or among specific diagnoses. This also includes allogenic HSCT when carried out with curative intent in an urgent indication (e.g., high-risk ALL or AML [173,175]). Autologous SCT may be delayed for no longer than 8 weeks in less urgent clinical settings (e.g., in eligible MM patients [175,176]). Where possible, highly immunosuppressive alternatives (e.g., schemes including bendamustine) should be avoided [173], and where possible, the lowest effective doses of agents, which may induce aplasia (e.g., methotrexate, cytarabine), should be administered [173]. Appropriate schemes that can be administered in outpatient settings may be preferred [173,175].

Preventive measures of SARS-CoV-2 acquisition should be strictly adhered to [172]. An occurrence of SARS-CoV-2 infection amidst active treatment generally mandates a pause of systemic anticancer therapy and/or delay of allogeneic HSCT until laboratory resolution (negative PCR test) [173,175], although there are isolated reports of continued modified systemic treatment despite SARS-CoV-2 infection, albeit of noncritical severity [177]. As is the case with any deviation from hematologic cancer treatment protocols, this decision should be weighed against the risk of therapy delay on a case-by-case basis [176]. Non-systemic antineoplastic administration (such as intrathecal chemotherapy) or non-cytotoxic, non-immunosuppressive systemic therapies such as tyrosine kinase inhibitors may be continued [173]. Evidently, the decision to administer any kind of anticancer treatment during the course of active COVID-19 warrants additional caution for the avoidance of interactions with anti-SARS-CoV-2 therapies and subsequent drug-related adverse events [173].

Despite general recommendations and development of guidelines that cover a broad range of clinical scenarios, the field of hematologic cancer therapy during the pandemic unavoidably includes a highly individualized component regarding clinical decision-making. A great degree of clinical readiness and experience is needed from the side of involved clinicians, in conjunction with adherence to local standard operating procedures and firm cooperation with hygiene and infectious disease specialists.

9. Lifestyle Changes (Diet and Exercise) and Cancer Survivorship in the Era of the COVID-19 Pandemic

Several studies have demonstrated a shift towards healthier behavior after cancer diagnosis or treatment [178–183]. Whereas the majority of evidence on lifestyle changes after cancer diagnosis or treatment has been drawn from female breast cancer survivor cohorts [180,183,184], several studies have focused on hematologic malignancies [180,185–188]. A recent cross-sectional study demonstrated that hematologic malignancy survivors exhibit a significant reduction in smoking behavior, with many patients quitting and nearly all patients limiting their smoking behavior after cancer diagnosis [180]. The researchers were not able to detect a significant change in exercise or dietary habits after diagnosis [180]. High post-diagnosis physical activity was associated with lower mortality among hematologic cancer survivors in a large retrospective analysis of 5182 patients [187]. Specifically, in a multivariate analysis including all hematologic cancer survivors, physical activity after diagnosis yielded an all-cause mortality hazard ratio of 0.61 (95% CI: 0.50–0.74), and the association remained significant in the subgroups of NHL, myeloma and leukemia survivors, respectively. A secondary analysis of a randomized controlled trial in allogeneic stem cell transplant patients compared the survival outcomes between patients assigned to an exercise intervention or a control group [180]. Total mortality (TM) but not non-relapse mortality (NRM) risk was reduced among the 103 allogeneic stem cell transplant patients with a combination of endurance and resistance exercise (TM: exercise vs. control group: 12.0 vs. 28.3%, $p = 0.03$) over a 2-year follow-up period. In a randomized controlled setting, the Healthy Exercise for Lymphoma Patients (HELP) trial randomized 122 lymphoma patients to either supervised aerobic training or no exercise [185]. The trial analysis did not detect a positive effect after 12 weeks of exercise on the progression-free survival of 122 lymphoma patients during a 61-month follow-up period. In a recent clinical trial, the researchers hypothesized that caloric restriction and increased exercise would not only decrease fat mass but would also lead to reduced post-induction minimal residual disease in patients with B-cell acute lymphoblastic leukemia [186]. The intervention consisted of caloric deficits of $\geq 20\%$ during induction, reduced fat intake, reduced glycemic load, and increased exercise; this led to a reduction in fat gain in the overweight and obese patients, and most importantly, it reduced minimal residual disease. Nevertheless, this single-arm intervention study utilized historical controls for comparative purposes and prospective randomized trials are eagerly needed for the validation of these findings.

In conclusion, several studies suggest that high physical activity levels are of potential benefit to the survivors of hematologic malignancies. However, physical activity levels can be affected by the overall condition of the patient, and the intensity of the treatment regimen or treatment-related complications; these factors can also directly affect survival outcomes. Larger, well-controlled clinical trials are required to unravel the potential causal relationship between behavioral changes and long-term outcomes in hematologic malignancy survivors.

The recently worldwide-imposed lockdowns during the COVID-19 pandemic had a dramatic impact on the lifestyle of the general population, including cancer survivors. An exploratory study in Northern Ireland reported the effects of the pandemic on several behavioral aspects of cancer survivors during the COVID-19 pandemic [189]. Interestingly, 52% of the patients reported reduced physical activity during restrictions, owing to isolation, declining health, lack of access to exercise facilities and motivation to exercise. Whereas 4% of participants had reported no physical activity before the pandemic, this number increased to 21% during the COVID-19 restrictions. In another observational study in France, 64% of the cancer survivors reported reduced physical activity and increased screen time during the COVID-19 lockdowns [190]. On the other hand, researchers from Italy effectively utilized tracker-based counselling and live-web exercise to engage breast cancer survivors in exercise and improve their sleep quality during the COVID-19 lockdowns [191]. The adherence of the participants to the exercise interventions, as well as the effectiveness of these programs in improving several sleep parameters, highlight the emerging value of modern technology in promoting the well-being of cancer survivors.

The off-label use of over-the-counter dietary supplements and nutraceuticals is highly prevalent among patients with cancer, especially in hematologic malignancies [192]; nonetheless, there is currently no solid evidence to justify this practice [178,193]. Among the available supplements, vitamin D has gathered interest for its potential benefits in hematologic cancer patients, considering the high deficiency prevalence and association with adverse prognosis in this population [194]. Interestingly, a likely multi-level relationship also exists between vitamin D deficiency and increased body adiposity, although the value of exogenous supplementation in obesity outcomes remains controversial [193]. Regarding COVID-19 outcomes, data on the role of vitamin D deficiency as a risk factor for adverse outcomes are equivocal, while exogenous supplementation, although safe, has not provided concrete evidence towards a clear benefit [195].

10. Conclusions and Perspectives

It is likely that multiple factors related to obesity, hematologic malignancy or their mutual pathogenetic attributes predispose people to a more adverse SARS-CoV-2 infection prognosis, thus, forming a complex intercorrelated relationship. Moreover, the co-existence of both obesity and hematologic abnormalities in the frame of the SARS-CoV-2 infection may theoretically further adversely affect prognosis through independent risk factors representative of each condition. In any case, the societal and health care system-related adaptations during the course of the pandemic brought about a variety of obstacles pertinent to the diagnosis, timely active treatment, and chronic management of patients with hematologic cancers, given the unique inherent and therapeutical features of this morbidity spectrum.

Unfortunately, it is likely that the pandemic may have already taken its toll on this vulnerable patient group; recent global-scale data indicate that they may have delayed or missed MM diagnoses in the early COVID-19 era compared with the previous year, in conjunction with a decreased survival among newly diagnosed cases (HR 0.61, 0.38–0.81 for diagnoses in 2020 compared with 2019) [196].

The field of hemato-oncology has already overcome the initial blow to a great degree and adjusted to the new reality brought forward by COVID-19. Nonetheless, there is a need for continued appraisal and update of numerous aspects of hematologic malignancy management. Moreover, the contribution of obesity and its severity as an additional risk factor for severe COVID-19 among those with hematologic malignancies has not yet been investigated. Additionally, other clinical, laboratory and treatment-related factors predisposing to severe disease should be identified to effectively stratify patients in susceptibility risk groups. Optimal timing of hemato-oncologic therapy initiation, post-treatment follow-up and timely therapeutical planning, including allogeneic HSCT in case of infections that emerge during active medical therapy, also need to be determined. Likewise, more evidence is needed to establish a potential superior efficacy of specific vaccine types among patients with hematologic cancer with or without obesity, as well as an effective vaccination schedule in the long term. Lastly, more data are needed regarding the optimal medical management of SARS-CoV-2 infections in this patient group, under the consideration of respective diagnoses and treatments which may individually affect the natural history of COVID-19.

Hopefully, all the above-mentioned parameters will help establish uniform international recommendations for hemato-oncologic management during and after the COVID-19 era. These could, in turn, be utilized in shaping national and regional guidelines considering the different aspects and unique challenges of this field.

Author Contributions: The corresponding author states that all authors meet authorship criteria and that no others meeting the criteria have been omitted. D.T. was involved in the literature research, writing of the draft, and editing of the final version. N.N.-A. created Figure 1 and was involved in writing and editing the final manuscript version. N.S. contributed to the literature research and writing of the manuscript. F.M. was involved in reviewing and editing the manuscript. M.D. conceived the idea and was involved in the literature research, writing and editing of the manuscript. All authors have read and agreed to the published version of the manuscript.

Funding: This research did not receive any specific grant from funding agencies in the public, commercial, or not-for-profit sectors.

Conflicts of Interest: The authors declare no conflict of interest.

References

1. Chudasama, Y.V.; Gillies, C.L.; Zaccardi, F.; Coles, B.; Davies, M.J.; Seidu, S.; Khunti, K. Impact of COVID-19 on routine care for chronic diseases: A global survey of views from healthcare professionals. *Diabetes Metab. Syndr.* **2020**, *14*, 965–967. [CrossRef] [PubMed]
2. Fekadu, G.; Bekele, F.; Tolossa, T.; Fetensa, G.; Turi, E.; Getachew, M.; Abdisa, E.; Assefa, L.; Afeta, M.; Demisew, W.; et al. Impact of COVID-19 pandemic on chronic diseases care follow-up and current perspectives in low resource settings: A narrative review. *Int. J. Physiol. Pathophysiol. Pharmacol.* **2021**, *13*, 86–93. [PubMed]
3. Dalamaga, M.; Christodoulatos, G.S.; Karampela, I.; Vallianou, N.; Apovian, C.M. Understanding the Co-Epidemic of Obesity and COVID-19: Current Evidence, Comparison with Previous Epidemics, Mechanisms, and Preventive and Therapeutic Perspectives. *Curr. Obes. Rep.* **2021**, *10*, 214–243. [CrossRef] [PubMed]
4. He, W.; Chen, L.; Chen, L.; Yuan, G.; Fang, Y.; Chen, W.; Wu, D.; Liang, B.; Lu, X.; Ma, Y.; et al. COVID-19 in persons with haematological cancers. *Leukemia* **2020**, *34*, 1637–1645. [CrossRef]
5. Huang, Y.; Lu, Y.; Huang, Y.M.; Wang, M.; Ling, W.; Sui, Y.; Zhao, H.L. Obesity in patients with COVID-19: A systematic review and meta-analysis. *Metabolism* **2020**, *113*, 154378. [CrossRef]
6. Vallianou, N.G.; Evangelopoulos, A.; Kounatidis, D.; Stratigou, T.; Christodoulatos, G.S.; Karampela, I.; Dalamaga, M. Diabetes Mellitus and SARS-CoV-2 Infection: Pathophysiologic Mechanisms and Implications in Management. *Curr. Diabetes Rev.* **2021**, *17*, e123120189797. [CrossRef]
7. Avgerinos, K.I.; Spyrou, N.; Mantzoros, C.S.; Dalamaga, M. Obesity and cancer risk: Emerging biological mechanisms and perspectives. *Metabolism* **2019**, *92*, 121–135. [CrossRef]
8. Dalamaga, M.; Christodoulatos, G.S. Adiponectin as a biomarker linking obesity and adiposopathy to hematologic malignancies. *Horm. Mol. Biol. Clin. Investig.* **2015**, *23*, 5–20. [CrossRef]
9. Lichtman, M.A. Obesity and the risk for a hematological malignancy: Leukemia, lymphoma, or myeloma. *Oncologist* **2010**, *15*, 1083–1101. [CrossRef]
10. Larsson, S.C.; Wolk, A. Body mass index and risk of non-Hodgkin's and Hodgkin's lymphoma: A meta-analysis of prospective studies. *Eur. J. Cancer* **2011**, *47*, 2422–2430. [CrossRef]
11. Strongman, H.; Brown, A.; Smeeth, L.; Bhaskaran, K. Body mass index and Hodgkin's lymphoma: UK population-based cohort study of 5.8 million individuals. *Br. J. Cancer* **2019**, *120*, 768–770. [CrossRef] [PubMed]
12. Larsson, S.C.; Wolk, A. Overweight and obesity and incidence of leukemia: A meta-analysis of cohort studies. *Int. J. Cancer* **2008**, *122*, 1418–1421. [CrossRef] [PubMed]
13. Mazzarella, L.; Botteri, E.; Matthews, A.; Gatti, E.; Di Salvatore, D.; Bagnardi, V.; Breccia, M.; Montesinos, P.; Bernal, T.; Gil, C.; et al. Obesity is a risk factor for acute promyelocytic leukemia: Evidence from population and cross-sectional studies and correlation with FLT3 mutations and polyunsaturated fatty acid metabolism. *Haematologica* **2020**, *105*, 1559–1566. [CrossRef] [PubMed]
14. Georgakopoulou, R.; Andrikopoulou, A.; Sergentanis, T.N.; Fiste, O.; Zagouri, F.; Gavriatopoulou, M.; Psaltopoulou, T.; Kastritis, E.; Terpos, E.; Dimopoulos, M.A. Overweight/Obesity and Monoclonal Gammapathy of Undetermined Significance. *Clin. Lymphoma Myeloma Leuk.* **2021**, *21*, 361–367. [CrossRef]
15. Landgren, O.; Rajkumar, S.V.; Pfeiffer, R.M.; Kyle, R.A.; Katzmann, J.A.; Dispenzieri, A.; Cai, Q.; Goldin, L.R.; Caporaso, N.E.; Fraumeni, J.F.; et al. Obesity is associated with an increased risk of monoclonal gammopathy of undetermined significance among black and white women. *Blood* **2010**, *116*, 1056–1059. [CrossRef]
16. Thordardottir, M.; Lindqvist, E.K.; Lund, S.H.; Costello, R.; Burton, D.; Korde, N.; Mailankody, S.; Eiriksdottir, G.; Launer, L.J.; Gudnason, V.; et al. Obesity and risk of monoclonal gammopathy of undetermined significance and progression to multiple myeloma: A population-based study. *Blood Adv.* **2017**, *1*, 2186–2192. [CrossRef]
17. Pylypchuk, R.D.; Schouten, L.J.; Goldbohm, R.A.; Schouten, H.C.; van den Brandt, P.A. Body mass index, height, and risk of lymphatic malignancies: A prospective cohort study. *Am. J. Epidemiol.* **2009**, *170*, 297–307. [CrossRef]
18. Calle, E.E.; Rodriguez, C.; Walker-Thurmond, K.; Thun, M.J. Overweight, obesity, and mortality from cancer in a prospectively studied cohort of U.S. adults. *N. Engl. J. Med.* **2003**, *348*, 1625–1638. [CrossRef]
19. Kyrgiou, M.; Kalliala, I.; Markozannes, G.; Gunter, M.J.; Paraskevaidis, E.; Gabra, H.; Martin-Hirsch, P.; Tsilidis, K.K. Adiposity and cancer at major anatomical sites: Umbrella review of the literature. *BMJ* **2017**, *356*, j477. [CrossRef]
20. Bhaskaran, K.; Douglas, I.; Forbes, H.; dos-Santos-Silva, I.; Leon, D.A.; Smeeth, L. Body-mass index and risk of 22 specific cancers: A population-based cohort study of 5.24 million UK adults. *Lancet* **2014**, *384*, 755–765. [CrossRef]
21. Ma, X.; Lim, U.; Park, Y.; Mayne, S.T.; Wang, R.; Hartge, P.; Hollenbeck, A.R.; Schatzkin, A. Obesity, lifestyle factors, and risk of myelodysplastic syndromes in a large US cohort. *Am. J. Epidemiol.* **2009**, *169*, 1492–1499. [CrossRef] [PubMed]
22. Schwabkey, Z.; Al Ali, N.; Sallman, D.; Kuykendall, A.; Talati, C.; Sweet, K.; Lancet, J.; Padron, E.; Komrokji, R. Impact of obesity on survival of patients with myelodysplastic syndromes. *Hematology* **2021**, *26*, 393–397. [CrossRef] [PubMed]
23. Leiba, A.; Duek, A.; Afek, A.; Derazne, E.; Leiba, M. Obesity and related risk of myeloproliferative neoplasms among israeli adolescents. *Obesity* **2017**, *25*, 1187–1190. [CrossRef] [PubMed]
24. Strom, S.S.; Yamamura, Y.; Kantarijian, H.M.; Cortes-Franco, J.E. Obesity, weight gain, and risk of chronic myeloid leukemia. *Cancer Epidemiol. Biomark. Prev.* **2009**, *18*, 1501–1506. [CrossRef] [PubMed]

25. Duncombe, A.S.; Anderson, L.A.; James, G.; de Vocht, F.; Fritschi, L.; Mesa, R.; Clarke, M.; McMullin, M.F. Modifiable Lifestyle and Medical Risk Factors Associated With Myeloproliferative Neoplasms. *Hemasphere* **2020**, *4*, e327. [CrossRef]
26. Leal, A.D.; Thompson, C.A.; Wang, A.H.; Vierkant, R.A.; Habermann, T.M.; Ross, J.A.; Mesa, R.A.; Virnig, B.A.; Cerhan, J.R. Anthropometric, medical history and lifestyle risk factors for myeloproliferative neoplasms in the Iowa Women's Health Study cohort. *Int. J. Cancer* **2014**, *134*, 1741–1750. [CrossRef]
27. Larsson, S.C.; Wolk, A. Obesity and risk of non-Hodgkin's lymphoma: A meta-analysis. *Int. J. Cancer* **2007**, *121*, 1564–1570. [CrossRef]
28. Willett, E.V.; Morton, L.M.; Hartge, P.; Becker, N.; Bernstein, L.; Boffetta, P.; Bracci, P.; Cerhan, J.; Chiu, B.C.; Cocco, P.; et al. Non-Hodgkin lymphoma and obesity: A pooled analysis from the InterLymph Consortium. *Int. J. Cancer* **2008**, *122*, 2062–2070. [CrossRef]
29. Carda, J.P.; Santos, L.; Mariz, J.M.; Monteiro, P.; Goncalves, H.M.; Raposo, J.; Gomes da Silva, M. Management of ibrutinib treatment in patients with B-cell malignancies: Clinical practice in Portugal and multidisciplinary recommendations. *Hematology* **2021**, *26*, 785–798. [CrossRef]
30. Da Cunha Junior, A.D.; Zanette, D.L.; Pericole, F.V.; Olalla Saad, S.T.; Barreto Campello Carvalheira, J. Obesity as a Possible Risk Factor for Progression from Monoclonal Gammopathy of Undetermined Significance Progression into Multiple Myeloma: Could Myeloma Be Prevented with Metformin Treatment? *Adv. Hematol.* **2021**, *2021*, 6615684. [CrossRef]
31. Bruno, D.S.; Berger, N.A. Impact of bariatric surgery on cancer risk reduction. *Ann. Transl. Med.* **2020**, *8*, S13. [CrossRef] [PubMed]
32. Look, A.R.G.; Yeh, H.C.; Bantle, J.P.; Cassidy-Begay, M.; Blackburn, G.; Bray, G.A.; Byers, T.; Clark, J.M.; Coday, M.; Egan, C.; et al. Intensive Weight Loss Intervention and Cancer Risk in Adults with Type 2 Diabetes: Analysis of the Look AHEAD Randomized Clinical Trial. *Obesity* **2020**, *28*, 1678–1686. [CrossRef]
33. Tao, W.; Santoni, G.; von Euler-Chelpin, M.; Ljung, R.; Lynge, E.; Pukkala, E.; Ness-Jensen, E.; Romundstad, P.; Tryggvadottir, L.; Lagergren, J. Cancer Risk After Bariatric Surgery in a Cohort Study from the Five Nordic Countries. *Obes. Surg.* **2020**, *30*, 3761–3767. [CrossRef] [PubMed]
34. Gurunathan, U.; Myles, P.S. Limitations of body mass index as an obesity measure of perioperative risk. *Br. J. Anaesth.* **2016**, *116*, 319–321. [CrossRef]
35. Liu, J.; Tsilingiris, D.; Dalamaga, M. The non-linear relationship between muscle mass and BMI calls into question the use of BMI as a major criterion for eligibility for bariatric surgery. *Metabol. Open* **2022**, *13*, 100164. [CrossRef]
36. Hagstrom, H.; Andreasson, A.; Carlsson, A.C.; Jerkeman, M.; Carlsten, M. Body composition measurements and risk of hematological malignancies: A population-based cohort study during 20 years of follow-up. *PLoS ONE* **2018**, *13*, e0202651. [CrossRef]
37. Dalamaga, M.; Crotty, B.H.; Fargnoli, J.; Papadavid, E.; Lekka, A.; Triantafilli, M.; Karmaniolas, K.; Migdalis, I.; Dionyssiou-Asteriou, A.; Mantzoros, C.S. B-cell chronic lymphocytic leukemia risk in association with serum leptin and adiponectin: A case-control study in Greece. *Cancer Causes Control* **2010**, *21*, 1451–1459. [CrossRef]
38. Dalamaga, M.; Karmaniolas, K.; Chamberland, J.; Nikolaidou, A.; Lekka, A.; Dionyssiou-Asteriou, A.; Mantzoros, C.S. Higher fetuin-A, lower adiponectin and free leptin levels mediate effects of excess body weight on insulin resistance and risk for myelodysplastic syndrome. *Metabolism* **2013**, *62*, 1830–1839. [CrossRef]
39. Dalamaga, M.; Karmaniolas, K.; Lekka, A.; Antonakos, G.; Thrasyvoulides, A.; Papadavid, E.; Spanos, N.; Dionyssiou-Asteriou, A. Platelet markers correlate with glycemic indices in diabetic, but not diabetic-myelodysplastic patients with normal platelet count. *Dis. Markers* **2010**, *29*, 55–61. [CrossRef]
40. Dalamaga, M.; Karmaniolas, K.; Matekovits, A.; Migdalis, I.; Papadavid, E. Cutaneous manifestations in relation to immunologic parameters in a cohort of primary myelodysplastic syndrome patients. *J. Eur. Acad. Dermatol. Venereol.* **2008**, *22*, 543–548. [CrossRef]
41. Dalamaga, M.; Karmaniolas, K.; Nikolaidou, A.; Chamberland, J.; Hsi, A.; Dionyssiou-Asteriou, A.; Mantzoros, C.S. Adiponectin and resistin are associated with risk for myelodysplastic syndrome, independently from the insulin-like growth factor-I (IGF-I) system. *Eur. J. Cancer* **2008**, *44*, 1744–1753. [CrossRef]
42. Dalamaga, M.; Karmaniolas, K.; Panagiotou, A.; Hsi, A.; Chamberland, J.; Dimas, C.; Lekka, A.; Mantzoros, C.S. Low circulating adiponectin and resistin, but not leptin, levels are associated with multiple myeloma risk: A case-control study. *Cancer Causes Control* **2009**, *20*, 193–199. [CrossRef] [PubMed]
43. Dalamaga, M.; Karmaniolas, K.; Papadavid, E.; Pelecanos, N.; Migdalis, I. Association of thyroid disease and thyroid autoimmunity with multiple myeloma risk: A case-control study. *Leuk. Lymphoma* **2008**, *49*, 1545–1552. [CrossRef] [PubMed]
44. Dalamaga, M.; Nikolaidou, A.; Karmaniolas, K.; Hsi, A.; Chamberland, J.; Dionyssiou-Asteriou, A.; Mantzoros, C.S. Circulating adiponectin and leptin in relation to myelodysplastic syndrome: A case-control study. *Oncology* **2007**, *73*, 26–32. [CrossRef] [PubMed]
45. Dalamaga, M.; Polyzos, S.A.; Karmaniolas, K.; Chamberland, J.; Lekka, A.; Triantafilli, M.; Migdalis, I.; Papadavid, E.; Mantzoros, C.S. Fetuin-A levels and free leptin index are reduced in patients with chronic lymphocytic leukemia: A hospital-based case-control study. *Leuk. Lymphoma* **2016**, *57*, 577–584. [CrossRef]
46. Li, B.; Jones, L.L.; Geiger, T.L. IL-6 Promotes T Cell Proliferation and Expansion under Inflammatory Conditions in Association with Low-Level RORgammat Expression. *J. Immunol.* **2018**, *201*, 2934–2946. [CrossRef]

47. Pronk, C.J.; Veiby, O.P.; Bryder, D.; Jacobsen, S.E. Tumor necrosis factor restricts hematopoietic stem cell activity in mice: Involvement of two distinct receptors. *J. Exp. Med.* **2011**, *208*, 1563–1570. [CrossRef]
48. Schuettpelz, L.G.; Link, D.C. Regulation of hematopoietic stem cell activity by inflammation. *Front. Immunol.* **2013**, *4*, 204. [CrossRef]
49. Tie, R.; Li, H.; Cai, S.; Liang, Z.; Shan, W.; Wang, B.; Tan, Y.; Zheng, W.; Huang, H. Interleukin-6 signaling regulates hematopoietic stem cell emergence. *Exp. Mol. Med.* **2019**, *51*, 1–12. [CrossRef]
50. Yamashita, M.; Passegue, E. TNF-alpha Coordinates Hematopoietic Stem Cell Survival and Myeloid Regeneration. *Cell Stem Cell* **2019**, *25*, 357–372. [CrossRef]
51. Gainsford, T.; Willson, T.A.; Metcalf, D.; Handman, E.; McFarlane, C.; Ng, A.; Nicola, N.A.; Alexander, W.S.; Hilton, D.J. Leptin can induce proliferation, differentiation, and functional activation of hemopoietic cells. *Proc. Natl. Acad. Sci. USA* **1996**, *93*, 14564–14568. [CrossRef] [PubMed]
52. Papathanassoglou, E.; El-Haschimi, K.; Li, X.C.; Matarese, G.; Strom, T.; Mantzoros, C. Leptin receptor expression and signaling in lymphocytes: Kinetics during lymphocyte activation, role in lymphocyte survival, and response to high fat diet in mice. *J. Immunol.* **2006**, *176*, 7745–7752. [CrossRef] [PubMed]
53. Konopleva, M.; Mikhail, A.; Estrov, Z.; Zhao, S.; Harris, D.; Sanchez-Williams, G.; Kornblau, S.M.; Dong, J.; Kliche, K.O.; Jiang, S.; et al. Expression and function of leptin receptor isoforms in myeloid leukemia and myelodysplastic syndromes: Proliferative and anti-apoptotic activities. *Blood* **1999**, *93*, 1668–1676. [CrossRef] [PubMed]
54. Hofmann, J.N.; Birmann, B.M.; Teras, L.R.; Pfeiffer, R.M.; Wang, Y.; Albanes, D.; Baris, D.; Colditz, G.A.; De Roos, A.J.; Giles, G.G.; et al. Low Levels of Circulating Adiponectin Are Associated with Multiple Myeloma Risk in Overweight and Obese Individuals. *Cancer Res.* **2016**, *76*, 1935–1941. [CrossRef]
55. Tamara, A.; Tahapary, D.L. Obesity as a predictor for a poor prognosis of COVID-19: A systematic review. *Diabetes Metab. Syndr.* **2020**, *14*, 655–659. [CrossRef]
56. Tsilingiris, D.; Dalamaga, M.; Liu, J. SARS-CoV-2 adipose tissue infection and hyperglycemia: A further step towards the understanding of severe COVID-19. *Metabol. Open* **2022**, *13*, 100163. [CrossRef]
57. Battisti, S.; Pedone, C.; Napoli, N.; Russo, E.; Agnoletti, V.; Nigra, S.G.; Dengo, C.; Mughetti, M.; Conte, C.; Pozzilli, P.; et al. Computed Tomography Highlights Increased Visceral Adiposity Associated With Critical Illness in COVID-19. *Diabetes Care* **2020**, *43*, e129–e130. [CrossRef]
58. Chandarana, H.; Dane, B.; Mikheev, A.; Taffel, M.T.; Feng, Y.; Rusinek, H. Visceral adipose tissue in patients with COVID-19: Risk stratification for severity. *Abdom. Radiol.* **2021**, *46*, 818–825. [CrossRef]
59. Watanabe, M.; Risi, R.; Tuccinardi, D.; Baquero, C.J.; Manfrini, S.; Gnessi, L. Obesity and SARS-CoV-2: A population to safeguard. *Diabetes Metab. Res. Rev.* **2020**, *36*, e3325. [CrossRef]
60. Gao, M.; Piernas, C.; Astbury, N.M.; Hippisley-Cox, J.; O'Rahilly, S.; Aveyard, P.; Jebb, S.A. Associations between body-mass index and COVID-19 severity in 6.9 million people in England: A prospective, community-based, cohort study. *Lancet Diabetes Endocrinol.* **2021**, *9*, 350–359. [CrossRef]
61. Kompaniyets, L.; Goodman, A.B.; Belay, B.; Freedman, D.S.; Sucosky, M.S.; Lange, S.J.; Gundlapalli, A.V.; Boehmer, T.K.; Blanck, H.M. Body Mass Index and Risk for COVID-19-Related Hospitalization, Intensive Care Unit Admission, Invasive Mechanical Ventilation, and Death—United States, March-December 2020. *MMWR Morb. Mortal. Wkly. Rep.* **2021**, *70*, 355–361. [CrossRef]
62. Sjogren, L.; Stenberg, E.; Thuccani, M.; Martikainen, J.; Rylander, C.; Wallenius, V.; Olbers, T.; Kindblom, J.M. Impact of obesity on intensive care outcomes in patients with COVID-19 in Sweden-A cohort study. *PLoS ONE* **2021**, *16*, e0257891. [CrossRef] [PubMed]
63. Jain, A.; Nayak, L.; Kulkarni, U.P.; Mehra, N.; Yanamandra, U.; Kayal, S.; Damodar, S.; John, J.M.; Mehta, P.; Singh, S.; et al. Outcomes of patients with hematologic malignancies and COVID-19 from the Hematologic Cancer Registry of India. *Blood Cancer J.* **2022**, *12*, 2. [CrossRef]
64. Pagano, L.; Salmanton-Garcia, J.; Marchesi, F.; Busca, A.; Corradini, P.; Hoenigl, M.; Klimko, N.; Koehler, P.; Pagliuca, A.; Passamonti, F.; et al. COVID-19 infection in adult patients with hematological malignancies: A European Hematology Association Survey (EPICOVIDEHA). *J. Hematol. Oncol.* **2021**, *14*, 168. [CrossRef]
65. Levy, I.; Lavi, A.; Zimran, E.; Grisariu, S.; Aumann, S.; Itchaki, G.; Berger, T.; Raanani, P.; Harel, R.; Aviv, A.; et al. COVID-19 among patients with hematological malignancies: A national Israeli retrospective analysis with special emphasis on treatment and outcome. *Leuk. Lymphoma* **2021**, *62*, 3384–3393. [CrossRef] [PubMed]
66. Garcia-Suarez, J.; de la Cruz, J.; Cedillo, A.; Llamas, P.; Duarte, R.; Jimenez-Yuste, V.; Hernandez-Rivas, J.A.; Gil-Manso, R.; Kwon, M.; Sanchez-Godoy, P.; et al. Impact of hematologic malignancy and type of cancer therapy on COVID-19 severity and mortality: Lessons from a large population-based registry study. *J. Hematol. Oncol.* **2020**, *13*, 133. [CrossRef] [PubMed]
67. Vijenthira, A.; Gong, I.Y.; Fox, T.A.; Booth, S.; Cook, G.; Fattizzo, B.; Martin-Moro, F.; Razanamahery, J.; Riches, J.C.; Zwicker, J.; et al. Outcomes of patients with hematologic malignancies and COVID-19: A systematic review and meta-analysis of 3377 patients. *Blood* **2020**, *136*, 2881–2892. [CrossRef]
68. Wang, Q.; Berger, N.A.; Xu, R. When hematologic malignancies meet COVID-19 in the United States: Infections, death and disparities. *Blood Rev.* **2021**, *47*, 100775. [CrossRef]

69. Lee, L.Y.W.; Cazier, J.B.; Starkey, T.; Briggs, S.E.W.; Arnold, R.; Bisht, V.; Booth, S.; Campton, N.A.; Cheng, V.W.T.; Collins, G.; et al. COVID-19 prevalence and mortality in patients with cancer and the effect of primary tumour subtype and patient demographics: A prospective cohort study. *Lancet Oncol.* **2020**, *21*, 1309–1316. [CrossRef]
70. Williamson, E.J.; Walker, A.J.; Bhaskaran, K.; Bacon, S.; Bates, C.; Morton, C.E.; Curtis, H.J.; Mehrkar, A.; Evans, D.; Inglesby, P.; et al. Factors associated with COVID-19-related death using OpenSAFELY. *Nature* **2020**, *584*, 430–436. [CrossRef]
71. Romero Starke, K.; Reissig, D.; Petereit-Haack, G.; Schmauder, S.; Nienhaus, A.; Seidler, A. The isolated effect of age on the risk of COVID-19 severe outcomes: A systematic review with meta-analysis. *BMJ Glob. Health* **2021**, *6*, e006434. [CrossRef] [PubMed]
72. Henkens, M.; Raafs, A.G.; Verdonschot, J.A.J.; Linschoten, M.; van Smeden, M.; Wang, P.; van der Hooft, B.H.M.; Tieleman, R.; Janssen, M.L.F.; Ter Bekke, R.M.A.; et al. Age is the main determinant of COVID-19 related in-hospital mortality with minimal impact of pre-existing comorbidities, a retrospective cohort study. *BMC Geriatr.* **2022**, *22*, 184. [CrossRef] [PubMed]
73. Bajaj, V.; Gadi, N.; Spihlman, A.P.; Wu, S.C.; Choi, C.H.; Moulton, V.R. Aging, Immunity, and COVID-19: How Age Influences the Host Immune Response to Coronavirus Infections? *Front. Physiol.* **2020**, *11*, 571416. [CrossRef] [PubMed]
74. Buikema, A.R.; Buzinec, P.; Paudel, M.L.; Andrade, K.; Johnson, J.C.; Edmonds, Y.M.; Jhamb, S.K.; Chastek, B.; Raja, H.; Cao, F.; et al. Racial and ethnic disparity in clinical outcomes among patients with confirmed COVID-19 infection in a large US electronic health record database. *EClinicalMedicine* **2021**, *39*, 101075. [CrossRef] [PubMed]
75. Fu, J.; Reid, S.A.; French, B.; Hennessy, C.; Hwang, C.; Gatson, N.T.; Duma, N.; Mishra, S.; Nguyen, R.; Hawley, J.E.; et al. Racial Disparities in COVID-19 Outcomes Among Black and White Patients With Cancer. *JAMA Netw. Open* **2022**, *5*, e224304. [CrossRef]
76. Arnautovic, J.; Mazhar, A.; Souther, B.; Mikhijan, G.; Boura, J.; Huda, N. Cardiovascular Factors Associated with Septic Shock Mortality Risks. *Spartan Med. Res. J.* **2018**, *3*, 6516. [CrossRef] [PubMed]
77. Mahalingam, M.; Moore, J.X.; Donnelly, J.P.; Safford, M.M.; Wang, H.E. Frailty Syndrome and Risk of Sepsis in the REasons for Geographic and Racial Differences in Stroke (REGARDS) Cohort. *J. Intensive Care Med.* **2019**, *34*, 292–300. [CrossRef]
78. Nunes, J.P. Arterial hypertension and sepsis. *Rev. Port. Cardiol.* **2003**, *22*, 1375–1379.
79. Papadimitriou-Olivgeris, M.; Aretha, D.; Zotou, A.; Koutsileou, K.; Zbouki, A.; Lefkaditi, A.; Sklavou, C.; Marangos, M.; Fligou, F. The Role of Obesity in Sepsis Outcome among Critically Ill Patients: A Retrospective Cohort Analysis. *BioMed. Res. Int.* **2016**, *2016*, 5941279. [CrossRef] [PubMed]
80. Wang, Z.; Ren, J.; Wang, G.; Liu, Q.; Guo, K.; Li, J. Association between Diabetes Mellitus and Outcomes of Patients with Sepsis: A Meta-Analysis. *Med. Sci. Monit.* **2017**, *23*, 3546–3555. [CrossRef]
81. Osuchowski, M.F.; Winkler, M.S.; Skirecki, T.; Cajander, S.; Shankar-Hari, M.; Lachmann, G.; Monneret, G.; Venet, F.; Bauer, M.; Brunkhorst, F.M.; et al. The COVID-19 puzzle: Deciphering pathophysiology and phenotypes of a new disease entity. *Lancet Respir. Med.* **2021**, *9*, 622–642. [CrossRef]
82. Andersen, C.J.; Murphy, K.E.; Fernandez, M.L. Impact of Obesity and Metabolic Syndrome on Immunity. *Adv. Nutr.* **2016**, *7*, 66–75. [CrossRef] [PubMed]
83. Silzle, T.; Blum, S.; Schuler, E.; Kaivers, J.; Rudelius, M.; Hildebrandt, B.; Gattermann, N.; Haas, R.; Germing, U. Lymphopenia at diagnosis is highly prevalent in myelodysplastic syndromes and has an independent negative prognostic value in IPSS-R-low-risk patients. *Blood Cancer J.* **2019**, *9*, 63. [CrossRef] [PubMed]
84. Ray-Coquard, I.; Cropet, C.; Van Glabbeke, M.; Sebban, C.; Le Cesne, A.; Judson, I.; Tredan, O.; Verweij, J.; Biron, P.; Labidi, I.; et al. Lymphopenia as a prognostic factor for overall survival in advanced carcinomas, sarcomas, and lymphomas. *Cancer Res.* **2009**, *69*, 5383–5391. [CrossRef]
85. Sewell, R.L. Lymphocyte abnormalities in myeloma. *Br. J. Haematol.* **1977**, *36*, 545–551. [CrossRef]
86. Tanaka, S.; Isoda, F.; Ishihara, Y.; Kimura, M.; Yamakawa, T. T lymphopaenia in relation to body mass index and TNF-alpha in human obesity: Adequate weight reduction can be corrective. *Clin. Endocrinol.* **2001**, *54*, 347–354. [CrossRef]
87. Huang, I.; Pranata, R. Lymphopenia in severe coronavirus disease-2019 (COVID-19): Systematic review and meta-analysis. *J. Intensive Care* **2020**, *8*, 36. [CrossRef]
88. Li, W.; Lin, F.; Dai, M.; Chen, L.; Han, D.; Cui, Y.; Pan, P. Early predictors for mechanical ventilation in COVID-19 patients. *Ther. Adv. Respir. Dis.* **2020**, *14*, 1753466620963017. [CrossRef]
89. Tan, L.; Wang, Q.; Zhang, D.; Ding, J.; Huang, Q.; Tang, Y.Q.; Wang, Q.; Miao, H. Lymphopenia predicts disease severity of COVID-19: A descriptive and predictive study. *Signal Transduct. Target Ther.* **2020**, *5*, 33. [CrossRef]
90. Rahimmanesh, I.; Kouhpayeh, S.; Azizi, Y.; Khanahmad, H. Conceptual Framework for SARS-CoV-2-Related Lymphopenia. *Adv. Biomed. Res.* **2022**, *11*, 16. [CrossRef]
91. Garbo, R.; Valent, F.; Gigli, G.L.; Valente, M. Pre-Existing Lymphopenia Increases the Risk of Hospitalization and Death after SARS-CoV-2 Infection. *Infect. Dis. Rep.* **2022**, *14*, 20–25. [CrossRef] [PubMed]
92. Goupil, R.; Brachemi, S.; Nadeau-Fredette, A.C.; Deziel, C.; Troyanov, Y.; Lavergne, V.; Troyanov, S. Lymphopenia and treatment-related infectious complications in ANCA-associated vasculitis. *Clin. J. Am. Soc. Nephrol.* **2013**, *8*, 416–423. [CrossRef] [PubMed]
93. Ortega-Loubon, C.; Cano-Hernandez, B.; Poves-Alvarez, R.; Munoz-Moreno, M.F.; Roman-Garcia, P.; Balbas-Alvarez, S.; de la Varga-Martinez, O.; Gomez-Sanchez, E.; Gomez-Pesquera, F.; Lorenzo-Lopez, M.; et al. The Overlooked Immune State in Candidemia: A Risk Factor for Mortality. *J. Clin. Med.* **2019**, *8*, 1512. [CrossRef] [PubMed]
94. Alahyari, S.; Rajaeinejad, M.; Jalaeikhoo, H.; Amani, D. Regulatory T Cells in Immunopathogenesis and Severity of COVID-19: A Systematic Review. *Arch. Iran. Med.* **2022**, *25*, 127–132. [CrossRef] [PubMed]

95. Banerjee, T.; Calvi, L.M.; Becker, M.W.; Liesveld, J.L. Flaming and fanning: The Spectrum of inflammatory influences in myelodysplastic syndromes. *Blood Rev.* **2019**, *36*, 57–69. [CrossRef]
96. Bosseboeuf, A.; Allain-Maillet, S.; Mennesson, N.; Tallet, A.; Rossi, C.; Garderet, L.; Caillot, D.; Moreau, P.; Piver, E.; Girodon, F.; et al. Pro-inflammatory State in Monoclonal Gammopathy of Undetermined Significance and in Multiple Myeloma Is Characterized by Low Sialylation of Pathogen-Specific and Other Monoclonal Immunoglobulins. *Front. Immunol.* **2017**, *8*, 1347. [CrossRef]
97. Craver, B.M.; El Alaoui, K.; Scherber, R.M.; Fleischman, A.G. The Critical Role of Inflammation in the Pathogenesis and Progression of Myeloid Malignancies. *Cancers* **2018**, *10*, 104. [CrossRef]
98. Purdue, M.P.; Hofmann, J.N.; Kemp, T.J.; Chaturvedi, A.K.; Lan, Q.; Park, J.H.; Pfeiffer, R.M.; Hildesheim, A.; Pinto, L.A.; Rothman, N. A prospective study of 67 serum immune and inflammation markers and risk of non-Hodgkin lymphoma. *Blood* **2013**, *122*, 951–957. [CrossRef]
99. Sanada, F.; Taniyama, Y.; Muratsu, J.; Otsu, R.; Shimizu, H.; Rakugi, H.; Morishita, R. Source of Chronic Inflammation in Aging. *Front. Cardiovasc. Med.* **2018**, *5*, 12. [CrossRef]
100. Pietrobon, A.J.; Teixeira, F.M.E.; Sato, M.N. Immunosenescence and Inflammaging: Risk Factors of Severe COVID-19 in Older People. *Front. Immunol.* **2020**, *11*, 579220. [CrossRef]
101. Nogueira, B.M.D.; Machado, C.B.; Montenegro, R.C.; MEA, D.E.M.; Moreira-Nunes, C.A. Telomere Length and Hematological Disorders: A Review. *In Vivo* **2020**, *34*, 3093–3101. [CrossRef] [PubMed]
102. Gielen, M.; Hageman, G.J.; Antoniou, E.E.; Nordfjall, K.; Mangino, M.; Balasubramanyam, M.; de Meyer, T.; Hendricks, A.E.; Giltay, E.J.; Hunt, S.C.; et al. Body mass index is negatively associated with telomere length: A collaborative cross-sectional meta-analysis of 87 observational studies. *Am. J. Clin. Nutr.* **2018**, *108*, 453–475. [CrossRef] [PubMed]
103. Johnscher, G.; Woenckhaus, C.; Nicolas, J.C.; Pons, M.; Descomps, B.; Crastes de Paulet, A. Specific modification of 17 beta-estradiol dehydrogenase from human placenta by nicotinamide- (5-bromoacetyl-4-methylimidazole) dinucleotide. *FEBS Lett.* **1976**, *61*, 176–179. [CrossRef]
104. Aviv, A. Telomeres and COVID-19. *FASEB J.* **2020**, *34*, 7247–7252. [CrossRef] [PubMed]
105. Tsilingiris, D.; Tentolouris, A.; Eleftheriadou, I.; Tentolouris, N. Telomere length, epidemiology and pathogenesis of severe COVID-19. *Eur. J. Clin. Investig.* **2020**, *50*, e13376. [CrossRef]
106. Sanchez-Vazquez, R.; Guio-Carrion, A.; Zapatero-Gaviria, A.; Martinez, P.; Blasco, M.A. Shorter telomere lengths in patients with severe COVID-19 disease. *Aging* **2021**, *13*, 1–15. [CrossRef]
107. Wang, Q.; Codd, V.; Raisi-Estabragh, Z.; Musicha, C.; Bountziouka, V.; Kaptoge, S.; Allara, E.; Angelantonio, E.D.; Butterworth, A.S.; Wood, A.M.; et al. Shorter leukocyte telomere length is associated with adverse COVID-19 outcomes: A cohort study in UK Biobank. *EBioMedicine* **2021**, *70*, 103485. [CrossRef]
108. Mongelli, A.; Barbi, V.; Gottardi Zamperla, M.; Atlante, S.; Forleo, L.; Nesta, M.; Massetti, M.; Pontecorvi, A.; Nanni, S.; Farsetti, A.; et al. Evidence for Biological Age Acceleration and Telomere Shortening in COVID-19 Survivors. *Int. J. Mol. Sci.* **2021**, *22*, 6151. [CrossRef]
109. Nie, M.; Yang, L.; Bi, X.; Wang, Y.; Sun, P.; Yang, H.; Liu, P.; Li, Z.; Xia, Y.; Jiang, W. Neutrophil Extracellular Traps Induced by IL8 Promote Diffuse Large B-cell Lymphoma Progression via the TLR9 Signaling. *Clin. Cancer Res.* **2019**, *25*, 1867–1879. [CrossRef]
110. Podaza, E.; Sabbione, F.; Risnik, D.; Borge, M.; Almejun, M.B.; Colado, A.; Fernandez-Grecco, H.; Cabrejo, M.; Bezares, R.F.; Trevani, A.; et al. Neutrophils from chronic lymphocytic leukemia patients exhibit an increased capacity to release extracellular traps (NETs). *Cancer Immunol. Immunother* **2017**, *66*, 77–89. [CrossRef]
111. D'Abbondanza, M.; Martorelli, E.E.; Ricci, M.A.; De Vuono, S.; Migliola, E.N.; Godino, C.; Corradetti, S.; Siepi, D.; Paganelli, M.T.; Maugeri, N.; et al. Increased plasmatic NETs by-products in patients in severe obesity. *Sci. Rep.* **2019**, *9*, 14678. [CrossRef] [PubMed]
112. Skendros, P.; Mitsios, A.; Chrysanthopoulou, A.; Mastellos, D.C.; Metallidis, S.; Rafailidis, P.; Ntinopoulou, M.; Sertaridou, E.; Tsironidou, V.; Tsigalou, C.; et al. Complement and tissue factor-enriched neutrophil extracellular traps are key drivers in COVID-19 immunothrombosis. *J. Clin. Investig.* **2020**, *130*, 6151–6157. [CrossRef] [PubMed]
113. Luo, S.; Wang, M.; Wang, H.; Hu, D.; Zipfel, P.F.; Hu, Y. How Does Complement Affect Hematological Malignancies: From Basic Mechanisms to Clinical Application. *Front. Immunol.* **2020**, *11*, 593610. [CrossRef]
114. Shim, K.; Begum, R.; Yang, C.; Wang, H. Complement activation in obesity, insulin resistance, and type 2 diabetes mellitus. *World J. Diabetes* **2020**, *11*, 1–12. [CrossRef] [PubMed]
115. WHO. Who Sage Roadmap for Prioritizing Uses of COVID-19 Vaccines in the Context of Limited Supply. Available online: https://www.who.int/docs/default-source/immunization/sage/covid/sage-prioritization-roadmap-covid19-vaccines.pdf (accessed on 11 February 2022).
116. Butsch, W.S.; Hajduk, A.; Cardel, M.I.; Donahoo, W.T.; Kyle, T.K.; Stanford, F.C.; Zeltser, L.M.; Kotz, C.M.; Jastreboff, A.M. COVID-19 vaccines are effective in people with obesity: A position statement from The Obesity Society. *Obesity* **2021**, *29*, 1575–1579. [CrossRef] [PubMed]
117. Townsend, M.J.; Kyle, T.K.; Stanford, F.C. COVID-19 Vaccination and Obesity: Optimism and Challenges. *Obesity* **2021**, *29*, 634–635. [CrossRef]
118. Stampfer, S.D.; Goldwater, M.S.; Jew, S.; Bujarski, S.; Regidor, B.; Daniely, D.; Chen, H.; Xu, N.; Li, M.; Green, T.; et al. Response to mRNA vaccination for COVID-19 among patients with multiple myeloma. *Leukemia* **2021**, *35*, 3534–3541. [CrossRef]

119. Malard, F.; Gaugler, B.; Gozlan, J.; Bouquet, L.; Fofana, D.; Siblany, L.; Eshagh, D.; Adotevi, O.; Laheurte, C.; Ricard, L.; et al. Weak immunogenicity of SARS-CoV-2 vaccine in patients with hematologic malignancies. *Blood Cancer J.* **2021**, *11*, 142. [CrossRef]
120. Teh, J.S.K.; Coussement, J.; Neoh, Z.C.F.; Spelman, T.; Lazarakis, S.; Slavin, M.A.; Teh, B.W. Immunogenicity of COVID-19 vaccines in patients with hematologic malignancies: A systematic review and meta-analysis. *Blood Adv.* **2022**, *6*, 2014–2034. [CrossRef]
121. Thakkar, A.; Gonzalez-Lugo, J.D.; Goradia, N.; Gali, R.; Shapiro, L.C.; Pradhan, K.; Rahman, S.; Kim, S.Y.; Ko, B.; Sica, R.A.; et al. Seroconversion rates following COVID-19 vaccination among patients with cancer. *Cancer Cell* **2021**, *39*, 1081–1090.e2. [CrossRef]
122. Greenberger, L.M.; Saltzman, L.A.; Senefeld, J.W.; Johnson, P.W.; DeGennaro, L.J.; Nichols, G.L. Antibody response to SARS-CoV-2 vaccines in patients with hematologic malignancies. *Cancer Cell* **2021**, *39*, 1031–1033. [CrossRef] [PubMed]
123. Le Bourgeois, A.; Coste-Burel, M.; Guillaume, T.; Peterlin, P.; Garnier, A.; Bene, M.C.; Chevallier, P. Safety and Antibody Response After 1 and 2 Doses of BNT162b2 mRNA Vaccine in Recipients of Allogeneic Hematopoietic Stem Cell Transplant. *JAMA Netw. Open* **2021**, *4*, e2126344. [CrossRef] [PubMed]
124. Salvini, M.; Maggi, F.; Damonte, C.; Mortara, L.; Bruno, A.; Mora, B.; Brociner, M.; Mattarucchi, R.; Ingrassia, A.; Sirocchi, D.; et al. Immunogenicity of anti-SARS-CoV-2 Comirnaty vaccine in patients with lymphomas and myeloma who underwent autologous stem cell transplantation. *Bone Marrow Transpl.* **2022**, *57*, 137–139. [CrossRef] [PubMed]
125. Rimar, D.; Slobodin, G.; Paz, A.; Henig, I.; Zuckerman, T. SARS-COV-2 vaccination after stem cell transplantation for scleroderma. *Ann. Rheum. Dis.* **2021**, *80*, 1354–1355. [CrossRef]
126. Tamariz-Amador, L.E.; Battaglia, A.M.; Maia, C.; Zherniakova, A.; Guerrero, C.; Zabaleta, A.; Burgos, L.; Botta, C.; Fortuno, M.A.; Grande, C.; et al. Immune biomarkers to predict SARS-CoV-2 vaccine effectiveness in patients with hematological malignancies. *Blood Cancer J.* **2021**, *11*, 202. [CrossRef]
127. Earle, K.A.; Ambrosino, D.M.; Fiore-Gartland, A.; Goldblatt, D.; Gilbert, P.B.; Siber, G.R.; Dull, P.; Plotkin, S.A. Evidence for antibody as a protective correlate for COVID-19 vaccines. *Vaccine* **2021**, *39*, 4423–4428. [CrossRef]
128. Khoury, D.S.; Cromer, D.; Reynaldi, A.; Schlub, T.E.; Wheatley, A.K.; Juno, J.A.; Subbarao, K.; Kent, S.J.; Triccas, J.A.; Davenport, M.P. Neutralizing antibody levels are highly predictive of immune protection from symptomatic SARS-CoV-2 infection. *Nat. Med.* **2021**, *27*, 1205–1211. [CrossRef]
129. CDC. COVID-19 Vaccines for Moderately or Severely Immunocompromised People. Available online: https://www.cdc.gov/coronavirus/2019-ncov/vaccines/recommendations/immuno.html (accessed on 2 March 2022).
130. Benotmane, I.; Bruel, T.; Planas, D.; Fafi-Kremer, S.; Schwartz, O.; Caillard, S. A fourth dose of the mRNA-1273 SARS-CoV-2 vaccine improves serum neutralization against the Delta variant in kidney transplant recipients. *Kidney Int.* **2022**, *101*, 1073–1076. [CrossRef]
131. Regev-Yochay, G.; Gonen, T.; Gilboa, M.; Mandelboim, M.; Indenbaum, V.; Amit, S.; Meltzer, L.; Asraf, K.; Cohen, C.; Fluss, R.; et al. 4th Dose COVID mRNA Vaccines' Immunogenicity & Efficacy Against Omicron VOC. *MedRxiv* **2022**. [CrossRef]
132. Re, D.; Seitz-Polski, B.; Brglez, V.; Carles, M.; Graca, D.; Benzaken, S.; Liguori, S.; Zahreddine, K.; Delforge, M.; Bailly-Maitre, B.; et al. Humoral and cellular responses after a third dose of SARS-CoV-2 BNT162b2 vaccine in patients with lymphoid malignancies. *Nat. Commun.* **2022**, *13*, 864. [CrossRef]
133. Wood, E.M.; McQuilten, Z.K. Outpatient transfusions for myelodysplastic syndromes. *Hematol. Am. Soc. Hematol. Educ. Program* **2020**, *2020*, 167–174. [CrossRef] [PubMed]
134. Bakkour, S.; Saa, P.; Groves, J.A.; Montalvo, L.; Di Germanio, C.; Best, S.M.; Grebe, E.; Livezey, K.; Linnen, J.M.; Strauss, D.; et al. Minipool testing for SARS-CoV-2 RNA in United States blood donors. *Transfusion* **2021**, *61*, 2384–2391. [CrossRef] [PubMed]
135. Cappy, P.; Candotti, D.; Sauvage, V.; Lucas, Q.; Boizeau, L.; Gomez, J.; Enouf, V.; Chabli, L.; Pillonel, J.; Tiberghien, P.; et al. No evidence of SARS-CoV-2 transfusion transmission despite RNA detection in blood donors showing symptoms after donation. *Blood* **2020**, *136*, 1888–1891. [CrossRef] [PubMed]
136. Cho, H.J.; Koo, J.W.; Roh, S.K.; Kim, Y.K.; Suh, J.S.; Moon, J.H.; Sohn, S.K.; Baek, D.W. COVID-19 transmission and blood transfusion: A case report. *J. Infect. Public. Health* **2020**, *13*, 1678–1679. [CrossRef]
137. Kwon, S.Y.; Kim, E.J.; Jung, Y.S.; Jang, J.S.; Cho, N.S. Post-donation COVID-19 identification in blood donors. *Vox. Sang.* **2020**, *115*, 601–602. [CrossRef]
138. Lee, C.K.; Leung, J.N.S.; Cheng, P.; Lung, D.C.; To, K.K.W.; Tsang, D.N.C. Absence of SARS-CoV-2 viraemia in a blood donor with COVID-19 post-donation. *Transfus. Med.* **2021**, *31*, 223–224. [CrossRef]
139. Liapis, K.; Papoutselis, M.; Vrachiolias, G.; Misidou, C.; Spanoudakis, E.; Bezirgiannidou, Z.; Pentidou, A.; Konstantinidis, T.; Kotsianidis, I. Blood and platelet transfusion from a donor with presymptomatic COVID-19. *Ann. Hematol.* **2021**, *100*, 2133–2134. [CrossRef]
140. Sekeres, M.A.; Steensma, D.P.; DeZern, A.; Roboz, G.; Garcia-Manero, G.; Komrokji, R. COVID-19 and Myelodysplastic Syndromes: Frequently Asked Questions. Available online: https://www.hematology.org/covid-19/covid-19-and-myelodysplastic-syndromes (accessed on 26 February 2022).
141. Carson, J.L.; Stanworth, S.J.; Dennis, J.A.; Trivella, M.; Roubinian, N.; Fergusson, D.A.; Triulzi, D.; Doree, C.; Hebert, P.C. Transfusion thresholds for guiding red blood cell transfusion. *Cochrane Database Syst. Rev.* **2021**, *12*, CD002042. [CrossRef]
142. Hammami, E.; Hadhri, M.; Fekih Salem, S.; Ben Lakhal, F.; El Borgi, W.; Gouider, E. COVID-19 induced blood supply shortage: A Tunisian blood deposit perspective. *Transfus Clin. Biol.* **2022**, *29*, 102–104. [CrossRef]
143. Delabranche, X.; Kientz, D.; Tacquard, C.; Bertrand, F.; Roche, A.C.; Tran Ba Loc, P.; Humbrecht, C.; Sirlin, F.; Pivot, X.; Collange, O.; et al. Impact of COVID-19 and lockdown regarding blood transfusion. *Transfusion* **2021**, *61*, 2327–2335. [CrossRef]

144. Tripathi, P.P.; Kumawat, V.; Patidar, G.K. Donor's Perspectives on Blood Donation during COVID-19 Pandemic. *Indian J. Hematol. Blood Transfus.* **2021**, *30*, 1–10. [CrossRef] [PubMed]
145. Velazquez-Kennedy, K.; Luna, A.; Sanchez-Tornero, A.; Jimenez-Chillon, C.; Jimenez-Martin, A.; Valles Carboneras, A.; Tenorio, M.; Garcia Garcia, I.; Lopez-Jimenez, F.J.; Moreno-Jimenez, G. Transfusion support in COVID-19 patients: Impact on hospital blood component supply during the outbreak. *Transfusion* **2021**, *61*, 361–367. [CrossRef] [PubMed]
146. Yuan, Z.; Chen, D.; Chen, X.; Wei, Y. Estimation of the number of blood donors during the COVID-19 incubation period across China and analysis of prevention and control measures for blood transfusion transmission. *Transfusion* **2020**, *60*, 1778–1784. [CrossRef] [PubMed]
147. Stanworth, S.J.; New, H.V.; Apelseth, T.O.; Brunskill, S.; Cardigan, R.; Doree, C.; Germain, M.; Goldman, M.; Massey, E.; Prati, D.; et al. Effects of the COVID-19 pandemic on supply and use of blood for transfusion. *Lancet Haematol.* **2020**, *7*, e756–e764. [CrossRef]
148. Al-Riyami, A.Z.; Abdella, Y.E.; Badawi, M.A.; Panchatcharam, S.M.; Ghaleb, Y.; Maghsudlu, M.; Satti, M.; Lahjouji, K.; Merenkov, Z.; Adwan, A.; et al. The impact of COVID-19 pandemic on blood supplies and transfusion services in Eastern Mediterranean Region. *Transfus. Clin. Biol.* **2021**, *28*, 16–24. [CrossRef] [PubMed]
149. Loua, A.; Kasilo, O.M.J.; Nikiema, J.B.; Sougou, A.S.; Kniazkov, S.; Annan, E.A. Impact of the COVID-19 pandemic on blood supply and demand in the WHO African Region. *Vox. Sang.* **2021**, *116*, 774–784. [CrossRef]
150. Osaro, E.; Charles, A.T. The challenges of meeting the blood transfusion requirements in Sub-Saharan Africa: The need for the development of alternatives to allogenic blood. *J. Blood Med.* **2011**, *2*, 7–21. [CrossRef]
151. Mirski, M.A.; Frank, S.M.; Kor, D.J.; Vincent, J.L.; Holmes, D.R., Jr. Restrictive and liberal red cell transfusion strategies in adult patients: Reconciling clinical data with best practice. *Crit. Care* **2015**, *19*, 202. [CrossRef]
152. Karampela, I.; Vallianou, N.G.; Tsilingiris, D.; Christodoulatos, G.S.; Muscogiuri, G.; Barrea, L.; Vitale, G.; Dalamaga, M. Could inhaled corticosteroids be the game changers in the prevention of severe COVID-19? A review of current evidence. *Panminerva Med.* **2021**. [CrossRef]
153. Vallianou, N.G.; Tsilingiris, D.; Christodoulatos, G.S.; Karampela, I.; Dalamaga, M. Anti-viral treatment for SARS-CoV-2 infection: A race against time amidst the ongoing pandemic. *Metabol. Open* **2021**, *10*, 100096. [CrossRef]
154. NIH. Prioritization of Anti-SARS-CoV-2 Therapies for the Treatment and Prevention of COVID-19 When There Are Logistical or Supply Constraints. Available online: https://www.covid19treatmentguidelines.nih.gov/therapies/statement-on-patient-prioritization-for-outpatient-therapies/ (accessed on 24 February 2022).
155. NHS. Who Is at High Risk from Coronavirus (COVID-19). Available online: https://www.nhs.uk/conditions/coronavirus-covid-19/people-at-higher-risk/who-is-at-high-risk-from-coronavirus/ (accessed on 25 February 2022).
156. Agarwal, A.; Rochwerg, B.; Lamontagne, F.; Siemieniuk, R.A.; Agoritsas, T.; Askie, L.; Lytvyn, L.; Leo, Y.S.; Macdonald, H.; Zeng, L.; et al. A living WHO guideline on drugs for covid-19. *BMJ* **2020**, *370*, m3379. [CrossRef] [PubMed]
157. Bathish, J.; Zabida, A.; Eisenberg, L.; Ben-Meir, L.C.; Zeidman, A. Steroid Treatment in Hematologic Patients with COVID-19: Experience of 2 cases. *Arch. Hematol. Case Rep. Rev.* **2020**, *5*, 028–033. [CrossRef]
158. Dell'Isola, G.B.; Felicioni, M.; Ferraro, L.; Capolsini, I.; Cerri, C.; Gurdo, G.; Mastrodicasa, E.; Massei, M.S.; Perruccio, K.; Brogna, M.; et al. Case Report: Remdesivir and Convalescent Plasma in a Newly Acute B Lymphoblastic Leukemia Diagnosis With Concomitant Sars-CoV-2 Infection. *Front. Pediatr.* **2021**, *9*, 712603. [CrossRef] [PubMed]
159. Klank, D.; Hoffmann, M.; Claus, B.; Zinke, F.; Bergner, R.; Paschka, P. Monoclonal Antibodies for the Prevention and Treatment of COVID-19 Disease in Patients with Hematological Malignancies: Two Case Reports and a Literature Review. *Hemasphere* **2021**, *5*, e651. [CrossRef]
160. Saultier, P.; Ninove, L.; Szepetowski, S.; Veneziano, M.; Visentin, S.; Barlogis, V.; Saba Villarroel, P.M.; Amroun, A.; Loosveld, M.; de Lamballerie, X.; et al. Monoclonal antibodies for the treatment of COVID-19 in a patient with high-risk acute leukaemia. *Br. J. Haematol.* **2022**, *196*, e1–e3. [CrossRef]
161. Biernat, M.M.; Kolasinska, A.; Kwiatkowski, J.; Urbaniak-Kujda, D.; Biernat, P.; Janocha-Litwin, J.; Szymczyk-Nuzka, M.; Bursy, D.; Kalicinska, E.; Simon, K.; et al. Early Administration of Convalescent Plasma Improves Survival in Patients with Hematological Malignancies and COVID-19. *Viruses* **2021**, *13*, 436. [CrossRef]
162. Jeyaraman, P.; Agrawal, N.; Bhargava, R.; Bansal, D.; Ahmed, R.; Bhurani, D.; Bansal, S.; Rastogi, N.; Borah, P.; Naithani, R.; et al. Convalescent plasma therapy for severe COVID-19 in patients with hematological malignancies. *Transfus. Apher. Sci.* **2021**, *60*, 103075. [CrossRef]
163. Thompson, M.A.; Henderson, J.P.; Shah, P.K.; Rubinstein, S.M.; Joyner, M.J.; Choueiri, T.K.; Flora, D.B.; Griffiths, E.A.; Gulati, A.P.; Hwang, C.; et al. Association of Convalescent Plasma Therapy With Survival in Patients With Hematologic Cancers and COVID-19. *JAMA Oncol.* **2021**, *7*, 1167–1175. [CrossRef]
164. Group, R.C. Convalescent plasma in patients admitted to hospital with COVID-19 (RECOVERY): A randomised controlled, open-label, platform trial. *Lancet* **2021**, *397*, 2049–2059. [CrossRef]
165. Sanchez-Ramon, S.; Dhalla, F.; Chapel, H. Challenges in the Role of Gammaglobulin Replacement Therapy and Vaccination Strategies for Hematological Malignancy. *Front. Immunol.* **2016**, *7*, 317. [CrossRef]
166. Kyriazopoulou, E.; Poulakou, G.; Milionis, H.; Metallidis, S.; Adamis, G.; Tsiakos, K.; Fragkou, A.; Rapti, A.; Damoulari, C.; Fantoni, M.; et al. Early treatment of COVID-19 with anakinra guided by soluble urokinase plasminogen receptor plasma levels: A double-blind, randomized controlled phase 3 trial. *Nat. Med.* **2021**, *27*, 1752–1760. [CrossRef] [PubMed]

167. Busca, A. Viral infections in patients with hematological malignancies. *Leuk. Suppl.* **2012**, *1*, S24–S25. [CrossRef] [PubMed]
168. Brudno, J.N.; Kochenderfer, J.N. Recent advances in CAR T-cell toxicity: Mechanisms, manifestations and management. *Blood Rev.* **2019**, *34*, 45–55. [CrossRef] [PubMed]
169. Chen, L.Y.C.; Quach, T.T.T. COVID-19 cytokine storm syndrome: A threshold concept. *Lancet Microbe* **2021**, *2*, e49–e50. [CrossRef]
170. Le, R.Q.; Li, L.; Yuan, W.; Shord, S.S.; Nie, L.; Habtemariam, B.A.; Przepiorka, D.; Farrell, A.T.; Pazdur, R. FDA Approval Summary: Tocilizumab for Treatment of Chimeric Antigen Receptor T Cell-Induced Severe or Life-Threatening Cytokine Release Syndrome. *Oncologist* **2018**, *23*, 943–947. [CrossRef]
171. Isidori, A.; de Leval, L.; Gergis, U.; Musto, P.; Porcu, P. Management of Patients With Hematologic Malignancies During the COVID-19 Pandemic: Practical Considerations and Lessons to Be Learned. *Front. Oncol.* **2020**, *10*, 1439. [CrossRef]
172. Hus, I.; Salomon-Perzynski, A.; Tomasiewicz, K.; Robak, T. The management of hematologic malignancies during the COVID-19 pandemic. *Expert Opin Pharm.* **2021**, *22*, 565–582. [CrossRef]
173. Ibrahim, A.; Noun, P.; Khalil, C.; Taher, A. Changing Management of Hematological Malignancies With COVID-19: Statement and Recommendations of the Lebanese Society of Hematology and Blood Transfusion. *Front. Oncol.* **2021**, *11*, 564383. [CrossRef]
174. Ljungman, P.; Mikulska, M.; de la Camara, R.; Basak, G.W.; Chabannon, C.; Corbacioglu, S.; Duarte, R.; Dolstra, H.; Lankester, A.C.; Mohty, M.; et al. The challenge of COVID-19 and hematopoietic cell transplantation; EBMT recommendations for management of hematopoietic cell transplant recipients, their donors, and patients undergoing CAR T-cell therapy. *Bone Marrow Transpl.* **2020**, *55*, 2071–2076. [CrossRef]
175. Zeidan, A.M.; Boddu, P.C.; Patnaik, M.M.; Bewersdorf, J.P.; Stahl, M.; Rampal, R.K.; Shallis, R.; Steensma, D.P.; Savona, M.R.; Sekeres, M.A.; et al. Special considerations in the management of adult patients with acute leukaemias and myeloid neoplasms in the COVID-19 era: Recommendations from a panel of international experts. *Lancet Haematol.* **2020**, *7*, e601–e612. [CrossRef]
176. Di Ciaccio, P.; McCaughan, G.; Trotman, J.; Ho, P.J.; Cheah, C.Y.; Gangatharan, S.; Wight, J.; Ku, M.; Quach, H.; Gasiorowski, R.; et al. Australian and New Zealand consensus statement on the management of lymphoma, chronic lymphocytic leukaemia and myeloma during the COVID-19 pandemic. *Intern. Med. J.* **2020**, *50*, 667–679. [CrossRef] [PubMed]
177. Wozniak, K.; Sachs, W.; Boguradzki, P.; Basak, G.W.; Stec, R. Chemotherapy during Active SARS-CoV2 Infection: A Case Report and Review of the Literature. *Front. Oncol.* **2021**, *11*, 662211. [CrossRef] [PubMed]
178. Bader-Larsen, K.S.; Larson, E.A.; Dalamaga, M.; Magkos, F. A Narrative Review of the Safety of Anti-COVID-19 Nutraceuticals for Patients with Cancer. *Cancers* **2021**, *13*, 6094. [CrossRef] [PubMed]
179. Blanchard, C.M.; Denniston, M.M.; Baker, F.; Ainsworth, S.R.; Courneya, K.S.; Hann, D.M.; Gesme, D.H.; Reding, D.; Flynn, T.; Kennedy, J.S. Do adults change their lifestyle behaviors after a cancer diagnosis? *Am. J. Health Behav.* **2003**, *27*, 246–256. [CrossRef]
180. Malalur, P.; Agastya, M.; Wahi-Gururaj, S.; Cross, C.L.; Deauna-Limayo, D.; Kingsley, E.C. Cancer survivorship in hematologic malignancies: Lifestyle changes after diagnosis. *Cancer Med.* **2021**, *10*, 1066–1073. [CrossRef]
181. Satia, J.A.; Walsh, J.F.; Pruthi, R.S. Health behavior changes in white and African American prostate cancer survivors. *Cancer Nurs.* **2009**, *32*, 107–117. [CrossRef]
182. Williams, K.; Steptoe, A.; Wardle, J. Is a cancer diagnosis a trigger for health behaviour change? Findings from a prospective, population-based study. *Br. J. Cancer* **2013**, *108*, 2407–2412. [CrossRef]
183. Yaw, Y.H.; Shariff, Z.M.; Kandiah, M.; Mun, C.Y.; Yusof, R.M.; Othman, Z.; Saibul, N.; Weay, Y.H.; Hashim, Z. Weight changes and lifestyle behaviors in women after breast cancer diagnosis: A cross-sectional study. *BMC Public Health* **2011**, *11*, 309. [CrossRef]
184. Ashing-Giwa, K.T.; Padilla, G.; Tejero, J.; Kraemer, J.; Wright, K.; Coscarelli, A.; Clayton, S.; Williams, I.; Hills, D. Understanding the breast cancer experience of women: A qualitative study of African American, Asian American, Latina and Caucasian cancer survivors. *Psychooncology* **2004**, *13*, 408–428. [CrossRef]
185. Courneya, K.S.; Friedenreich, C.M.; Franco-Villalobos, C.; Crawford, J.J.; Chua, N.; Basi, S.; Norris, M.K.; Reiman, T. Effects of supervised exercise on progression-free survival in lymphoma patients: An exploratory follow-up of the HELP Trial. *Cancer Causes Control.* **2015**, *26*, 269–276. [CrossRef]
186. Orgel, E.; Framson, C.; Buxton, R.; Kim, J.; Li, G.; Tucci, J.; Freyer, D.R.; Sun, W.; Oberley, M.J.; Dieli-Conwright, C.; et al. Caloric and nutrient restriction to augment chemotherapy efficacy for acute lymphoblastic leukemia: The IDEAL trial. *Blood Adv.* **2021**, *5*, 1853–1861. [CrossRef] [PubMed]
187. Schmid, D.; Behrens, G.; Arem, H.; Hart, C.; Herr, W.; Jochem, C.; Matthews, C.E.; Leitzmann, M.F. Pre- and post-diagnosis physical activity, television viewing, and mortality among hematologic cancer survivors. *PLoS ONE* **2018**, *13*, e0192078. [CrossRef] [PubMed]
188. Wiskemann, J.; Kleindienst, N.; Kuehl, R.; Dreger, P.; Schwerdtfeger, R.; Bohus, M. Effects of physical exercise on survival after allogeneic stem cell transplantation. *Int. J. Cancer* **2015**, *137*, 2749–2756. [CrossRef] [PubMed]
189. Brown, M.; O'Connor, D.; Murphy, C.; McClean, M.; McMeekin, A.; Prue, G. Impact of COVID-19 on an established physical activity and behaviour change support programme for cancer survivors: An exploratory survey of the Macmillan Move More service for Northern Ireland. *Support. Care Cancer* **2021**, *29*, 6135–6143. [CrossRef]
190. Motton, S.; Vergriete, K.; VanPhi, L.N.; Lambaudie, E.; Berthoumieu, A.; Pous, J.; Delannes, M.; Piscione, J.; Cornou, C.; Bataille, B.; et al. Evaluation of the impact of the COVID-19 lockdown on the quality of life of patients monitored for cancer who practice an adapted physical activity: Rugby for health. *J. Cancer Res. Clin. Oncol.* **2022**, *148*, 425–439. [CrossRef]

191. Di Blasio, A.; Morano, T.; Lancia, F.; Viscioni, G.; Di Iorio, A.; Grossi, S.; Cianchetti, E.; Pippi, R.; Gobbo, S.; Bergamin, M.; et al. Effects of activity tracker-based counselling and live-web exercise on breast cancer survivors' sleep and waking time during Italy's COVID-19 lockdown. *Home Health Care Serv. Q.* **2022**, *41*, 1–19. [CrossRef]
192. Tank, M.; Franz, K.; Cereda, E.; Norman, K. Dietary supplement use in ambulatory cancer patients: A survey on prevalence, motivation and attitudes. *J. Cancer Res. Clin. Oncol.* **2021**, *147*, 1917–1925. [CrossRef]
193. Karampela, I.; Sakelliou, A.; Vallianou, N.; Christodoulatos, G.S.; Magkos, F.; Dalamaga, M. Vitamin D and Obesity: Current Evidence and Controversies. *Curr. Obes. Rep.* **2021**, *10*, 162–180. [CrossRef]
194. Kulling, P.M.; Olson, K.C.; Olson, T.L.; Feith, D.J.; Loughran, T.P., Jr. Vitamin D in hematological disorders and malignancies. *Eur. J. Haematol.* **2017**, *98*, 187–197. [CrossRef]
195. Barnes, P.R.; Williams, C.B.; Davies, R.L.; Childs, C.S.; Hedges, A.; Graham, D. The use of intravenous meptazinol for analgesia in colonoscopy. *Postgrad. Med. J.* **1985**, *61*, 221–224. [CrossRef]
196. Martinez-Lopez, J.; Hernandez-Ibarburu, G.; Alonso, R.; Sanchez-Pina, J.M.; Zamanillo, I.; Lopez-Munoz, N.; Iniguez, R.; Cuellar, C.; Calbacho, M.; Paciello, M.L.; et al. Impact of COVID-19 in patients with multiple myeloma based on a global data network. *Blood Cancer J.* **2021**, *11*, 198. [CrossRef] [PubMed]

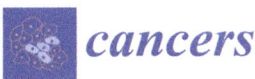 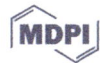

Perspective

Where Enhanced Recovery after Surgery (ERAS) Protocols Meet the Three Major Current Pandemics: COVID-19, Obesity and Malignancy

Anastasia Prodromidou [1,*], Aristotelis-Marios Koulakmanidis [1], Dimitrios Haidopoulos [1], Gregg Nelson [2], Alexandros Rodolakis [1] and Nikolaos Thomakos [1]

[1] Gynaecologic Oncology Unit, 1st Department of Obstetrics and Gynaecology, Alexandra Hospital, National and Kapodistrian University of Athens, 11528 Athens, Greece; aristoteliskoulak@gmail.com (A.-M.K.); dimitrioshaidopoulos@gmail.com (D.H.); a.rodolaki@gmail.com (A.R.); thomakir@hotmail.com (N.T.)
[2] Department of Obstetrics and Gynecology, University of Calgary, Calgary, AB T2N 1N4, Canada; gregg.nelson@albertahealthservices.ca
* Correspondence: a.prodromidou@hotmail.com; Tel.: +30-6972751000

Simple Summary: The SARS-CoV-2 (COVID-19) pandemic has significantly modified the medical services provided for patients that receive care either for COVID-19 or for those that need care for benign diseases, including obesity, or for malignant ones, such as gynecological cancer. We sought to investigate the association among three major worldwide health issues (COVID-19, obesity, and malignancy) and how ERAS protocols can potentially provide optimal management of patients with obesity and malignancy during the COVID-19 pandemic, with special attention to patients who required surgery for gynecologic oncology. We strongly believe that the application of ERAS protocols could play a key role during these unprecedented COVID-19 times.

Abstract: The outbreak of the SARS-CoV-2 (COVID-19) pandemic has transformed the provision of medical services for both patients that receive care for COVID-19 and for those that need care either for benign diseases, including obesity, or for malignancies, such as gynecological cancer. In this perspective article, we focus on the association among three major worldwide health issues and how ERAS protocols can potentially provide optimal management of patients with obesity and malignancy during the COVID-19 pandemic, with special attention to patients who required surgery for gynecologic oncology. A thorough search of the literature on the respective topics was performed. Patients with malignancy and obesity presented with increased vulnerability to COVID-19 infection. However, the management of their disease should not be withheld. Protective measures should be established to reduce exposure of patients with oncological diseases to SARS-CoV-2 while simultaneously enabling their access to vaccination. Since ERAS protocols have proved to be efficient in many surgical fields, including gynecologic oncology, general surgery, and orthopedics, we strongly believe that ERAS protocols may play a significant role in this effort. The end of the COVID-19 pandemic cannot be accurately predicted. Nevertheless, we have to ensure the appropriate and efficient management of certain groups of patients.

Keywords: COVID-19; gynecologic oncology; obesity; SARS-CoV-2; malignancy; cancer

Citation: Prodromidou, A.; Koulakmanidis, A.-M.; Haidopoulos, D.; Nelson, G.; Rodolakis, A.; Thomakos, N. Where Enhanced Recovery after Surgery (ERAS) Protocols Meet the Three Major Current Pandemics: COVID-19, Obesity and Malignancy. *Cancers* **2022**, *14*, 1660. https://doi.org/10.3390/cancers14071660

Academic Editors: Maria Dalamaga, Narjes Nasiri-Ansari and Nikolaos Spyrou

Received: 6 February 2022
Accepted: 21 March 2022
Published: 25 March 2022

Publisher's Note: MDPI stays neutral with regard to jurisdictional claims in published maps and institutional affiliations.

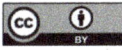

Copyright: © 2022 by the authors. Licensee MDPI, Basel, Switzerland. This article is an open access article distributed under the terms and conditions of the Creative Commons Attribution (CC BY) license (https://creativecommons.org/licenses/by/4.0/).

1. Introduction

The outbreak of SARS-CoV-2 (COVID-19) and its subsequent declaration by the World Health Organization (WHO) as a pandemic on 11th March 2020 has transformed the provision of medical services for both patients that receive care for COVID-19 and those that need care for other benign or malignant diseases. The pandemic has had significant professional and psychological consequences for healthcare providers. During the year 2021, the introduction of vaccines has brought significant hope for immunity against the disease for society as a whole; however it is still markedly uneven due to the inequity of vaccine access and the emergence of novel viral variants [1]. Furthermore, the different immune susceptibilities of the new variants has raised concerns regarding the amount of viral load in the community and the expansion of disease transmission [1].

Pandemics and cancer present similarities in growth and risk models and are both leading causes of mortality worldwide [2]. Despite the significant advances in modern therapies and quality of treatment, malignant diseases are among the most fatal conditions globally. A rise of approximately 50% in cancer cases is expected in 2040 compared with in 2020 [3]. According to the WHO, cancer is the second leading cause of death worldwide, with an estimate of 9.6 million cancer-related deaths in 2018; that can be translated to one in six deaths [3,4]. Cancer exerts significant psychological, physical, and economic burdens on individuals, societies, and healthcare systems. Gynecologic malignancies, including mainly cervical, endometrial, and ovarian cancer, are associated with significant morbidity and mortality among the gynecologic population [5]. A variety of clinicopathological characteristics have shown effects on the prognosis of gynecologic oncology patients [5]. Obesity not only is considered a risk factor for the development of certain types of gynecologic malignancies but also has been associated with poorer surgical outcomes [6].

Obesity has reached pandemic proportions worldwide, with estimated overweight and obese populations of approximately 39% and 13%, respectively [7]. Obesity is a major global health concern because of its overwhelming effect on an individual's health, which correlates with high rates of morbidity, including elevated risk of infection, respiratory and cardiometabolic diseases, as well as the development of malignancy [7]. Furthermore, the socioeconomic impact of obesity constitutes a huge burden, related not only to an excess of healthcare expenditure but also to critical loss of public productivity as a result of increased mortality and permanent disability [8]. Especially during the COVID-19 pandemic, patients with obesity suffered from a number of penalties that affected both populations with and without infections [9]. In particular, patients with obesity and a COVID-19 infection have a worse prognosis, which is mainly related to their comorbidities and impaired immune system [9]. Furthermore, patients with obesity require special care by qualified medical staff and using equipment that are not always available [9]. Patients without COVID-19 infections, on the other hand, are isolated at home during the pandemic; have limited access to potential planned surgical procedures; and are restricted in their choice of physical activity, which can worsen their already fragile medical condition [9].

During recent decades, Enhanced Recovery After Surgery (ERAS) protocols have been applied in a variety of surgical subspecialties. They were initially proposed for patients who underwent surgery for colorectal cancer and aimed to hasten postoperative recovery while simultaneously decreasing postoperative morbidity and readmissions [10,11]. By introducing a variety of standardized pre-, intra-, and postoperative modalities, the ERAS protocols have shown expedited functional recovery through attenuation of the stress response [11].

In this perspective article, we focus on the association among three major worldwide health issues and how ERAS protocols can potentially provide optimal management of patients with obesity and malignancy during the COVID-19 pandemic. We specifically focus on patients with gynecologic malignancies who underwent surgery, which represents a specific population of patients with cancer.

2. COVID-19 and Malignancy

The ongoing COVID-19 pandemic has dramatically changed the characteristics of medical care for patients with malignant diseases. A variety of unknown and difficult-to-solve problems have arisen, especially in daily surgical clinical practice. After an interval of about 6–8 months of almost total cancellation of all elective surgeries, the surgical community was called upon to take effective measures in preventing in-hospital SARS-CoV-2 spread so as to resume elective surgical procedures with the greatest safety for the patient [12]. Patients with oncological diseases have faced significant delays in their cancer diagnoses and treatments during the COVID-19 pandemic era. In particular, the diagnostic workflow of patients suspected of having cancer has been withheld due to the limited access of those patients to healthcare services and diagnostic procedures during the COVID-19 pandemic. Consequently, this has resulted in significant delays in cancer diagnosis, which advanced the stage of disease at diagnosis and the number of potentially avoidable cancer-related deaths [13]. This is also reflected in the decreased number of new cancer diagnoses during the COVID-19 pandemic due to the restrictions and alterations in health-seeking guidelines [13]. Decisions about the management of patients with oncological diseases should balance the need for proceeding with cancer treatment with the reported elevated susceptibility to COVID-19 infection and with the subsequent potentially poor outcomes of patients with COVID-19 infections and cancer [14]. In order to proceed with the surgical management of patients with oncological diseases, a plethora of preventative measures have been proposed by several surgical societies. Among them, restrictions regarding hospital visits unless absolutely necessary, limitations in the number of family members accompanying the patient, pre-operative SARS-CoV-2 screening before admission to the hospital and frequently thereafter during hospital stay, isolation of patients for a couple of days before surgery, and attempts to reduce hospital stays after surgery have been proposed. Some ongoing studies aim to elucidate the exact role of preoperative SARS-CoV-2 testing and remote prehabilitation in patients who are scheduled for elective surgeries [15]. In any case, all appropriate measures should be taken to ensure the availability of an operating theatre, surgeons, hospital staff, and resources in order for the cancer surgery to be prioritized [16]. Consequently, there is a need to establish perioperative pathways to hasten recovery and to increase hospital capacity [16]. ERAS protocols could serve as a major tool in helping combat this problem [16].

Furthermore, special attention should be paid to the characteristics and care of patients with cancer who are diagnosed with SARS-CoV-2. According to some studies, patients with malignancies are at higher risk of developing a COVID-19 infection [17]. However, no firm conclusion can be derived based on the current literature regarding the exact interaction between SARS-CoV-2 and cancer since there are many cofounders that can influence the course of those patients including age, comorbidities, smoking, and obesity. The potential suppression of the immune system of patients with cancer who undergo anti-cancer therapy explains the vulnerability of this group of patients with malignant diseases [17,18]. However, this could not be the case for all patients with cancer. Furthermore, cancer-related hypercoagulopathy could further increase the morbidity of these patients [18]. Therefore, prevention, early recognition, and appropriate management of thrombosis cases could be an important tool in reducing patients' morbidity.

We identified three studies in the literature that compared the differences in characteristics and outcomes among 5542 COVID-19 infected patients with (n = 398) and without malignancies (n = 5144) [19–21]. Their outcomes are summarized in Table 1.

The presence of comorbidities was more prevalent in patients with cancer who were infected with SARS-CoV-2. As shown in Table 1, mortality rates were controversial among the included studies. The multivariate analysis performed by Dai et al. revealed that the elevated risk of mortality, the presence of severe symptoms, ICU admission, and mechanical ventilation remained significant for patients with cancer who were infected by COVID-19 [19]. The same authors performed a separate analysis among patients with metastatic and non-metastatic cancer and proved that, concerning the aforementioned parameters, significance was only retained for patients with metastasis [19]. Additionally, patients who received surgery and immunotherapy presented with elevated mortality and increased incidence of severe symptoms, while this was not observed for those under radiotherapy [19]. Finally, Aboueshia et al. detected no difference in mortality rates among patients with cancer who were currently under treatment (active) and those who were not (non-active) [21].

Table 1. Studies reporting characteristics and outcomes of patients with COVID-19 with malignancy versus without malignancy.

Year; Author	2021; Aboueshia	2021; Mohamed	2020; Dai
Country	USA, Egypt	USA	China, USA
Type of study	RS	RS	MS-PS
Study period	February 2017–April 2020	March 2020–April 2020	January 2020–February 2020
Inclusion criteria	Adult patients hospitalized with COVID-19	Patients who are positive for COVID-19 who had testing due to fever or signs/symptoms suggestive of respiratory illness, history of travel to affected areas, direct contact with a person who was confirmed as having a COVID-19 infection	Patients with or without cancer who were infected with COVID-19 matched by age
Evaluated outcomes	Relationship between cancer and severe COVID-19 illness with adverse outcomes/in-hospital mortality, ICU admission, risk of intubation, duration of mechanical ventilation, LOS	Difference between patients with COVID-19 and with and without cancer in demographics, clinical and behavioral characteristics; prediction of mortality in patients with cancer	Death; ICU admission; severe clinical symptoms; acute kidney injury; disseminated intravascular coagulation; rhabdomyolysis
Patient No	57 vs. 203	236 vs. 4405	105 vs. 536
Age (years)	63.6 ± 12.5 [a] vs. 58.7 ± 14.6 [a] $p = 0.023$	69 (61–78) vs. 57 (40–70) $p < 0.001$	64 (14) [b] vs. 63.5(14) [b] $p = 0.25$
Most common type of cancer	Breast and prostate	N/A	Lung cancer
ICU admission (%)	22.2% vs. 16.1% $p = 0.07$	N/A	OR 2.84 95% CI 1.59–5.08 $p < 0.01$
Complications (%)	78.8% vs. 79.9% $p = 0.84$	N/A	N/A
Mechanical ventilation N (%)	12 (26.1%) vs. 52 (32.9%) $p = 0.47$ (closed cases)	N/A	11(10.48%) vs. 47 (8.77%) $p = 0.58$ (non-invasive) 11(10.48%) vs. 15(2.79%) $p < 0.001$
Mortality (%)	12.3% vs. 16.3% $p = 0.53$	29 (12.3%) vs. 357 (8.1%) $p = 0.023$	OR 2.34 95% CI 1.15–4.77 $p = 0.03$
Discharged patients N (%)	42/49 (85.7%) vs. 142/175 (81.1%)	75 (31.8%) vs. 2026 (46%) $p < 0.001$	N/A
LOS	12.8 ± 11.4 [a] vs. 8.58 ± 6.5 [a] $p = 0.002$	N/A	27.01 ± 9.52 vs. 17.75 ± 8.64 $p < 0.01$

RS: Retrospective; MS: multicenter; ICU: intensive care unit; LOS: length of stay, [a] mean ± SD, [b] median (IQR).

The management of patients with malignancy during the COVID-19 pandemic is of critical importance. However, the available guidelines by existing committees are not yet clear on the optimal approach regarding patients with malignancy who were or were not infected with COVID-19 during the pandemic. Further trials and audits from high-volume centers are warranted to elucidate whether COVID-19 infection and malignancy correlate with higher mortality, and to identify potential biomarkers used to stratify the risk of mortality and development of severe complications in those patients. The establishment of strategies and modalities to protect patients with cancer from SARS-CoV-2 infection during their treatment and to adjust their management against cancer during a COVID-19 episode would be beneficial for this evidently high-risk group of patients.

3. COVID-19 and Obesity

The restrictions to physical activity and the potentially unhealthy eating habits that have been adopted during the COVID-19 pandemic could be considered as additional risk factors that predispose a person to obesity. Similar to other infectious diseases, a COVID-19 infection has been claimed to induce obesity. The potential mechanisms that have been proposed include the increase in adipogenesis and in chronic inflammation that promote fatty tissue angiogenesis [22]. Finally, the pandemic has paused elective bariatric procedures, and thus, the management of obesity in patients was withheld, leading to a significant expansion of the adverse consequences of obesity including cardiovascular complications, diabetes mellitus, and cancer [22]. However, the outcomes from a single high-volume center in Canada showed that the application of ERAS protocols kept the bariatric program fully functional during the pandemic, allowing for discharges on the first postoperative day [23].

As mentioned above, patients with obesity can have compromised immune systems with a low-grade inflammatory state as well as respiratory dysfunction, indicating a potential relationship between obesity and the severity of SARS-CoV-2 disease. A recent meta-analysis by Cai et al. showed that patients with obesity and SARS-CoV-2 were more likely to be hospitalized, to suffer from more severe disease, to be admitted to the ICU, and to receive mechanical ventilation more often compared with patients without obesity [7]. The mortality rates of those patients were accordingly elevated [7]. Susceptibility to acute respiratory distress syndrome (ARDS), which constitutes the primary cause of mortality due to SARS-CoV-2, is considerably greater among patients with obesity. There is strong evidence suggesting that a higher body mass index (BMI) is greatly associated with COVID-19 infection, with an estimated risk increase of about 5–10% of hospitalization due to SARS-CoV-2 for every kg/m^2 excess of BMI [24]. In addition, patients with obesity are at a higher risk for reduced effectiveness of COVID-19 vaccination, which can be potentially attributed to metabolic dysfunction, leading to a weakened immune response [25].

4. The Triangle of Pandemic Doom

As previously highlighted, appropriate clinical decision-making for patients undergoing surgery during these unprecedented times is of paramount importance in order to achieve optimal outcomes, while a dangerous triangle of doom is forming (Figure 1). Patients with obesity undergoing surgery for cancer and imperiled by COVID-19 infection find themselves at a very high risk for perioperative complications and mortality. At this point, the implementation of ERAS protocols may serve as a life jacket for patients who find themselves within this deleterious triangle.

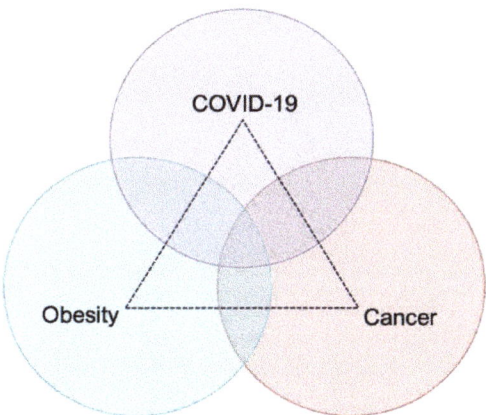

Figure 1. The triangle of pandemic doom.

5. ERAS and Surgical Oncology

The application of ERAS fast-track protocols has been proposed as a tool for improving the perioperative care of patients and aiming to decrease postoperative morbidity, hospital stay, and hospitalization costs. The main goal of applying ERAS protocols is to hasten the return of patients to normal activity. It is known that surgical operations and hospital stays can interfere with normal homeostasis, a phenomenon that is called the surgical stress response (SSR) and involves the immune and neuroendocrine systems [26]. The decrease in SSR could lead to an optimal postoperative course with significant reduction in postoperative morbidity [26]. In that context, the application of ERAS protocols could contribute to protection against SSR. This can be achieved by encompassing strategies to eliminate perioperative opioid use and to introduce early oral food intake and ambulation, as well as prudent fluid administration. The components of ERAS protocols are classified into pre-, intra-, and postoperative components [27]. There is a significant interaction among the ERAS components, with one affecting the other [28]. Some of the main components of ERAS protocols in gynecologic oncology are shown in Table 2.

Table 2. Key principles of ERAS protocols in gynecologic/oncology.

- Thorough preoperative counseling.
- Preoperative prehabilitation and optimization (cessation of smoking and alcohol abuse, and correction of possible anemia).
- No mechanical bowel preparation.
- Clear fluids consumption (oral carbohydrate drinks): until 2 h preoperatively and a light meal 6 h prior to the introduction of anesthesia.
- No administration of preoperative sedatives for anxiety reduction.
- For surgery > 30 min, dual VTE prophylaxis administration: including mechanical and either LMWH or heparin.
- Administration of first-generation cephalosporins and anaerobic prophylaxis (in case of bowel resection) 60 min prior to incision.
- Short-acting anesthetics and local anesthesia wound infiltration.
- Use > 2 antiemetic agents for PONV prevention.
- No routine use of nasogastric intubation. If inserted during surgery, remove immediately after surgery.
- No use of surgical drains.
- Preservation of normothermia and euvolemia intra-operatively.
- Early discontinuation of intravenous fluids postoperatively (once tolerating oral fluids) and simultaneous return to regular diet within the first 24 h postoperatively.
- Maintenance of blood glucose levels < 180–200 mg/dL, and if glucose levels surpass this range, use insulin infusions.
- Opioid sparing strategies with multimodal analgesia.
- Remove bladder catheter at <24 h postoperatively.
- Active mobilization from the first postoperative day.

VTE: venous thromboembolism; LMWH: low molecular weight heparin; PONV: postoperative nausea and vomiting.

The cooperation of a multidisciplinary team consisting of surgeons, anesthesiologists, nutrition specialists, nursing staff, and physiotherapists is of critical importance to achieve the optimal postoperative care [28]. To that end, the proper education of all these specialties could lead to the successful application of ERAS protocols. A plethora of original studies and reviews have demonstrated the superiority of ERAS protocols in many surgical fields in ameliorating short-term outcomes including a significant reduction in complication rates and hospital stays with no impact in reoperation and readmission rates [29,30]. However, less is known about the long-term efficacy of ERAS protocols in patients with malignancy. According to the findings by Gustafsson et al., the application of ERAS protocols in patients with colorectal cancer undergoing surgery was shown to be associated with improved 5 year disease specific survival [31]. Interestingly, the maintenance of fluid balance, the prevention of fluid overload, and monitoring of calories by oral intake at the day of surgery were considered the ERAS components that were independently related to improved 5 year survival outcomes [31]. ERAS can be applied in all patients who have been selected to receive surgical management for their disease.

5.1. ERAS and Gastrointestinal Surgery

The use of ERAS-based clinical pathways for patients who had pancreatoduodenectomy due to pancreatic cancer has been shown to be effective for both increased patient care and reduced hospital costs according to the meta-analysis by Karunakaran et al. [32]. The authors recorded a significant decrease in hospital stays, complications, and overall hospital costs through the ERAS arm of care compared with standard care [32]. The respective benefits have also been seen in patients with gastric cancer who underwent surgery with preoperative education, early rehabilitation with mobilization, and first postoperative day oral feeding [33]. In liver surgery, the application of ERAS resulted in a significant reduction in complications and length of stay with no impact to mortality and re-admission rates [34]. Furthermore, for patients with colorectal cancer who had laparoscopic surgery, the application of ERAS was associated with shorter hospital stays, and earlier time to first flatus and defecation, based on the outcomes of a meta-analysis of 13 randomized clinical trials [35].

5.2. ERAS and Gynecologic Oncology Surgery

ERAS protocols have also been used in patients with gynecologic cancers. According to a recent meta-analysis by Bisch et al., the application of ERAS protocols in patients with gynecologic malignancy has been associated with significant benefits for the patients' postoperative course by reducing the length of hospital stays and postoperative complications with no impact in readmission rates and mortality [36]. Additionally, Tankou et al. compared the postoperative outcomes of patients with advanced ovarian cancer who had interval debulking surgery after the application of neoadjuvant chemotherapy before and after ERAS [10]. They showed a significantly elevated proportion of patients that resumed chemotherapy at 28 days after surgery in the post-ERAS group compared with those in the pre-ERAS group (80% vs. 64%, odds ratios 2.29, $p = 0.002$) [10]. The ERAS Society has issued and updated guidelines on the optimal perioperative care of patients with gynecologic malignancy that aimed to improve patients' postoperative outcomes [37].

5.3. ERAS and Urological Surgery

The use of ERAS has also been extensively investigated in patients who had surgery due to urological indications. More specifically, for patients with bladder cancer who had radical cystectomy, those who were managed under ERAS protocols had a shorter time to first bowel movement and a shorter hospital stay compared with the group without ERAS management. No difference was observed in the 30-day readmission and complication rates [38]. ERAS protocols were also shown to be beneficial in terms of time to first flatus, increasing safety in catheter removal and reducing hospital stay in patients who had radical prostatectomy [39].

5.4. ERAS and Head and Neck Surgery

The current literature also presents encouraging perioperative outcomes in the use of ERAS in patients with head and neck cancers. In particular, there is growing evidence for the clinical and financial benefits of ERAS in major head and neck surgery [40]. Early oral intake and trachea-stoma closure have been recorded as the key beneficial components of ERAS in these surgeries [41]. However, data are still limited in the field and further, larger, well-designed trials are required to validate the safety and feasibility of ERAS protocols in head and neck surgery [41,42].

6. Key Role of ERAS in Gynecologic Oncology

Patients with malignant diseases are more susceptible to SARS-CoV-2 due to cancer-related immunosuppression. Therefore, there is an urgent need to develop strategies to reduce exposure to COVID-19 in patients with cancer in need of surgical intervention. ERAS protocols have been proposed as valuable tools in the surgical management of patients with malignancy during the SARS-CoV-2 era [16]. These protocols maintain homeostasis during the perioperative period, aiming to minimize the prevalence and severity of complications after complex gynecologic oncology surgeries even during the COVID-19 pandemic [12]. More specifically, strategies for the reduction in the length of hospital stays and readmissions are among the preventative measures of transmission of SARS-CoV-2 [43]. Moreover, a shorter length of hospitalization can improve the mental well-being not only of patients after surgery but also of their care providers and relatives, who are restricted from hospital visits, and can thus result in more favorable postoperative outcomes [43]. Finally, the implementation of ERAS protocols also seems to be cost-effective: the increase in total savings per cancer patient allows for the opportunity to redistribute these savings to other areas of the healthcare system. It is obvious that the combination of obesity and malignancy expands the risks of suffering from SARS-CoV-2 and the severe complications of the disease. During this unknown and difficult period, there is an increased need for the development of perioperative care pathways that will ensure the safety of patients with obesity and gynecologic malignancies.

The use of ERAS protocols in gynecologic oncology has shown reduced lengths of hospital stays, which can also minimize the risk of COVID-19 infection. Additionally, in patients with obesity and gynecologic malignancies, the use of ERAS protocols has been proven to be safe and efficient, with comparable perioperative outcomes to patients without obesity [44]. The implementation of ERAS protocols in patients who required surgery for gynecologic oncology and who had minimally invasive hysterectomy was associated with significantly increased same-day discharge rates: 75% following ERAS protocols as compared with 29% during the pre-implementation era, with no impact in complication and readmission rates [45]. Interestingly, the mean BMI of the study population was 32, with no observable difference in BMI among the pre-ERAS and post-ERAS intervention groups [45]. This clearly indicates the applicability of the suggested, minimally invasive ERAS program in patients with obesity that can also facilitate better hospital management of patients with obesity who require surgery for malignancy during the COVID-19 pandemic. In addition, ERAS protocols promote early functional recovery after surgery, resulting in lower rates of complications and a faster return to the intended oncology treatment, compared with traditional methods in patients with a high risk of postoperative morbidity, such as those with obesity. Therefore, the application of the main components of ERAS, such as those mentioned in Table 2, with further special consideration to some specific elements, can contribute to the optimal management of patients with obesity, COVID-19 infections, and oncologic diseases. Moreover, emphasis should be given to prehabilitation strategies that promote weight loss and exercise; the application of a preoperative low-calorie diet and improvements in general fitness and respiratory capacity are of paramount importance. Postoperative dietary and nutritional support is equally important in providing early nutritional care to patients with oncological diseases during the immediate postoperative period. As for the anesthesiology part, the anesthesiologist should be aware of the challenges of intubation of patients with obesity and adopt lung protective strategies with adjustment in ventilation parameters and positioning that can improve gas exchange and pulmonary mechanisms. ERAS protocols enable safe and effective treatment options for patients with obesity, while human and institutional resources are preserved for patients with SARS-CoV-2 requiring hospitalization. Women with obesity represent a significant proportion of patients with gynecologic malignancies and the postponement or the cancellation of their management will lead to a further peak of cancer-related deaths added to those due to COVID-19 infection.

7. Conclusions

No one can accurately predict when the COVID-19 pandemic will end. However, we have to ensure the appropriate and efficient management of patients with oncological diseases during these unprecedented times. Greater attention should be paid to patients with obesity, which constitute a high-risk group of patients. Consequently, there is a strong need to establish strategies to eliminate the adverse outcomes that can arise from the combination of malignancy, obesity, and COVID-19 infection. Despite the increased vulnerability of patients with obesity and cancer to COVID-19 infection, the management of their disease should not be withheld. To that end, we should ensure that management strategies consist of protective measures to reduce their exposure to SARS-CoV-2, and unfettered access to vaccination. Since ERAS fast-track protocols have been proven to be effective in gynecologic oncology surgery and other surgical oncology disciplines, we strongly believe that ERAS fast-track protocols may play a significant role in efforts to combat the serious "triangle of pandemic doom".

Author Contributions: Conceptualization: N.T.; Methodology: N.T., G.N. and A.P.; Validation: N.T. and G.N.; Formal analysis: A.P. and A.-M.K.; Investigation: N.T., G.N. and A.P.; Data curation: A.P. and A.-M.K.; Writing—Original Draft Preparation: N.T., G.N., A.P. and A.-M.K.; Writing—Review and Editing: N.T., G.N., D.H. and A.P.; Supervision: A.R. and N.T. All authors have read and agreed to the published version of the manuscript.

Funding: This research received no external funding.

Conflicts of Interest: The authors declare no conflict of interest.

References

1. Pappas, G.; Saloustros, E.; Boutis, A.; Tsoukalas, N.; Nikolaou, M.; Christopoulou, A.; Agelaki, S.; Boukovinas, I.; Ardavanis, A.; Saridaki, Z. Vaccine third dose and cancer patients: Necessity or luxury? *ESMO Open* **2021**, *6*, 100306. [CrossRef] [PubMed]
2. Vandamme, L.K.J.; de Hingh, I.H.J.T.; Fonseca, J.; Rocha, P.R.F. Similarities between pandemics and cancer in growth and risk models. *Sci. Rep.* **2021**, *11*, 349. [CrossRef] [PubMed]
3. Sung, H.; Ferlay, J.; Siegel, R.L.; Laversanne, M.; Soerjomataram, I.; Jemal, A.; Bray, F. Global Cancer Statistics 2020: GLOBOCAN Estimates of Incidence and Mortality Worldwide for 36 Cancers in 185 Countries. *CA Cancer J. Clin.* **2021**, *71*, 209–249. [CrossRef] [PubMed]
4. Ferlay, J.; Ervik, M.; Lam, F.; Colombet, M.; Mery, L.; Piñeros, M.; Znaor, A.; Soerjomataram, I.; Bray, F. *Global Cancer Observatory: Cancer Today*; International Agency for Research on Cancer: Lyon, France, 2020. Available online: https://gco.iarc.fr/today (accessed on 1 February 2022).
5. Yamagami, W.; Nagase, S.; Takahashi, F.; Ino, K.; Hachisuga, T.; Aoki, D.; Katabuchi, H. Clinical statistics of gynecologic cancers in Japan. *J. Gynecol. Oncol.* **2017**, *28*, e32. [CrossRef]
6. Modesitt, S.C.; Van Nagell, J.R., Jr. The impact of obesity on the incidence and treatment of gynecologic cancers: A review. *Obstet. Gynecol. Surv.* **2005**, *60*, 683–692. [CrossRef]
7. Cai, Z.; Yang, Y.; Zhang, J. Obesity is associated with severe disease and mortality in patients with coronavirus disease 2019 (COVID-19): A meta-analysis. *BMC Public Health* **2021**, *21*, 1505. [CrossRef]
8. Fallah-Fini, S.; Adam, A.; Cheskin, L.J.; Bartsch, S.M.; Lee, B.Y. The Additional Costs and Health Effects of a Patient Having Overweight or Obesity: A Computational Model. *Obesity* **2017**, *25*, 1809–1815. [CrossRef]
9. Slim, K.; Boirie, Y. The quintuple penalty of obese patients in the COVID-19 pandemic. *Surg. Obes. Relat. Dis.* **2020**, *16*, 1163–1164. [CrossRef]
10. Tankou, J.I.; Foley, O.; Falzone, M.; Kalyanaraman, R.; Elias, K.M. Enhanced recovery after surgery protocols improve time to return to intended oncology treatment following interval cytoreductive surgery for advanced gynecologic cancers. *Int. J. Gynecol. Cancer* **2021**, *31*, 1145–1153. [CrossRef]

11. Ljungqvist, O.; de Boer, H.D.; Balfour, A.; Fawcett, W.J.; Lobo, D.N.; Nelson, G.; Scott, M.J.; Wainwright, T.W.; Demartines, N. Opportunities and Challenges for the Next Phase of Enhanced Recovery After Surgery: A Review. *JAMA Surg.* **2021**, *156*, 775–784. [CrossRef]
12. Stone, R.; Scheib, S. Advantages of, and Adaptations to, Enhanced Recovery Protocols for Perioperative Care during the COVID-19 Pandemic. *J. Minim. Invasive Gynecol.* **2021**, *28*, 481–489. [CrossRef] [PubMed]
13. Popovic, M.; Fiano, V.; Moirano, G.; Chiusa, L.; Conway, D.I.; Garzino Demo, P.; Gilardetti, M.; Iorio, G.C.; Moccia, C.; Ostellino, O.; et al. The Impact of the COVID-19 Pandemic on Head and Neck Cancer Diagnosis in the Piedmont Region, Italy: Interrupted Time-Series Analysis. *Front. Public Health* **2022**, *10*, 809283. [CrossRef] [PubMed]
14. Garcia, D.; Siegel, J.B.; Mahvi, D.A.; Zhang, B.; Mahvi, D.M.; Camp, E.R.; Graybill, W.; Savage, S.J.; Giordano, A.; Giordano, S.; et al. What is Elective Oncologic Surgery in the Time of COVID-19? A Literature Review of the Impact of Surgical Delays on Outcomes in Patients with Cancer. *Clin. Oncol. Res.* **2020**, *2020*, 1–11. [CrossRef]
15. Charlesworth, M.; Grossman, R. Pre-operative SARS-CoV-2 testing, isolation, vaccination and remote prehabilitation—The road to 'COVID-19 secure' elective surgery. *Anaesthesia* **2021**, *76*, 1439–1441. [CrossRef]
16. Butler, J.; Finley, C.; Norell, C.H.; Harrison, S.; Bryant, H.; Achiam, M.P.; Altman, A.D.; Baxter, N.; Bentley, J.; Cohen, P.A.; et al. New approaches to cancer care in a COVID-19 world. *Lancet Oncol.* **2020**, *21*, e339–e340. [CrossRef]
17. van Dam, P.A.; Huizing, M.; Mestach, G.; Dierckxsens, S.; Tjalma, W.; Trinh, X.B.; Papadimitriou, K.; Altintas, S.; Vermorken, J.; Vulsteke, C.; et al. SARS-CoV-2 and cancer: Are they really partners in crime? *Cancer Treat. Rev.* **2020**, *89*, 102068. [CrossRef]
18. Šálek, T.; Slopovský, J.; Pörsök, Š.; Pazderová, N.; Mináriková, Z.; Zomborská, E.; Špánik, B. COVID-19 and oncological disease. *Klin. Onkol.* **2021**, *34*, 211–219. [CrossRef]
19. Dai, M.; Liu, D.; Liu, M.; Zhou, F.; Li, G.; Chen, Z.; Zhang, Z.; You, H.; Wu, M.; Zheng, Q.; et al. Patients with cancer appear more vulnerable to SARS-COV-2: A multicenter study during the COVID-19 outbreak. *Cancer Discov.* **2020**, *10*, 783–791. [CrossRef]
20. Mohamed, N.E.; Benn, E.K.; Astha, V.; Shah, Q.N.; Gharib, Y.; Kata, H.E.; Honore-Goltz, H.; Dovey, Z.; Kyprianou, N.; Tewari, A.K. COVID-19 in patients with and without cancer: Examining differences in patient characteristics and outcomes. *J. Cancer Biol.* **2021**, *2*, 25–32. [CrossRef]
21. Aboueshia, M.; Hussein, M.H.; Attia, A.S.; Swinford, A.; Miller, P.; Omar, M.; Toraih, E.A.; Saba, N.; Safah, H.; Duchesne, J.; et al. Cancer and COVID-19: Analysis of patient outcomes. *Futur. Oncol.* **2021**, *17*, 3499–3510. [CrossRef]
22. Zakka, K.; Chidambaram, S.; Mansour, S.; Mahawar, K.; Salminen, P.; Almino, R.; Schauer, P.; Kinross, J.; Purkayastha, S.; on behalf of the PanSurg Collaborative. SARS-CoV-2 and Obesity: "CoVesity"—A Pandemic Within a Pandemic. *Obes. Surg.* **2021**, *31*, 1745–1754. [CrossRef] [PubMed]
23. Abu-Omar, N.; Marcil, G.; Mocanu, V.; Dang, J.T.; Switzer, N.; Kanji, A.; Birch, D.; Karmali, S. The effect of the COVID-19 pandemic on bariatric surgery delivery in Edmonton, Alberta: A single-centre experience. *Can. J. Surg.* **2021**, *64*, E307–E309. [CrossRef] [PubMed]
24. Sattar, N.; Valabhji, J. Obesity as a Risk Factor for Severe COVID-19: Summary of the Best Evidence and Implications for Health Care. *Curr. Obes. Rep.* **2021**, *10*, 282–289. [CrossRef]
25. Popkin, B.M.; Du, S.; Green, W.D.; Beck, M.A.; Algaith, T.; Herbst, C.H.; Alsukait, R.F.; Alluhidan, M.; Alazemi, N.; Shekar, M. Individuals with obesity and COVID-19: A global perspective on the epidemiology and biological relationships. *Obes. Rev.* **2020**, *21*, e13128. [CrossRef] [PubMed]
26. Mari, G.; Costanzi, A.; Crippa, J.; Falbo, R.; Miranda, A.; Rossi, M.; Berardi, V.; Maggioni, D. Surgical Stress Reduction in Elderly Patients Undergoing Elective Colorectal Laparoscopic Surgery within an ERAS Protocol. *Chirurgia* **2016**, *111*, 476–480. [CrossRef] [PubMed]
27. Altman, A.D.; Helpman, L.; McGee, J.; Samouëlian, V.; Auclair, M.-H.; Brar, H.; Nelson, G.S. Enhanced recovery after surgery: Implementing a new standard of surgical care. *Can. Med Assoc. J.* **2019**, *191*, E469–E475. [CrossRef]
28. Manso, M.; Schmelz, J.; Aloia, T. ERAS-Anticipated outcomes and realistic goals. *J. Surg. Oncol.* **2017**, *116*, 570–577. [CrossRef]
29. Zhou, J.; Du, R.; Wang, L.; Wang, F.; Li, D.; Tong, G.; Wang, W.; Ding, X.; Wang, D. The Application of Enhanced Recovery After Surgery (ERAS) for Patients Undergoing Bariatric Surgery: A Systematic Review and Meta-analysis. *Obes. Surg.* **2021**, *31*, 1321–1331. [CrossRef]
30. Mao, F.; Huang, Z. Enhanced Recovery After Surgery for Patients Undergoing Cytoreductive Surgery and Hyperthermic Intraperitoneal Chemotherapy: A Systematic Review and Meta-Analysis. *Front. Surg.* **2021**, *8*, 713171. [CrossRef]
31. Gustafsson, U.O.; Oppelstrup, H.; Thorell, A.; Nygren, J.; Ljungqvist, O. Adherence to the ERAS protocol is Associated with 5-Year Survival After Colorectal Cancer Surgery: A Retrospective Cohort Study. *World J. Surg.* **2016**, *40*, 1741–1747. [CrossRef]
32. Karunakaran, M.; Jonnada, P.K.; Chandrashekhar, S.H.; Vinayachandran, G.; Kaambwa, B.; Barreto, S.G. Enhancing the cost-effectiveness of surgical care in pancreatic cancer: A systematic review and cost meta-analysis with trial sequential analysis. *HPB* **2021**, *24*, 309–321. [CrossRef] [PubMed]
33. Rosa, F.; Longo, F.; Pozzo, C.; Strippoli, A.; Quero, G.; Fiorillo, C.; Mele, M.C.; Alfieri, S. Enhanced recovery after surgery (ERAS) versus standard recovery for gastric cancer patients: The evidences and the issues. *Surg. Oncol.* **2022**, *41*, 101727. [CrossRef] [PubMed]
34. Noba, L.; Rodgers, S.; Chandler, C.; Balfour, A.; Hariharan, D.; Yip, V.S. Enhanced Recovery After Surgery (ERAS) Reduces Hospital Costs and Improve Clinical Outcomes in Liver Surgery: A Systematic Review and Meta-Analysis. *J. Gastrointest. Surg.* **2020**, *24*, 918–932. [CrossRef] [PubMed]

35. Ni, X.; Jia, D.; Chen, Y.; Wang, L.; Suo, J. Is the Enhanced Recovery After Surgery (ERAS) Program Effective and Safe in Laparoscopic Colorectal Cancer Surgery? A Meta-Analysis of Randomized Controlled Trials. *J. Gastrointest. Surg.* **2019**, *23*, 1502–1512. [CrossRef]
36. Bisch, S.P.; Jago, C.A.; Kalogera, E.; Ganshorn, H.; Meyer, L.A.; Ramirez, P.T.; Dowdy, S.C.; Nelson, G. Outcomes of enhanced recovery after surgery (ERAS) in gynecologic oncology—A systematic review and meta-analysis. *Gynecol. Oncol.* **2021**, *161*, 46–55. [CrossRef]
37. Nelson, G.; Bakkum-Gamez, J.; Kalogera, E.; Glaser, G.; Altman, A.; Meyer, L.A.; Taylor, J.S.; Iniesta, M.; Lasala, J.; Mena, G.; et al. Guidelines for perioperative care in gynecologic/oncology: Enhanced Recovery After Surgery (ERAS) Society recommendations—2019 update. *Int. J. Gynecol. Cancer* **2019**, *29*, 651–668. [CrossRef]
38. Peerbocus, M.; Wang, Z.-J. Enhanced Recovery After Surgery and Radical Cystectomy: A Systematic Review and Meta-Analysis. *Res. Rep. Urol.* **2021**, *13*, 535–547. [CrossRef]
39. Xing, J.; Wang, J.; Liu, G.; Jia, Y. Effects of enhanced recovery after surgery on robotic radical prostatectomy: A systematic review and meta-analysis. *Gland Surg.* **2021**, *10*, 3264–3271. [CrossRef]
40. Huber, G.F.; Dort, J.C. Reducing morbidity and complications after major head and neck cancer surgery: The (future) role of enhanced recovery after surgery protocols. *Curr. Opin. Otolaryngol. Head Neck Surg.* **2018**, *26*, 71–77. [CrossRef]
41. Watson, L.-J.; Ewers, C. Enhanced recovery after head and neck cancer surgery: A review of current literature. *Curr. Opin. Otolaryngol. Head Neck Surg.* **2020**, *28*, 161–164. [CrossRef]
42. Low, G.M.I.; Kiong, K.L.; Amaku, R.; Kruse, B.; Zheng, G.; Weber, R.S.; Lewis, C.M. Feasibility of an Enhanced Recovery After Surgery (ERAS) pathway for major head and neck oncologic surgery. *Am. J. Otolaryngol.* **2020**, *41*, 102679. [CrossRef] [PubMed]
43. Thomakos, N.; Pandraklakis, A.; Bisch, S.P.; Rodolakis, A.; Nelson, G. ERAS protocols in gynecologic oncology during COVID-19 pandemic. *Int. J. Gynecol. Cancer* **2020**, *30*, 728–729. [CrossRef] [PubMed]
44. Harrison, R.; Iniesta, M.D.; Pitcher, B.; Ramirez, P.T.; Cain, K.; Siverand, A.M.; Mena, G.; Lasala, J.; Meyer, L.A. Enhanced recovery for obese patients undergoing gynecologic cancer surgery. *Int. J. Gynecol. Cancer* **2020**, *30*, 1595–1602. [CrossRef] [PubMed]
45. Kim, S.R.; Laframboise, S.; Nelson, G.; McCluskey, S.A.; Avery, L.; Kujbid, N.; Zia, A.; Spenard, E.; Bernardini, M.Q.; Ferguson, S.E.; et al. Enhanced recovery after minimally invasive gynecologic oncology surgery to improve same day discharge: A quality improvement project. *Int. J. Gynecol. Cancer* **2022**, ijgc-2021-003065. [CrossRef] [PubMed]

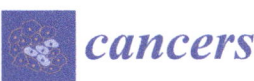

Review

Breast Cancer and COVID-19: Challenges in Surgical Management

Zoe Petropoulou *[ID], Nikolaos Arkadopoulos and Nikolaos V. Michalopoulos

4th Department of Surgery, Medical School, "Attikon" University Hospital, University of Athens, 12462 Athens, Greece
* Correspondence: zoegpetr@gmail.com

Simple Summary: The COVID-19 pandemic imposed serious strain on healthcare services and patient management, affecting almost every medical field. Cancer patients underwent and are still facing major modifications and turbulences with regard to their therapeutic courses, with the medical community awkwardly balancing the disease's menacing nature and their increased vulnerability to novel infection. As the cancer with the highest incidence and prevalence, breast-cancer patients and caregivers were widely affected by the healthcare crisis in multiple domains and ways, leading to rapid adjustments in response, maintaining one aim: to provide safe and uninterrupted cancer care regardless of the resource and communication shortages. This review summarizes the challenges in breast-cancer management and the subsequent alterations in clinical practice. The reflexes and adaptability of the medical community under this massive pressure provide a glimmer of optimism, but the impact of these forced changes and their contribution to this goal still need to be evaluated.

Abstract: The harsh healthcare reality imposed by the COVID-19 pandemic resulted in wide clinical practice alterations, postponements, and shortages, affecting both patients and caregivers. Breast-cancer management, from diagnosis to treatment and follow up, was a field that did not escape such changes, facing a challenging set of obstacles in order to maintain adequate cancer care services while diminishing viral spread among patients and personnel. In this review article, we discuss the impact of the COVID-19 pandemic on several aspects of breast-cancer management, and the subsequent modifications adopted by clinicians, scientific groups, and governments as a response to the novel conditions. Screening and diagnosis, as well as breast-cancer treatment paths—especially surgical interventions—were the most affected domains, while patients' psychological burden also emerged as a notable consequence. The aftermath of diagnostic and surgical delays is yet to be assessed, while the treatment alterations and the introduction of new therapeutic schemes might signify the opening of a novel era in breast-cancer management.

Keywords: breast cancer; COVID-19; cancer care; screening; surgery; psychological distress

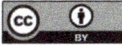

1. Introduction

The COVID-19 pandemic has imposed significant strain on healthcare services, including cancer-care providers. The struggle mostly concerns the fine balance between the risk of virus transmission among vulnerable oncological patients and valuable healthcare personnel, the preservation of human and material resources, the alleviation of facilities' overload, and the ensuring of high-quality cancer care.

Restrictive measures and social distancing; the redeployment of human resources; and limitations in personal protective equipment, material, and hospital beds revealed the need for adapting to a new, hostile clinical setting, both for patients and clinicians, with subsequent inevitable modifications, delays, or even postponements in many aspects of clinical practice. More specifically, concerning breast-cancer patients, many national committees responded to these unprecedented conditions with omissions of screening and follow-up programs during the overload phases of the pandemic, as well as alterations in the execution of diagnostic and treatment procedures. Major health organizations and professional bodies issued recommendations to provide some of the much needed guidance regarding demanding breast-cancer-patient management from diagnosis to treatment and follow-up during this overwhelming period.

In addition to healthcare systems' dysfunctions, patients' psychology and behavior were not spared from the devastating effects of the pandemic, leading to further delays and cancellations in screening or in diagnostic, therapeutic, or follow-up appointments, further compromising the achievement of delivering adequate cancer care in such a rough setting.

In this review article, we identify, summarize, and eventually assess the impact of the COVID-19 pandemic on several stages of breast-cancer management.

2. Main Text

2.1. Challenges in Diagnosis

To minimize COVID-19 spread, several social distancing measures and transport limitations were imposed in most countries. Compliance with these measures, as well as the fear of getting infected, led a significant number of women to postpone or cancel medical appointments and breast-cancer screening examinations, even in cases where symptoms were present, with a subsequent reduction in the number of patient referrals and overall breast-cancer diagnoses [1–4]. In addition to the reluctance of the population eligible for screening, many screening programs worldwide were temporarily halted, and primary care appointments, diagnostic imaging, and breast biopsies were reduced in response to augmented clinical demands and a shortage of human and material resources [1,2,4–8]. This practice was also favored by the recommendations published by experts' consortia [9–11]. As expected, the losses in screening and primary care appointments were translated into a significant decrease in breast-cancer incidence and diagnoses during the intense phases of the pandemic, especially for in situ ductal carcinomas (DCIS), early-stage disease, and women aged over 50 years old (the cutoff age for some screening programs), according to some studies [2,5].

The consequences of these diagnostic delays are not yet extensively known, but estimation models based on well-monitored populations predict a possible increase in breast-cancer-related deaths, proportional to the duration of screening cessation [4,8]. Long-term studies should be conducted in order to shed light on this assumption.

Providing screening programs and non-urgent primary and specialized breast-cancer diagnostic services during periods of such overload may not be feasible, but a number of alternatives and modifications can contribute to the effort to stay close to the standard of care. Notably, the use of telemedicine emerged as a useful referral alternative that spares medical resources and provides the opportunity to avoid unnecessary in-person visits, advantages that made it a preferable option among physicians [7]. Furthermore, instead of complete screening and diagnostic-program cessation, detailed planning and information on safety protocols during diagnostic imaging and procedures, as well as the modification of the number of women per screening session, can ease the execution of these programs, achieving safer procedures and fewer patient cancellations.

2.2. Challenges in Treatment

Saving valuable medical and facility resources, and mitigating the spread of SARS-CoV-2 while offering breast-cancer patients high-quality treatment close to the standard care, was again the main struggle regarding breast-cancer treatment and decision making. At the beginning of the pandemic, cancer patients, including breast-cancer patients, were considered high-risk patients for COVID-19-related morbidity and mortality, due to disease and chemotherapy-induced immunosuppression [7]. From this point of view, minimizing the risk of COVID-19 exposure by reducing in-person appointments and sessions, avoiding long hospital stays, and limiting the probability of treatment complications and adverse effects and subsequent readmissions was of paramount importance. Additionally, in the context of the healthcare crisis, immense operating-room schedule redistribution and elective-surgery volume reduction occurred, creating another therapeutic obstacle for a significant portion of breast-cancer patients [6,12]. In this setting, the avoidance of undertreatment and providing safe and timely therapeutic options without compromising the outcomes becomes a quite challenging task. A series of therapeutic modifications emerged as a response to the new conditions, rapidly included in breast cancer decision-making guidelines and recommendations issued especially for clinical practice during the pandemic, which were mostly characterized by a shift from surgical and hospitalization-requiring therapies towards conservative, at-home treatments. Notably, the COVID-19 pandemic era was intensely marked by the broad use of neoadjuvant hormonal therapy for hormonal receptor (HR)-positive tumors, both early-stage and locally advanced breast cancer or even DCIS, as a first-line, surgery-sparing treatment for every age group, serving as a major contributor to surgical-load reduction [2,5,6,8,9,12–16].

Surgical practice and treatment were highly affected during the pandemic and especially during the confinement periods, facing a trend that called for operation omissions, careful preoperative patient selection, and surgical-management modifications [5,12].

Non-urgent surgical procedures were postponed, a decision also supported by several professional group recommendations (ACR, ESMO, ACCN, ASBrS, NAPBC, and CoC) [5–8,10–12,14,17–19]. Studies stating that surgery delays of up to 12 weeks have no impact on patients' long-term survival and the rise in neoadjuvant therapies allowed this direction to be implemented in several countries, with 13.6% of surveyed US breast surgeons declaring to have had all of their operations stopped and 100% reporting a reduction in the number of elective surgeries [3,6,12]. In a survey conducted by Rocco et al., including breast surgeons from various countries worldwide, only 4% of the participants reported retaining unchanged operating schedules. From the affected portion, 62% declared reducing their sessions and 34% performing only emergency breast operations [12]. To achieve this reduction, a primary systemic treatment was offered as an alternative to surgery in 48% of the cases diagnosed during the pandemic [12].

To aid patient selection, multidisciplinary team cooperation and patient triaging are necessary. Many health systems, following the management recommendations, used a patient-selection system, usually dividing breast-cancer patients into three or four surgical-time groups, from high (<2 weeks) to low surgical priority (>4 or up to >8 weeks), according to surgery urgency. Patients facing surgical complications (hematomas, abscesses, and flap ischemia) are of high surgical priority regardless of the COVID-19 urgency setting [10,11,19]. Patients completing neoadjuvant chemotherapy, breast cancer during pregnancy, T2 or N1 HR+/HER2- tumors, and triple-negative or HER2+ patients range from high to intermediate surgical priority, taking into consideration the COVID-19 urgency setting and alternative treatment options [8–12,14,15,18,19]. The excision of malignant recurrence, clinically low-risk primary disease, discordant biopsies likely to be malignant, and patients unable to receive neoadjuvant treatment are considered of intermediate priority [8–12,14,15,18,19]. All high-risk benign lesions, DCIS cases, discordant biopsies likely to be benign, re-excision surgeries, prophylactic operations, delayed sentinel lymph node biopsies, and primary-systemic-treatment-eligible patients are classified as low priority [10,11,19].

The type of surgical approach was also affected, with an increase in minimal, breast-conserving operations in order to avoid extensive surgeries and thereupon the risk of major complications, patient revisits, unnecessary hospitalizations, and prolonged hospital stay [6,8,9,14,16]. When mastectomy was performed, immediate breast reconstruction (IBR) was not the reconstructive method of choice; instead, delayed reconstruction was preferred in order to reduce surgical time and the risk of complications in many cases [12,16]. The axillary surgical approach does not seem to have been affected, although some technical considerations arose regarding the COVID-19 vaccination site and timing or the feasibility of dual tracer sentinel lymph node (SLN) mapping, creating space for possible alternatives [16,20,21].

Regarding radiotherapy and systemic therapy, following the same principles of in-person appointment and hospitalization reductions and resource retaining, several alterations were applied. Current practices and literature support that adjuvant radiotherapy initiation can be delayed for up to 3–6 months for selected patients, and hypofractionated radiotherapy schedules are preferred during periods of health-system overload since there seems to be no difference in terms of the therapeutic effect [7,9,10,13,15,22]. In general, radiation treatment was preserved for high-risk breast-cancer patients postoperatively and as palliative treatment for local or metastatic disease presenting with urgent or otherwise uncontrollable symptoms (bleeding mass, spinal cord compression, and symptomatic brain lesions), in addition to patients already on treatment [10,11].

Both adjuvant and neoadjuvant hormonal therapy (NET) for every stage HR positive tumors became widely suggested, as well as HER2-directed therapy for HER2+ disease, facilitating the delay of surgical treatment [2,6,8,9,13,14,16]. More specifically, primary hormonal therapy was considered acceptable in most of HR+/HER2- cases, especially post-menopausal women, in some countries, including those with N1 axillary disease, accompanied by neoadjuvant chemotherapy in high-risk patients, the selection of whom was facilitated by the use of genomic testing [5,6,9,12–14]. This practice can delay surgical treatment up to 6–12 months [11]. Wilke et al. report an additional 31% of the patients in their database receiving NET due to COVID-19, in contradiction to 6.9% receiving NET as the usual approach, highlighting the impact of the pandemic on this particular type of treatment [6]. Chemotherapeutic protocols were modified in order to avoid toxicity and chemotherapy (CMT)-related adverse effects (most importantly immunosuppression), with complete avoidance of CMT in selected patients, the use of longer interval regimens, universal-growth-factor support, and limited anthracycline and steroid use [9–11,13,15]. Genomic testing, even on biopsy specimens, was strongly encouraged for patient selection [6,9,13].

2.3. Challenges in Follow-Up

Managing patient visits after treatment initiation was also a field affected by the pandemic, as this part of caregiving is not considered as urgent and therefore was subject to limitations. In the absence of symptoms, routine follow-up and breast-imaging appointments were deferred, with a reduction in in-person visits up to 49.4% in some countries [10,12,13,23]. Telemedicine came up again as a solution to some cases, filling part of this void and cutting down the necessity for face-to-face appointments, while providing adequate healthcare services [10,23]. It was included as the recommended method for established cases without new issues, psychological support visits, and newly diagnosed non-invasive breast-cancer patients [11].

2.4. Challenges for the Patients

While healthcare personnel have often been found crushed under the pandemic's suffocating burden, patients were not at all spared the psychological pressure imposed by this new threat either. The pandemic brought additional stressors to an already psychologically vulnerable population group, such as the fear of infection, especially for immunosuppressed patients; the fear of disease undertreatment and recurrence due to delays and changes in cancer therapies; and the logistics of scheduling and attending a screening, treatment, or follow-up appointment [1,17,24]. In addition, through restrictive measures and isolation, it deprived them of several supporting mechanisms: in-person communication and interaction, participation in group activities, and even receiving specialized help and care. Breast-cancer patients' life became gloomier, as a Canadian study shows, with 63.9% of the participants declaring having experienced at least one COVID-19-related stressor and almost 40% showing clinical levels of concerns such as anxiety, insomnia, and depressive symptoms [24]. Promoting mental health and emotional stability for these patients is a principal priority per se but also serves as a way to ensure better compliance and engagement, avoiding screening or treatment drop outs that jeopardize patients' outcomes [1,24]. Communication is key to overcoming these psychological obstacles, alleviating the frustration deriving from management alterations and providing needed information, counseling, and support, creating a safe environment for the patient, even when it is accomplished remotely or with the use of informational material [1,17].

2.5. Challenges in Breast-Surgery Education

The pandemic-induced shift from surgical to non-surgical breast-cancer treatments left breast surgical training in crisis too. The inevitable changes in clinical practice affected surgical trainees worldwide regardless of their training program duration or setting. Breast-surgery fellowships in particular, due to the short-time programs (usually 1 year), faced major interruptions.

The alterations that most affected postgraduate surgical education include the dramatic decrease in elective operations, the missing cases due to diagnostic delays, the reduced clinic and outpatient unit hours, and the trainees' redeployment to COVID-19 related units [25–28]. The main result of these changes was a significant gap in hands-on, operative, and in-patient exposure. As stated by Kilgore et al., 43% of breast-surgery trainees incurred partial or complete deprivation of their time in the operating room [26]. In a prospective study conducted by a COVID-STAR collaborative study group among trainees of several surgical subspecialties, including breast surgery, the respondents reported a complete or >50% loss of their training regarding elective operating, emergency operating, and outpatient activity in 69.5%, 48%, and 67.3% of respondents, respectively, which affected their progression and perception of competence in their fields [28]. Moreover, reduced contact and communication with physicians of the same or relevant specialties in the context of COVID-19 risk-reduction measures hindered mentorship and peer guidance, further limiting gained experience.

Apart from the clinical aspects of surgical education, delays in clinical research; cancellations and disabled attendance in conferences; and postponements of certification or qualifying exams posed a threat to academic development [25,26,29].

As a result of educational and professional uncertainty, along with a fear of COVID-19 infection and transmission, stress levels were heightened; 81% of surgical trainees declared that their mental health was affected by the situation, and 93% of breast-surgery fellows admitted having faced increased stress [26,28]. The educational challenges hide a long-term breast-cancer management challenge since the deficient training at the present could lead to insufficient surgeons in the future, imperiling patients' safety and outcomes [27].

3. Discussion

The ongoing COVID-19 pandemic has been a burdensome situation for healthcare systems, clinicians, and patients worldwide. Breast-cancer management is facing several obstacles inflicted by this pandemic in all of its aspects. Screening, patient diagnosis, treatment and follow-up are all parts of this multifaceted challenge and the most important questions arising concern how these difficulties are to be overcome and what will be the impact of our decisions be—its extent and its contribution—on breast-cancer patients' course.

In such unprecedented conditions, providing high-quality cancer care with compromised material, human, and even psychological reserves requires cautious and thorough decision making, which can be achieved only when based on well founded, evidence-based knowledge and uninterrupted multidisciplinary coordination. Consultations and guidelines elaborated by scientific groups aid this process and provide a base for consonant clinical practice, without limiting the opportunity for personalized care. Furthermore, establishing and supporting communication between caregivers and patients with detailed and comprehensible information about their disease, options, and COVID-19 risks seems to be an important step towards a safe and effective therapeutic plan.

It is apparent that the impact of the current situation and its subsequent alterations in breast-cancer management is still unknown, and further investigation is essential. Screening and diagnostic delays due to suspended screening programs and reduced referrals, as well as patient hesitancy, could contribute to a shift towards higher stage disease at the time of diagnosis, losses in diagnoses, and ultimately an increase in breast cancer mortality, a hypothesis that needs to be assessed. Treatment modifications, such as the rapid increase in neoadjuvant hormonal therapy use, surgery and radiotherapy delays, and systemic therapy regimen alterations, are another field of evaluation, in order to define the safety and efficacy of COVID-19-driven management decisions and acquire valuable data on the impact of the pandemic on breast-cancer patients' outcomes. Finally, although the changes implemented are considered as resource-sparing, the aftermath of breast-cancer screening and treatment distortions may still not favor health systems' sustainability. It is of value to take into consideration whether missing early-stage disease, delaying surgery and performing two-step surgeries instead of one (as in the case of avoided immediate breast reconstruction operations) could ultimately increase the cost of breast-cancer care.

Another topic yet to be clarified is the actual relationship between COVID-19 and breast cancer in order to define the level of patients' risk and include it in decision making. The existing literature suggests that breast cancer per se is not a major contributor to COVID-19 mortality, nor is its treatment, and COVID-19 infection outcomes in these patients are mostly affected by patient's comorbidities [7,14,30]. Thus, it would be reasonable to redefine the existing modifications or the population that they concern, considering their application only for high-risk patients.

Despite being a first-line therapy for many cases, breast-cancer surgery is one of the fields receiving the most extensive changes and reductions for the sake of hospital operations and resource preservation. It should be noted though that the majority of oncological breast surgeries require short operation times and a limited hospital stay and have almost no need for ICU beds [12]. The rates of complication and hospital readmissions are low, especially when an IBR is not performed, and postoperative follow-up is usually not demanding [12]. Therefore, the need for strict surgery avoidance may be questioned, and the possibility of breast-cancer surgery regaining its place is a topic to be discussed.

Within difficulty lies opportunity, and this dire situation seems to be no exception to that. The urgent and massive need for clinical practice rescheduling received an immediate response from the scientific community, adjusting to the new setting effectively and responsibly in order to maintain the standard of care. The readiness and responsiveness are a promising sign, as are some of the decisions that the pandemic forced us to dare to make, including instituting the new therapeutic approaches and alternative ways of caregiving, such as the establishment of telemedicine, a tool that is going to be useful in the post-COVID era too. A careful interpretation of the new data acquired during this period could hopefully fructify in terms of progress.

4. Conclusions

The COVID-19 pandemic and the induced healthcare crisis enforced an era of shortages in caregiving, due to the massive needs in human and material resources and hospital beds, as well as in patients' wellbeing and mental health as a result of the restrictive measures imposed. In this hostile setting, breast-cancer management faced challenges at multiple levels; from screening and prevention, to diagnosis, treatment, and follow-up, struggling at each step to deliver the highest possible quality of care. Responding to these conditions included delays and postponements, mostly for the diagnostic part and considerable or minor alterations for the therapeutic plans, with two major points regarding this field: the rise and extensive use of neoadjuvant hormonal therapy and the significant reduction in the first-line surgical approach. These changes in therapeutic strategy remain to be evaluated.

Author Contributions: Conceptualization, N.A.; methodology, Z.P., N.V.M.; writing—original draft preparation, Z.P., N.V.M.; writing—review and editing, Z.P., N.V.M., N.A.; supervision, N.A. All authors have read and agreed to the published version of the manuscript.

Funding: This research received no external funding.

Conflicts of Interest: The authors declare no conflict of interest.

References

1. Schifferdecker, K.E.; Vaclavik, D.; Wernli, K.J.; Buist, D.S.M.; Kerlikowske, K.; Sprague, B.L.; Henderson, L.M.; Johnson, D.; Budesky, J.; Jackson-Nefertiti, G.; et al. Women's considerations and experiences for breast cancer screening and surveillance during the COVID-19 pandemic in the United States: A focus group study. *Prev. Med.* 2021, *151*, 106542. [CrossRef] [PubMed]
2. Gathani, T.; Clayton, G.; MacInnes, E.; Horgan, K. The COVID-19 pandemic and impact on breast cancer diagnoses: What happened in England in the first half of 2020. *Br. J. Cancer* 2020, *124*, 710–712. [CrossRef] [PubMed]
3. Gosset, M.; Gal, J.; Schiappa, R.; Dejode, M.; Fouché, Y.; Alazet, F.; Roux, E.; Delpech, Y.; Barranger, E. Impact de la pandémie de COVID-19 sur les prises en charge pour cancer du sein et gynécologique. Impact of COVID-19 pandemic on breast and gynecologic cancers management. Experience of the Surgery Department in the Nice Anticancer Center. *Bull. Cancer* 2020, *108*, 3–11. [CrossRef] [PubMed]
4. Figueroa, J.D.; Gray, E.; Pashayan, N.; Deandrea, S.; Karch, A.; Vale, D.B.; Elder, K.; Procopio, P.; van Ravesteyn, N.T.; Mutabi, M.; et al. Breast Screening Working Group (WG2) of the COVID-19 and Cancer Global Modelling Consortium. The impact of the COVID-19 pandemic on breast cancer early detection and screening. *Prev. Med.* 2021, *151*, 106585. [CrossRef]
5. Eijkelboom, A.H.; de Munck, L.; Vrancken Peeters, M.T.F.D.; Broeders, M.J.M.; Strobbe, L.J.A.; Bos, M.E.M.M.; Schmidt, M.K.; Guerrero Paez, C.; Smidt, M.L.; Bessems, M.; et al. Impact of the COVID-19 pandemic on diagnosis, stage, and initial treatment of breast cancer in the Netherlands: A population-based study. *J. Hematol. Oncol.* 2021, *14*, 64. [CrossRef]
6. Wilke, L.G.; Nguyen, T.T.; Yang, Q.; Hanlon, B.M.; Wagner, K.A.; Strickland, P.; Brown, E.; Dietz, J.R.; Boughey, J.C. Analysis of the Impact of the COVID-19 Pandemic on the Multidisciplinary Management of Breast Cancer: Review from the American Society of Breast Surgeons COVID-19 and Mastery Registries. *Ann. Surg. Oncol.* 2021, *28*, 5535–5543. [CrossRef]
7. Mathelin, C.; Ame, S.; Anyanwu, S.; Avisar, E.; Boubnider, W.M.; Breitling, K.; Anie, H.A.; Conceição, J.C.; Dupont, V.; Elder, E.; et al. Breast Cancer Management during the COVID-19 Pandemic: The Senologic International Society Survey. *Eur. J. Breast Health* 2021, *17*, 188–196, Erratum in *Eur. J. Breast Health* 2021, *17*, 296. [CrossRef]
8. Tonneson, J.E.; Hoskin, T.L.; Day, C.N.; Durgan, D.M.; Dilaveri, C.A.; Boughey, J.C. Impact of the COVID-19 Pandemic on Breast Cancer Stage at Diagnosis, Presentation, and Patient Management. *Ann. Surg. Oncol.* 2021, *23*, 1–9. [CrossRef]
9. Curigliano, G.; Cardoso, M.J.; Poortmans, P.; Gentilini, O.; Pravettoni, G.; Mazzocco, K.; Houssami, N.; Pagani, O.; Senkus, E.; Cardoso, F.; et al. Recommendations for triage, prioritization and treatment of breast cancer patients during the COVID-19 pandemic. *Breast* 2020, *52*, 8–16. [CrossRef]
10. Dietz, J.R.; Moran, M.S.; Isakoff, S.J.; Kurtzman, S.H.; Willey, S.C.; Burstein, H.J.; Bleicher, R.J.; Lyons, J.A.; Sarantou, T.; Baron, P.L.; et al. Recommendations for prioritization, treatment, and triage of breast cancer patients during the COVID-19 pandemic. the COVID-19 pandemic breast cancer consortium. *Breast Cancer Res. Treat.* 2020, *181*, 487–497. [CrossRef]
11. de Azambuja, E.; Trapani, D.; Loibl, S.; Delaloge, S.; Senkus, E.; Criscitiello, C.; Poortmans, P.; Gnant, M.; Di Cosimo, S.; Cortes, J.; et al. ESMO Management and treatment adapted recommendations in the COVID-19 era: Breast Cancer. *ESMO Open* 2020, *5* (Suppl. 3), e000793. [CrossRef] [PubMed]
12. Rocco, N.; Montagna, G.; Di Micco, R.; Benson, J.; Criscitiello, C.; Chen, L.; Di Pace, B.; Esgueva Colmenarejo, A.J.; Harder, Y.; Karakatsanis, A.; et al. The Impact of the COVID-19 Pandemic on Surgical Management of Breast Cancer: Global Trends and Future Perspectives. *Oncologist* 2021, *26*, e66–e77. [CrossRef] [PubMed]
13. Freedman, R.A.; Sedrak, M.S.; Bellon, J.R.; Block, C.C.; Lin, N.U.; King, T.A.; Minami, C.; VanderWalde, N.; Jolly, T.A.; Muss, H.B.; et al. Weathering the Storm: Managing Older Adults With Breast Cancer Amid COVID-19 and Beyond. *J. Natl. Cancer Inst.* 2021, *113*, 355–359. [CrossRef] [PubMed]
14. Brenes Sánchez, J.M.; Picado, A.L.; Olivares Crespo, M.E.; García Sáenz, J.Á.; De La Plata Merlo, R.M.; De La Muela, M.H. Breast Cancer Management During COVID-19 Pandemic in Madrid: Surgical Strategy. *Clin. Breast Cancer* 2021, *21*, e128–e135. [CrossRef]
15. Spicer, J.; Chamberlain, C.; Papa, S. Provision of cancer care during the COVID-19 pandemic. *Nat. Rev. Clin. Oncol.* 2020, *17*, 329–331. [CrossRef]
16. Romics, L.; Doughty, J.; Stallard, S.; Mansell, J.; Blackhall, V.; Lannigan, A.; Elgammal, S.; Reid, J.; McGuigan, M.-C.; Savioli, F.; et al. A prospective cohort study of the safety of breast cancer surgery during COVID-19 pandemic in the West of Scotland. *Breast* 2021, *55*, 1–6. [CrossRef]
17. Sokas, C.; Kelly, M.; Sheu, C.; Song, J.; Welch, H.G.; Bergmark, R.; Minami, C.; Trinh, Q.D. Cancer in the Shadow of COVID: Early-Stage Breast and Prostate Cancer Patient Perspectives on Surgical Delays Due to COVID-19. *Ann. Surg. Oncol.* 2021, *28*, 8688–8696. [CrossRef]
18. Johnson, B.A.; Waddimba, A.C.; Ogola, G.O.; Fleshman JWJr Preskitt, J.T. A systematic review and meta-analysis of surgery delays and survival in breast, lung and colon cancers: Implication for surgical triage during the COVID-19 pandemic. *Am. J. Surg.* 2021, *222*, 311–318. [CrossRef]
19. American College of Surgeons. COVID-19 Guidelines for Triage of Breast Cancer Patients. Available online: https://www.facs.org/COVID-19/clinical-guidance/elective-case/breast-cancer (accessed on 20 February 2022).
20. Ko, G.; Hota, S.; Cil, T.D. COVID-19 Vaccination and Breast Cancer Surgery Timing. *Breast Cancer Res. Treat* 2021, *188*, 825–826. [CrossRef]
21. Cocco, D.; Valente, S.A. Sentinel Lymph Node Mapping and Biopsy in Breast Cancer Patients During the COVID-19 Pandemic. *Ann. Surg. Oncol.* 2021, *28*, 4056–4057. [CrossRef]

22. Fortunato, L.; d'Amati, G.; Taffurelli, M.; Tinterri, C.; Marotti, L.; Cataliotti, L. Severe Impact of COVID-19 Pandemic on Breast Cancer Care in Italy: A Senonetwork National Survey. *Clin. Breast Cancer* **2021**, *21*, e165–e167. [CrossRef] [PubMed]
23. Sonagli, M.; Cagnacci Neto, R.; Leite, F.P.M.; Makdissi, F.B.A. The use of telemedicine to maintain breast cancer follow-up and surveillance during the COVID-19 pandemic. *J. Surg. Oncol.* **2021**, *123*, 371–374. [CrossRef]
24. Massicotte, V.; Ivers, H.; Savard, J. COVID-19 Pandemic Stressors and Psychological Symptoms in Breast Cancer Patients. *Curr. Oncol.* **2021**, *28*, 294–300. [CrossRef] [PubMed]
25. Friedrich, A.U.; DiComo, J.A.; Golshan, M. The Impact of COVID-19 on Breast Surgery Fellowships. *Curr. Breast Cancer Rep.* **2021**, *13*, 235–240. [CrossRef] [PubMed]
26. Kilgore, L.J.; Murphy, B.L.; Postlewait, L.M.; Liang, D.H.; Bedrosian, I.; Lucci, A.; Kuerer, H.M.; Hunt, K.K.; Teshome, M. Impact of the early COVID-19 pandemic on Breast Surgical Oncology fellow education. *J Surg Oncol.* **2021**, *124*, 989–994. [CrossRef]
27. Munro, C.; Burke, J.; Allum, W.; Mortensen, N. COVID-19 leaves surgical training in crisis. *BMJ* **2021**, *372*, n659. [CrossRef]
28. COVID-STAR Collaborative Study Group. COVID-19 impact on Surgical Training and Recovery Planning (COVID-STAR)—A cross-sectional observational study. *Int. J. Surg.* **2021**, *88*, 105903. [CrossRef]
29. Daodu, O.; Panda, N.; Lopushinsky, S.; Varghese TKJr Brindle, M. COVID-19—Considerations and Implications for Surgical Learners. *Ann. Surg.* **2020**, *272*, e22–e23. [CrossRef]
30. Vuagnat, P.; Frelaut, M.; Ramtohul, T.; Basse, C.; Diakite, S.; Noret, A.; Bellesoeur, A.; Servois, V.; Hequet, D.; Laas, E.; et al. COVID-19 in breast cancer patients: A cohort at the Institut Curie hospitals in the Paris area. *Breast Cancer Res.* **2020**, *22*, 55. [CrossRef]

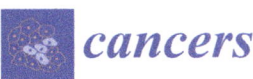 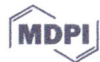

Systematic Review

Colorectal Surgery in the COVID-19 Era: A Systematic Review and Meta-Analysis

Nikolaos Pararas, Anastasia Pikouli, Dimitrios Papaconstantinou *, Georgios Bagias, Constantinos Nastos, Andreas Pikoulis, Dionysios Dellaportas, Panagis Lykoudis and Emmanouil Pikoulis

3rd Department of Surgery, Attikon University Hospital, National and Kapodistrian University of Athens Medical School, Rimini 1, 12462 Chaidari, Greece; npararas@gmail.com (N.P.); anastasiapikouli@gmail.com (A.P.); georgebagias@live.com (G.B.); kosnastos@yahoo.gr (C.N.); crisismed@outlook.com (A.P.); dellapdio@gmail.com (D.D.); p.lykoudis@ucl.ac.uk (P.L.); mpikoul@med.uoa.gr (E.P.)
* Correspondence: dimpapa7@hotmail.com; Tel.: +30-210-5832373

Simple Summary: The rapid spread of the new Coronavirus-19 disease (COVID-19) has led to the implementation of unprecedented confinement measures, while healthcare systems were restructured in order to confront the pandemic; these radical measures have prevented people from seeking medical advice. At the same time, oncology and surgery societies altered treatment guidelines, favoring postponement of surgery. The aim of the present study is to determine the impact of the pandemic in the management of colorectal cancer patients. We confirmed that during the pandemic, patients were more likely to present with metastatic cancer, often requiring emergent or palliative interventions. In addition, neoadjuvant therapy and conventional open surgery utilization rates were increased in the pandemic era. These observed changes in clinical practice may be associated with tumor upstaging, which carries significant implications regarding the long-term oncologic survival of patients with colorectal neoplasias.

Abstract: (1) Background: To determine the impact of the COVID-19 pandemic in the management of colorectal cancer patients requiring surgery and to examine whether the restructuring of healthcare systems led to cancer stage upshifting or adverse treatment outcomes; (2) Methods: A systematic literature search of the MedLine, Scopus, Web of Science, and CNKI databases was performed (PROSPERO ID: CRD42021288432). Data were summarized as odds ratios (OR) or weighted mean differences (WMDs) with 95% confidence intervals (95% CIs); (3) Results: Ten studies were examined, including 26,808 patients. The number of patients presenting with metastases during the pandemic was significantly increased (OR 1.65, 95% CI 1.02–2.67, $p = 0.04$), with no differences regarding the extent of the primary tumor (T) and nodal (N) status. Patients were more likely to have undergone neoadjuvant therapy (OR 1.22, 95% CI 1.09–1.37, $p < 0.001$), while emergency presentations (OR 1.74, 95% CI 1.07–2.84, $p = 0.03$) and palliative surgeries (OR 1.95, 95% CI 1.13–3.36, $p = 0.02$) were more frequent during the pandemic. There was no significant difference recorded in terms of postoperative morbidity; (4) Conclusions: Patients during the pandemic were more likely to undergo palliative interventions or receive neoadjuvant treatment.

Keywords: cancer; colorectal; COVID-19; pandemic; meta-analysis

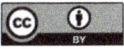

1. Introduction

The rapid worldwide spread of the new SARS-CoV 19 virus led to the implementation of unprecedented confinement measures in order to minimize the dissemination of the Coronavirus-19 disease (COVID-19). At the same time, healthcare systems around the world were restructured in order to confront the pandemic; hospitals were closed or were repurposed into COVID-19 treatment centers, most prominently by suspending outpatient clinics and elective surgeries [1]. These radical measures have prevented people from carrying out annual medical screening or seeking medical advice [1,2]. Newly diagnosed cancer cases were significantly lower in 2020 compared to the pre-pandemic era [3,4], while cancer-related deaths were also significantly increased during the same time period [5].

Management of colorectal cancer, the third most common cancer worldwide [6], was consequently affected by the pandemic. The number of colonoscopies and colorectal cancer screening tests was markedly reduced in 2020 [7]; as a result, many colorectal cancer cases remained either undiagnosed or were diagnosed at an advanced stage with significant implications regarding the long-term oncologic outcomes of these patients [8]. At the same time, oncology and surgery societies altered treatment guidelines, favoring postponement of surgery [9,10]. Reports from different institutions around the world highlight the increasing number of patients presenting late, with symptoms of bowel obstruction or bowel perforation, which carry higher postoperative morbidity and mortality rates [11].

The aim of the present systematic review and meta-analysis is to determine the impact of the pandemic in the management of colorectal cancer patients requiring surgery and to assess whether the reduced accessibility to healthcare resources caused by COVID-19 led to cancer stage upshifting or adverse treatment outcomes.

2. Materials and Methods

A systematic literature search of the MedLine, Scopus, Web of Science, and China National Knowledge Infrastructure (CNKI) databases and clinicaltrials.gov register was conducted using a combination of the search terms "COVID-19", "coronavirus", "pandemic", "colorectal cancer", and "surgery" using the Boolean operators AND/OR as appropriate for each database. After removing duplicated studies, the titles and abstracts generated by the search algorithm were screened independently by two authors (GB, AP), and after the removal of obviously irrelevant studies, the remaining were evaluated in full-text. The reference lists were further manually checked using the snowballing technique to identify additional potentially relevant studies. Any discrepancies and disagreements ensuing during the initial screening process of the systematic literature search were resolved either by common consensus or by the mediation of a third reviewer (DD).

Studies were eligible for inclusion if they provided comparative data on tumor stage and treatment outcomes for patients managed during the pre-pandemic and pandemic time periods. The predetermined study exclusion criteria were: (1) case reports, reviews, or non-clinical studies, (2) studies published in non-English languages, (3) studies with non-surgically treated patients, (4) studies not reporting tumor or treatment-related outcomes, (5) studies not providing comparative data between pre-pandemic and pandemic patient cohorts or comparing different patient populations, and (6) studies including patients with pathologies other than colorectal cancer.

2.1. Data Extraction and Outcomes Evaluated and Definitions

Data from included studies were extracted by two authors (GB, AP) and were entered into standardized excel spreadsheets (Microsoft, Redmond, Washington, DC, USA) for data tabulation. Data of primary importance were the time interval of data collection for the pre-pandemic and pandemic cohorts, the the tumor, node, and metastasis (TNM) classification (TNM) stage (AJCC 8th edition) [12] of the involved colorectal tumors, the number of total patients, the emergency presentation rates, neoadjuvant utilization rates, minimally invasive technique utilization rates, palliative-intent surgery rates, mortality/morbidity rates, and the length of hospital stay.

Secondary data were the patient demographics, the location of the tumors, the rates of stoma formation, the number of tumors complicated by obstruction or perforation, and the number of lymph nodes retrieved by surgery.

Minimally invasive surgery is defined as either laparoscopic or robotic abdominal surgery. Palliative intent surgery refers to palliative ostomy or by-pass procedures in cases in which tumor removal was either not possible or contraindicated. Tumors complicated by obstruction, perforation, or acute bleeding are referred to as complicated tumors throughout this analysis. Finally, stoma formation corresponds to the number of ostomies performed either for palliative reasons or for intentional diversion in cases of rectal surgery.

The present study was registered in the "International Prospective Register of Systematic Review" in 2021 (PROSPERO ID: CRD42021288432) and was conducted according to PRISMA guidelines [13].

2.2. Methodological Quality Assessment

Assessment of included studies for methodological integrity and accuracy of data reporting was performed using the Newcastle–Ottawa scale (NOS). The NOS is an 8-item scale evaluating the adequacy of the patient selection process (score of 0 to 4 stars), the comparability of the involved groups (0 to 2 stars), and the ascertainment of the reported exposure (0 to 3 stars). Each study is awarded a score of 0 to 9 stars, quantifying its methodological quality, with studies scoring 7 to 9 being of high quality, studies with scores from 5 to 6 being of mediocre quality, and studies with a score of 4 or less being of poor quality.

2.3. Statistical Analysis

Odds Ratios (OR) were calculated for the pooled analysis of dichotomous outcomes and Weighted Mean Differences (WMD) for continuous outcomes. The random-effects model was a priori selected to calculate ORs, WMDs, 95% Confidence Intervals (CI), and relevant p-values due to expected clinical heterogeneity in terms of geography, regional covid prevalence, and the extent of elective service disruption by Covid. The Higgin's I^2 statistic and relevant p-values were calculated to assess existing statistical heterogeneity between the sampled studies. All analyses were performed with the Revman v 5.4.1 (The Cochrane Collaboration, 2020) software. Funnel plots were constructed for each outcome (Figures S19–S36); however, statistical testing for publication bias was not possible due to the small number of included studies. All p-values less than 0.05 were considered statistically significant.

Leave-one-out sensitivity analysis was performed for those outcomes in which the Higgin's I^2 test for heterogeneity was statistically significant or demonstrated a statistically significant effect size. The analysis was performed by iteratively removing one study at a time in order to identify outliers that contributed to the increased heterogeneity and evaluate the robustness of the analysis after the outliers were removed.

3. Results

After screening 283 abstracts generated by the search algorithm, 10 studies were deemed eligible for inclusion in the final quantitative analysis (Figure 1). In total, 26,808 patients were incorporated in the analysis (19,152 in the pre-pandemic cohort and 7656 in the pandemic cohort), with five studies being from east Asia (one from Japan [14], two from China [15,16], and two from Korea [17,18]) and the remaining five from Europe (two from the United Kingdom [11,19], one from Italy [20], one from Ireland [3], and one from Serbia [21]). The size of the pandemic cohorts in each study was compared to that of the pre-pandemic cohorts after matching for the time duration of the data collection in the pandemic cohorts (in months).

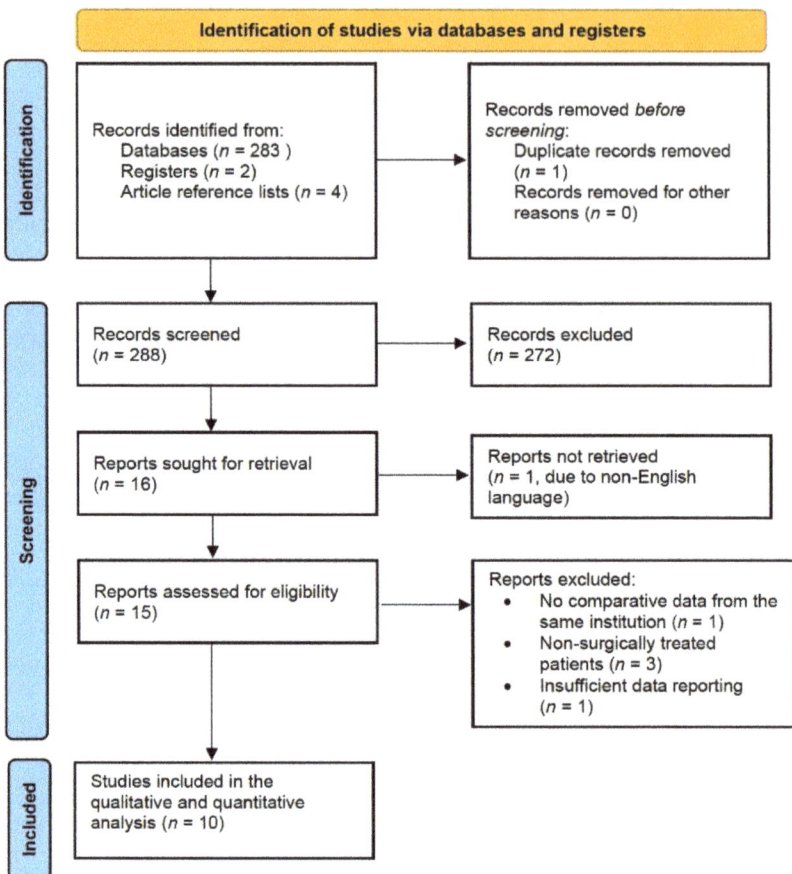

Figure 1. Prisma flowchart of study selection.

When analyzed for methodological quality, eight studies had an NOS score of 7 to 9 and were deemed of high methodological quality, and two studies had a score of 5 or 6 and were deemed of mediocre methodological quality. The median score of the obtained NOS scores was 7.5 (Table 1).

Table 1. Included study characteristics.

Study	Country	Time Interval of Data Collection	Total Patients	Age (Mean ± SD)	Sex (Male/Female)	Newcastle–Ottawa Scale Score
		Pre-pandemic versus Pandemic cohorts, n (%)				
Donlon [3]	Ireland	March 2019–March 2020 vs. March 2020–March 2021	1631 vs. 1093	N/a	N/a	7
Peltrini [20]	Italy	October 2019–February 2020 vs. January 2021–May 2021	41 vs. 43	N/a	N/a	5
Lim [18]	Korea	January–July 2017–2019 vs. January–July 2020	2514 vs. 715	61 (18–90) vs. 61 (17–97) *	1484 (59%)/1030 (41%) vs. 415 (58%)/300(42%)	8
Shinkwin [11]	UK	January–December /2018–2019 vs. January–December 2020	539 vs. 267	70 ± 12.5 vs. 70 ± 14	308 (57.1%)/231 (42.9%) vs. 151 (56.6%)/116 (43.4%)	8
Kuryba [19]	UK	Six weeks before 23 March 2020 vs. nine weeks after	11703 vs. 3227	N/a	6586 (56.2%)/5117 (43.8%) vs. 1793 (55.5%)/1434 (44.5%)	9
Choi [17]	Korea	March-September 2018–2019 vs. March–September 2020	1985 vs. 916	62.6 ± 12.2 vs. 61.7 ± 12.1	1160 (58.4%)/825 (41.6%) vs. 524 (57.2%)/392 (42.8%)	9
Radulovic [21]	Serbia	January–December 2019 vs. March 2020–April 2021	152 vs. 49	67.11 ± 11.62 vs. 67.41 ± 10.37	87 (57.2%)/65 (42.8%) vs. 22 (44.9%)/27 (55.1%)	6
Xu [15]	China	January–May 2019 vs. January–May 2020	828 vs. 710	N/a	518 (62.6%)/310 (37.4%) vs. 438 (61.7%)/272 (38.3%)	7
Cui [16]	China	February-May 2018–2019 vs. February–May 2020	205 vs. 67	65.6 ± 11.65 vs. 67.1 ± 11.4	111 (54.1%)/94 (45.9%) vs. 44 (65.7%)/23 (34.3%)	9
Mizuno [14]	Japan	December 2018–April 2020 vs. April 2020–August 2020	92 vs. 31	72.91 ± 10.58 vs. 72 ± 10.7	54 (58.7%)/38 (51.3%) vs. 25 (80.6%)/16 (19.4%)	9

N/a = Not available. * Data presented as median (range).

3.1. Tumor-Related Factors

Overall, the T3 stage was the most commonly encountered, both in the pre-pandemic (14.5%) and the pandemic (20%) cohorts. No statistically significant differences were encountered between the compared patient populations regarding the tumor extent (T) or nodal (N) stages of the involved tumors (Table 2). On the contrary, the number of patients presenting with metastases was found to be significantly increased in the pandemic cohort (OR 1.65, 95% CI 1.02–2.67, p = 0.04), with high interstudy heterogeneity (I^2 = 91%).

Table 2. Pooled analysis outcomes.

Outcome	Number of Studies	Total Patients	Patients in the Prepandemic Cohort n(%)	Patients in the Pandemic Cohort n(%)	OR/WMD	95% Confidence Intervals	p-Value	I^2	I^2 p-Value
			Tumor-Related Factors						
Tis-T1 stage	5	7301	628 (4.1)	276 (6.3)	1.14	0.87–1.48	0.34	41%	0.15
T2 stage	5	7301	703 (4.6)	255 (5.9)	0.91	0.78–1.06	0.2	0%	0.6
T3 stage	5	7301	2198 (14.5)	883 (20)	1.18	0.82–1.7	0.38	88%	<0.001
T4 stage	6	7385	736 (4.2)	290 (5.7)	1.19	0.79–1.8	0.4	80%	<0.001
N + stage	6	7385	1797 (10.2)	720 (14.3)	1	0.89–1.11	0.96	0%	0.54
M + stage	6	19,414	2020 (11.8)	711 (13.5)	1.65	1.02–2.67	0.04	91%	<0.001
Right-sided tumors	7	19,893	5294 (37.5)	1834 (37.4)	0.88	0.51–1.52	0.66	99%	<0.001
Left-sided tumors	7	19,893	4946 (35)	1759 (35.9)	0.91	0.56–1.5	0.72	96%	<0.001
Rectal tumors	8	22,794	4794 (29.8)	1934 (33.2)	0.93	0.63–1.37	0.71	95%	<0.001
			Presentation-Related Factors						
Emergency presentation	3	18,965	2851 (19.3)	1149 (27.3)	1.74	1.07–2.84	0.03	95%	<0.001
Complicated tumor	3	4562	113 (3.9)	84 (5.1)	1.72	0.78–3.78	0.18	82%	0.004
			Treatment-Related Factors						
Neoadjuvant therapy	3	7668	1459 (27.4)	656 (30.6)	1.22	1.09–1.37	<0.001	0%	0.4
Palliative intent surgery	4	4795	114 (6.6)	126 (7.3)	1.95	1.13–3.36	0.02	54%	0.09
Minimally Invasive Surgery	6	22,584	7680 (48.1)	2056 (34.9)	0.68	0.37–1.24	0.2	98%	<0.001
Stoma Formation	5	19,683	1425 (10.2)	479 (8.4)	0.91	0.51–1.62	0.74	94%	<0.001
			Treatment Outcome Factors						
Mortality	1	13,060	163 (1.6)	74 (2.6)	N/a	N/a	N/a	N/a	N/a
Morbidity	2	1810	63 (6.1)	37 (4.8)	0.92	0.55–1.55	0.76	25%	0.25
Length of hospital stay	3	2011	N/a	N/a	0.51	−0.93–1.94	0.49	79%	0.008
Lymph node harvest	3	1894	N/a	N/a	1.57	−1.99–5.13	0.39	64%	0.06

Tis = T in situ, OR = Odds Ratio, WMD = Weighted Mean Difference, I^2 = Higgin's I^2 statistic, N/a = Not available.

Data on the distribution of tumors throughout the hindgut were available in eight studies, reporting similar patterns of distribution in both the pandemic and the pre-pandemic cohorts, with right-sided tumors (of the cecum, ascending, and transverse colons) being the most common tumor type in both the pre-pandemic (37.5%) and the pandemic (37.4%) cohorts. Forest plots are available for review in the Supplementary Material, Figures S1–S9.

3.2. Presentation-Related Factors

Data from three studies encompassing 18,965 patients indicated a statistically significant increase of emergency presentations during the pandemic (OR 1.74, 95% CI 1.07–2.84, p = 0.03, Figure S10), from 19.3% in the pre-pandemic group of patients to 27.3% in the pandemic group. Study heterogeneity was high (I^2 = 95%). Although there was a trend towards increased number of complicated tumors (by perforation or obstruction) in the pandemic group of patients (5.1% versus 3.9% in the pre-pandemic group), the difference was not statistically significant (Table 2, Figure S11).

3.3. Treatment-Related Factors

Neoadjuvant therapy utilization rates were significantly higher during the pandemic era, administered to 30.6% of the group population versus 27.4% of the group population during the pre-pandemic era (OR 1.22, 95% CI 1.09–1.37, $p < 0.001$, Figure S12), with no encountered interstudy heterogeneity ($I^2 = 0$%). Similarly, patients in the pandemic group were more likely to be treated with palliative intent (OR 1.95, 95% CI 1.13–3.36, $p = 0.02$, $I^2 = 54$%, Figure S13).

Minimally invasive approaches were more commonly used in the pre-pandemic group (48.1% versus 34.9% in the pandemic group, Figure S14), albeit without attaining statistical significance ($p = 0.2$). The same was evident for the stoma formation rates as well, with the pre-pandemic stoma rates being 10.2% and the pandemic being 8.4% ($p = 0.74$, Table 2, Figure S15).

3.4. Treatment Outcome Factors

There was no statistically significant difference recorded in terms of length of hospital stay ($p = 0.49$, Figure S17), lymph node yield ($p = 0.39$, Figure S18), or postoperative morbidity ($p = 0.76$, Figure S16). Mortality rates were only reported in a single study on 13,060 patients, indicating mortality rates of 1.6% in the pre-pandemic patient population and 2.6% in the pandemic one (Table 2).

3.5. Sensitivity Analysis

No single study was found to be the cause of the increased statistical heterogeneity observed for the T3/T4 stage, right-sided, left-sided, rectal tumor location, complicated tumor presentation, palliative intent surgery, minimally invasive surgery, and stoma formation outcomes. The study by Shinkwin et al. [11] was responsible for the encountered heterogeneity in the metastatic tumor (M+) outcome, while the study by Lim et al. [18] was responsible for the observed heterogeneity in the emergency presentation outcome. In both cases, after removal of the outlier studies, the recalculated OR failed to retain their statistical significance, therefore suggesting the presence of a type I statistical error. Finally, the heterogeneity encountered in the length of hospital stay outcome was attributed solely to the study by Cui et al. [16]; however, removal of the study, the significance of the obtained OR, was not influenced.

4. Discussion

The COVID-19 pandemic has significantly decreased the availability of health services for non-covid patients [22]. With regard to colorectal neoplasias, the unprecedented burden of the pandemic on healthcare systems has led to a considerable reduction in the number of diagnostic and surveillance endoscopic procedures performed in the general population [23,24]. Recent reports indicate that such drastic changes in clinical practice are projected to lead to increased incidence and tumor stage upshifting as missed cancer cases keep accumulating, in turn increasing colorectal cancer-associated mortality [25]. The problem is further compounded by the encountered delays and postponements of elective colorectal surgical procedures [2], carrying severe implications regarding the long-term impact of the pandemic in the survival of colorectal cancer patients.

Patient demographics and location of the tumors in the pandemic group of patients did not exhibit any significant differences when compared to the pre-pandemic group. Similarly, no differences were registered regarding the T and N staging of involved tumors; however, there was a significant increase in the number of patients presenting with metastatic neoplasms during the pandemic. In fact, patients operated for colorectal cancer during the pandemic were 65% more likely to be affected by metastatic colorectal tumors ($p = 0.04$). This implies that diagnostic and treatment delays may have led to significant tumor upstaging as has been previously postulated [26,27]. Although this explanation is both worrying and compelling, it should be examined in the context of reduced elective, but not emergent, operations during the pandemic era.

More specifically, results obtained from the present meta-analysis demonstrate that the odds of performing an emergency operation were significantly increased (by 74%, $p = 0.03$) during the pandemic, similarly to the odds for palliative-intent surgery (by 95%, $p = 0.02$). Both of these findings suggest that patients with advanced, symptomatic tumors comprised a larger percentage of the patient pool treated surgically during the pandemic, indicating that surgical healthcare accessibility was preferentially maintained for this particular patient subset. However, when patients with complicated tumors (by perforation or obstruction) were assessed, no statistically significant differences were encountered (Table 1, $p = 0.18$), although it is plausible that this is the result of a type II statistical error due to the small number of patients involved in this outcome.

Another finding of the pooled data analysis is the increased rate of neoadjuvant therapy utilization. Patients receiving surgical treatment for colorectal cancer during the pandemic were 22% more likely to have undergone neoadjuvant therapy ($p < 0.001$). Deferral of surgery in favor of neoadjuvant therapy appears to provide an effective solution while waiting for the resumption of normal elective surgical practice. Morris et al. in a population-based study in England reported a 44% increase in the rate of neoadjuvant therapy utilization for rectal cancer during the pandemic era, with long-course regimens being preferred over short-course ones [2]. In our pooled patient cohort, neoadjuvant therapy rates rose form 27.4% in the pre-pandemic group to 30.6% in the pandemic group, clearly indicating a shift in clinical practice brought upon by the COVID-19 pandemic, which appears to be consistent across different included studies ($I^2 = 0\%$) and falls within the general underlying trend favoring surgery deferral.

Surgical practices did not significantly differ, although there was a clear trend towards less minimally invasive surgery in the pandemic cohort (34.8% of cases vs. 48.1% in the pre-pandemic cohort). This change in practice is directly attributable to fear of COVID-19 spread via aerosolization during pneumoperitoneum evacuation, a concern that has controversially led to opposition of minimally invasive techniques during the initial phase of the pandemic [28,29]. Subsequently published guidelines from surgical societies have proposed reinstatement of minimally invasive techniques in both elective and emergency surgical practice, provided that precautionary protective practices, such as use of personal protective equipment, pneumoperitoneum release filters, and liberal preoperative COVID-19 molecular testing are followed [30,31]. Despite the reduced rates of minimally invasive technique utilization in the pandemic cohort, the length of hospital stay—although inconsistently reported in included studies—remained comparable between the two evaluated groups. The same holds true for stoma formation rates as well, despite the evidently increased rates of emergency surgery, suggesting that the employed surgical strategies remained roughly unchanged.

Lymph node yield, morbidity, and mortality rates could rationally represent metrics of surgical safety and efficacy; however, they were seldom reported. A eta-analysis of two studies [15,16] revealed a combined morbidity rate of 6.1% in pre-pandemic patients versus 4.8% in their pandemic counterparts, without any statistically significant difference. Similarly, lymph node yield was equivalent in the two groups based on pooled outcomes from three studies [16,20,21]. Although the paucity of data precludes any concrete assumptions to be made, safety of surgical practice appears to be maintained in the pandemic era despite the looming threat of COVID-19 infection, with oncologic surgical benchmarks being seemingly comparable to the pre-pandemic controls.

The study by Kuryba et al. [19] was the only study to report data on mortality, derived from a large UK-based population registry, revealing 2.6% mortality rates in the pandemic cohort versus 1.6% in the pre-pandemic one. The encountered marginal increase in mortality was mainly attributable to emergency surgery cases (OR 1.74, $p = 0.003$) and was especially pronounced in so-called "hot-sites", i.e., centers that accommodated COVID-19 positive patients as well as elective and emergency colorectal cancer cases. More importantly, COVID-19 superinfection in patients undergoing surgery resulted in a tenfold increase in mortality rates in both elective and emergency cases and was accompanied by prolongation of hospital stay that reached a median of 17 to 20 days, highlighting the detrimental effects of COVID-19 infection in such patients.

One major limitation of the present study is that the evaluated outcomes were inconsistently reported amongst included studies reporting on widely varying number of patients as is exhibited in Table 2. Moreover, differences in the local prevalence of COVID-19, the type of confinement and social distancing measures imposed by governmental authorities, and the extent of surgical service disruption could not be accounted for, given that the majority of included studies are single-center reports. This fact renders the obtained results highly susceptible to the possibility of selection and sampling biases. Another caveat of the meta-analysis is the inability to assess the impact of the pandemic on disease-free and overall survival, which remain as yet uncertain. Finally, there was high interstudy statistical heterogeneity encountered for the metastatic tumors and emergency surgery outcomes, coupled together with the results of the sensitivity analysis that demonstrated the presence of single study outliers, whose subsequent removal altered the significance of the obtained cumulative results. As such, no concrete conclusions can be reached for these particular outcomes, and they should be interpreted with caution.

5. Conclusions

The COVID-19 pandemic has resulted in demonstrable changes in the surgical practice involving colorectal malignancies. Patients during the pandemic were more likely to undergo palliative interventions as opposed to pre-pandemic controls. In addition, neoadjuvant therapy utilization rates were increased in the pandemic era as a means of safe postponement of surgery in select cases. These evident changes in practice recorded during the initial months of the pandemic are rational, taking into account the severe sequelae of COVID-19 infection during the perioperative period. However, they may be alarmingly associated with tumor upstaging, with significant implications regarding the long-term oncologic survival of patients with colorectal neoplasias.

Supplementary Materials: The following supporting information can be downloaded at: https://www.mdpi.com/article/10.3390/cancers14051229/s1, Figure S1: Tis-T1 stage forest plot; Figure S2: T2 stage forest plot; Figure S3: T3 stage forest plot; Figure S4: T4 stage forest plot; Figure S5: Node positive tumors forest plot; Figure S6: Metastatic tumors forest plot; Figure S7: Right-sided tumors forest plot; Figure S8: Left-sided tumors forest plot; Figure S9: Rectal tumors forest plot; Figure S10: Emergency presentation forest plot; Figure S11: Complicated tumors forest plot; Figure S12: Neoadjuvant utilization forest plot; Figure S13: Palliative intent surgery forest plot; Figure S14: Minimally invasive surgery forest plot; Figure S15: Stoma formation forest plot; Figure S16: Morbidity forest plot; Figure S17: Length of hospital stay forest plot; Figure S18: Lymph node harvest forest plot; Figure S19: Tis-T1 stage funnel plot; Figure S20: T2 stage funnel plot; Figure S21: T3 stage funnel plot; Figure S22: T4 stage funnel plot; Figure S23: Node positive tumors funnel plot; Figure S24: Metastatic tumors funnel plot; Figure S25: Right-sided tumors funnel plot; Figure S26: Left-sided tumors funnel plot; Figure S27: Rectal tumors funnel plot; Figure S28: Emergency presentation funnel plot; Figure S29: Funnel plot of complicated tumors; Figure S30: Neoadjuvant utilization funnel plot; Figure S31: Palliative intent surgery funnel plot; Figure S32: Minimally invasive surgery funnel plot; Figure S33: Stoma formation funnel plot; Figure S34: Morbidity funnel plot; Figure S35: Length of hospital stay funnel plot; Figure S36: Lymph node harvest funnel plot.

Author Contributions: Conceptualization E.P. and D.P.; methodology N.P. and D.P.; literature search/data extraction G.B. and A.P. (Anastasia Pikouli); statistical analysis G.B., D.P. and P.L.; writing—original draft C.N. and A.P. (Andreas Pikoulis); supervision/data validation E.P. and D.D.; manuscript revision; D.P., N.P. and P.L. All authors have read and agreed to the published version of the manuscript.

Funding: This research received no external funding.

Conflicts of Interest: The authors declare no conflict of interest.

References

1. Alam, W.; Bouferraa, Y.; Haibe, Y.; Mukherji, D.; Shamseddine, A. Management of colorectal cancer in the era of COVID-19: Challenges and suggestions. *Sci. Prog.* **2021**, *104*, 368504211010626. [CrossRef] [PubMed]
2. Morris, E.J.A.; Goldacre, R.; Spata, E.; Mafham, M.; Finan, P.J.; Shelton, J.; Richards, M.; Spencer, K.; Emberson, J.; Hollings, S.; et al. Impact of the COVID-19 pandemic on the detection and management of colorectal cancer in England: A population-based study. *Lancet Gastroenterol. Hepatol.* **2021**, *6*, 199–208. [CrossRef]
3. Donlon, N.E.; Hayes, C.; Davern, M.; Bolger, J.C.; Irwin, S.C.; Butt, W.T.; McNamara, D.A.; Mealy, K. Impact of COVID-19 on the Diagnosis and Surgical Treatment of Colorectal Cancer: A National Perspective. *Dis. Colon Rectum* **2021**, *64*, 1305–1309. [CrossRef]
4. De Vincentiis, L.; Carr, R.A.; Mariani, M.P.; Ferrara, G. Cancer diagnostic rates during the 2020 "lockdown", due to COVID-19 pandemic, compared with the 2018-2019: An audit study from cellular pathology. *J. Clin. Pathol.* **2021**, *74*, 187–189. [CrossRef] [PubMed]
5. Maringe, C.; Spicer, J.; Morris, M.; Purushotham, A.; Nolte, E.; Sullivan, R.; Rachet, B.; Aggarwal, A. The impact of the COVID-19 pandemic on cancer deaths due to delays in diagnosis in England, UK: A national, population-based, modelling study. *Lancet Oncol.* **2020**, *21*, 1023–1034. [CrossRef]
6. Siegel, R.L.; Miller, K.D.; Goding Sauer, A.; Fedewa, S.A.; Butterly, L.F.; Anderson, J.C.; Cercek, A.; Smith, R.A.; Jemal, A. Colorectal cancer statistics, 2020. *CA Cancer J. Clin.* **2020**, *70*, 145–164. [CrossRef] [PubMed]
7. Tinmouth, J.; Dong, S.; Stogios, C.; Rabeneck, L.; Rey, M.; Dubé, C. Estimating the Backlog of Colonoscopy due to Coronavirus Disease 2019 and Comparing Strategies to Recover in Ontario, Canada. *Gastroenterology* **2021**, *160*, 1400–1402.e1. [CrossRef]
8. Grass, F.; Behm, K.T.; Duchalais, E.; Crippa, J.; Spears, G.M.; Harmsen, W.S.; Hübner, M.; Mathis, K.L.; Kelley, S.R.; Pemberton, J.H.; et al. Impact of delay to surgery on survival in stage I-III colon cancer. *Eur. J. Surg. Oncol. J. Eur. Soc. Surg. Oncol. Br. Assoc. Surg. Oncol.* **2020**, *46*, 455–461. [CrossRef]
9. Vecchione, L.; Stintzing, S.; Pentheroudakis, G.; Douillard, J.-Y.; Lordick, F. ESMO management and treatment adapted recommendations in the COVID-19 era: Colorectal cancer. *ESMO Open* **2020**, *5*, e000826. [CrossRef]
10. O'Connor, J.M.; Esteso, F.; Chacón, M. Official French SARS-CoV-2 guidelines for cancer patients, a triage solution with precision medicine. *Color. Cancer* **2020**, *9*, CRC21. [CrossRef]
11. Shinkwin, M.; Silva, L.; Vogel, I.; Reeves, N.; Cornish, J.; Horwood, J.; Davies, M.M.; Torkington, J.; Ansell, J. COVID-19 and the emergency presentation of colorectal cancer. *Color. Dis. Off. J. Assoc. Coloproctol. Gt. Br. Irel.* **2021**, *23*, 2014–2019. [CrossRef] [PubMed]
12. Weiser, M.R. AJCC 8th Edition: Colorectal Cancer. *Ann. Surg. Oncol.* **2018**, *25*, 1454–1455. [CrossRef] [PubMed]
13. Page, M.J.; McKenzie, J.E.; Bossuyt, P.M.; Boutron, I.; Hoffmann, T.C.; Mulrow, C.D.; Shamseer, L.; Tetzlaff, J.M.; Akl, E.A.; Brennan, S.E.; et al. The PRISMA 2020 statement: An updated guideline for reporting systematic reviews. *PLoS Med.* **2021**, *18*, e1003583. [CrossRef]
14. Mizuno, R.; Ganeko, R.; Takeuchi, G.; Mimura, K.; Nakahara, H.; Hashimoto, K.; Hinami, J.; Shimomatsuya, T.; Kubota, Y. The number of obstructive colorectal cancers in Japan has increased during the COVID-19 pandemic: A retrospective single-center cohort study. *Ann. Med. Surg.* **2020**, *60*, 675–679. [CrossRef] [PubMed]
15. Xu, Y.; Huang, Z.-H.; Zheng, C.Z.-L.; Li, C.; Zhang, Y.-Q.; Guo, T.-A.; Liu, F.-Q.; Xu, Y. The impact of COVID-19 pandemic on colorectal cancer patients: A single-center retrospective study. *BMC Gastroenterol.* **2021**, *21*, 185. [CrossRef] [PubMed]
16. Cui, J.; Li, Z.; An, Q.; Xiao, G. Impact of the COVID-19 Pandemic on Elective Surgery for Colorectal Cancer. *J. Gastrointest. Cancer* **2021**, 1–7. [CrossRef] [PubMed]
17. Choi, J.Y.; Park, I.J.; Lee, H.G.; Cho, E.; Kim, Y., II; Kim, C.W.; Yoon, Y.S.; Lim, S.-B.; Yu, C.S.; Kim, J.C. Impact of the COVID-19 Pandemic on Surgical Treatment Patterns for Colorectal Cancer in a Tertiary Medical Facility in Korea. *Cancers* **2021**, *13*, 2221. [CrossRef]
18. Lim, J.H.; Lee, W.Y.; Yun, S.H.; Kim, H.C.; Cho, Y.B.; Huh, J.W.; Park, Y.A.; Shin, J.K. Has the COVID-19 Pandemic Caused Upshifting in Colorectal Cancer Stage? *Ann. Coloproctol.* **2021**, *37*, 253–258. [CrossRef]
19. Kuryba, A.; Boyle, J.M.; Blake, H.A.; Aggarwal, A.; van der Meulen, J.; Braun, M.; Walker, K.; Fearnhead, N.S. Surgical Treatment and Outcomes of Colorectal Cancer Patients During the COVID-19 Pandemic: A National Population-based Study in England. *Ann. Surg. Open Perspect. Surg. Hist. Educ. Clin. Approaches* **2021**, *2*, e071. [CrossRef]
20. Peltrini, R.; Imperatore, N.; Di Nuzzo, M.M.; D'Ambra, M.; Bracale, U.; Corcione, F. Effects of the first and second wave of the COVID-19 pandemic on patients with colorectal cancer: What has really changed in the outcomes? *Br. J. Surg.* **2021**, *108*, e365–e366. [CrossRef]
21. Radulovic, R.S.; Cuk, V.V.; Juloski, J.T.; Arbutina, D.D.; Krdžic, I.D.; Milic, L.V.; Kenic, M.V.; Karamarkovic, A.R. Is Colorectal Cancer Stage Affected by COVID-19 Pandemic? *Chirurgia* **2021**, *116*, 331–338. [CrossRef]
22. Moynihan, R.; Sanders, S.; Michaleff, Z.A.; Scott, A.M.; Clark, J.; To, E.J.; Jones, M.; Kitchener, E.; Fox, M.; Johansson, M.; et al. Impact of COVID-19 pandemic on utilisation of healthcare services: A systematic review. *BMJ Open* **2021**, *11*, e045343. [CrossRef]
23. Mazidimoradi, A.; Tiznobaik, A.; Salehiniya, H. Impact of the COVID-19 Pandemic on Colorectal Cancer Screening: A Systematic Review. *J. Gastrointest. Cancer* **2021**, 1–15. [CrossRef] [PubMed]
24. Issaka, R.B.; Feld, L.D.; Kao, J.; Hegarty, E.; Snailer, B.; Kalra, G.; Tomizawa, Y.; Strate, L. Real-World Data on the Impact of COVID-19 on Endoscopic Procedural Delays. *Clin. Transl. Gastroenterol.* **2021**, *12*, e00365. [CrossRef] [PubMed]

25. Harber, I.; Zeidan, D.; Aslam, M.N. Colorectal Cancer Screening: Impact of COVID-19 Pandemic and Possible Consequences. *Life* **2021**, *11*, 1297. [CrossRef] [PubMed]
26. Suárez, J.; Mata, E.; Guerra, A.; Jiménez, G.; Montes, M.; Arias, F.; Ciga, M.A.; Ursúa, E.; Ederra, M.; Arín, B.; et al. Impact of the COVID-19 pandemic during Spain's state of emergency on the diagnosis of colorectal cancer. *J. Surg. Oncol.* **2021**, *123*, 32–36. [CrossRef] [PubMed]
27. Santoro, G.A.; Grossi, U.; Murad-Regadas, S.; Nunoo-Mensah, J.W.; Mellgren, A.; Di Tanna, G.L.; Gallo, G.; Tsang, C.; Wexner, S.D. DElayed COloRectal cancer care during COVID-19 Pandemic (DECOR-19): Global perspective from an international survey. *Surgery* **2021**, *169*, 796–807. [CrossRef]
28. Chadi, S.A.; Guidolin, K.; Caycedo-Marulanda, A.; Sharkawy, A.; Spinelli, A.; Quereshy, F.A.; Okrainec, A. Current Evidence for Minimally Invasive Surgery During the COVID-19 Pandemic and Risk Mitigation Strategies: A Narrative Review. *Ann. Surg.* **2020**, *272*, e118–e124. [CrossRef]
29. Di Saverio, S.; Khan, M.; Pata, F.; Ietto, G.; De Simone, B.; Zani, E.; Carcano, G. Laparoscopy at all costs? Not now during COVID-19 outbreak and not for acute care surgery and emergency colorectal surgery: A practical algorithm from a hub tertiary teaching hospital in Northern Lombardy, Italy. *J. Trauma Acute Care Surg.* **2020**, *88*, 715–718. [CrossRef]
30. Francis, N.; Dort, J.; Cho, E.; Feldman, L.; Keller, D.; Lim, R.; Mikami, D.; Phillips, E.; Spaniolas, K.; Tsuda, S.; et al. SAGES and EAES recommendations for minimally invasive surgery during COVID-19 pandemic. *Surg. Endosc.* **2020**, *34*, 2327–2331. [CrossRef]
31. De Simone, B.; Chouillard, E.; Sartelli, M.; Biffl, W.L.; Di Saverio, S.; Moore, E.E.; Kluger, Y.; Abu-Zidan, F.M.; Ansaloni, L.; Coccolini, F.; et al. The management of surgical patients in the emergency setting during COVID-19 pandemic: The WSES position paper. *World J. Emerg. Surg.* **2021**, *16*, 14. [CrossRef] [PubMed]

MDPI
St. Alban-Anlage 66
4052 Basel
Switzerland
Tel. +41 61 683 77 34
Fax +41 61 302 89 18
www.mdpi.com

Cancers Editorial Office
E-mail: cancers@mdpi.com
www.mdpi.com/journal/cancers

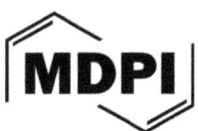

www.ingramcontent.com/pod-product-compliance
Lightning Source LLC
LaVergne TN
LVHW070409100526
838202LV00014B/1418